DIET

A

NEW

FOR

JOHN ROBBINS

AMERICA

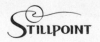

STILLPOINT

STILLPOINT PUBLISHING

Books that explore the expanding frontiers of human consciousness

For a free catalog or ordering information
write:
Stillpoint Publishing, Box 640, Walpole, NH 03608 USA
or call
1-800-847-4014 TOLL FREE
(Continental US, except NH)
1-603-756-9281
(Foreign and NH)

This book is manufactured in the United States of America.
Text and cover design by Eismont Design.
Graphics by Deo Robbins.
Typesetting by Batsch Spectracomp.
Published by Stillpoint Publishing, a division of Stillpoint International, Inc.,
Box 640, Meetinghouse Road, Walpole, NH 03608.

Library of Congress Card Catalog Number: 87-061157
Robbins, John
Diet for a New America

ISBN 0-913299-54-5 Trade Paper Edition

25   26   27   28   29   30

DIET FOR A NEW AMERICA

ACKNOWLEDGMENTS

MY GRATITUDE AND THANKS TO:
Deo Robbins, who nursed the book and me through thick and thin, her utterly unique wit providing me a continual source of renewal. Her example is a living demonstration that health comes through love.

Don Rosenthal, whose keen eye and high editorial standards helped sharpen the focus of my thoughts.

Ocean Robbins, whose love for all of life is a continuous inspiration to all who know him.

Salima Cobb and Martha Rosenthal, who believed in my ability to do this book, even when my faith flickered.

Kali Rae, for her support in the original inspiration for the book.

Anton Grosz, Errol Sowers, and all the people at Stillpoint International, for their ongoing dedication to world spiritual awakening.

All the animals I've been fortunate enough to know. Simply by being themselves they have encouraged me to be a voice for the voiceless.

My thanks also to the numerous physicians, nutritionists, environmentalists, researchers, and other concerned people who read and criticized the book as it took shape.

And to all those yet to be inspired by the vision of DIET FOR A NEW AMERICA.

MAY ALL BE FED; MAY ALL BE HEALED; MAY ALL BE LOVED.

FOREWORD

By Joanna Macy, author
Despair and Personal Power
in the Nuclear Age

AFTER READING THIS book for the second time, I took a walk on the beach below the oil refineries on San Francisco Bay. Seagulls careened in the afternoon sun. A tanker hooked up a half-mile out on the jetty. As I watched idly, my thoughts still occupied with the book, a strange fantasy arose in my mind.

It was a scenario of what would happen if Americans no longer found animal products attractive. Say they simply woke up one day and found meat and poultry and dairy products unappealing. Given U.S. eating habits, that speculation borders on the absurd, I know. But suppose some magical transformation took place that would diminish our attraction to animal-based foods, and at the same time increase our appetite and enjoyment for other foods which really nourish, and are far better for us.

What would happen? What would it mean for our lives and our world? Would that tanker, for example, still be making its deliveries of imported oil? Would those refineries stretch back for as many miles as they do now? Would there be as much DDT in the gulls overhead or in my own body? Would they and I be likely to live longer and healthier?

The research that John Robbins has done for us in this book, gathering and distilling an extraordinary amount of little known but vital information, allows us to deduce what would happen in such a scenario. From the evidence accrued in hundreds of recent medical, agricultural, economic and environmental studies, which he presents in terms easy for the lay person to grasp, we can indeed estimate the results if Americans were to change their eating habits and kick the habit of over-consuming animal proteins and animal fats.

I imagine then the scenario, as I walk along the water's edge.

The effects on our physical health are immediate. The incidence of cancer and heart attack, the nation's biggest killers, drops precipitously. So do many other diseases now demonstrably and causally linked to consumption of animal proteins and fats, such as osteoporosis, a major affliction among older women; my mother suffers from it; I fear it. The hormonal imbalances causing miscarriages and increasing aberrations of sexual development similarly drop away, as we cease ingesting with our meat, poultry and milk the drugs pumped into our livestock. So do the neurological disorders and birth defects due to pesticides and other chemicals, as we begin to eat lower on the food chain where these poisons are far less concentrated. Mother's milk, where they concentrate in greatest intensity, becomes safe again; we can nurse our babies without fear. Since these toxins attack the gene pool itself, causing irreversible damage, the change in diet improves the health of my children's children's children and generations to come.

The social, ecological and economic consequences, as we Americans turn away from animal food products, are equally remarkable. We find that the grain we previously fed to fatten livestock can now feed five times the U.S. population; so we have become able to alleviate malnutrition and hunger on a worldwide scale. We discover what it is like for us to sit down to eat without feeling guilt. Once relieved of it, we realize how great was that burden, that unspoken sense of being watched and judged by those who were hungry. We find ourselves also relieved of fear. For on a semiconscious level we knew all along that the old disparities in consumption were turning our planet into a tinder box, breeding resentments and desperations that could only eventuate in war. We breathe easier, letting ourselves be emotionally in touch again with *all* our brothers and sisters.

The great forests of the world, that we had been decimating for grazing purposes (that was, we discover, the major cause of deforestation), begin to grow again. Oxygen-producing trees are no longer sacrificed for cholesterol—producing steaks.

The water crisis eases. As we stop raising and grinding up cattle for hamburgers, we discover that ranching and farm factories had been the major drain on our water resources. The amount now available for irrigation and hydroelectric power doubles. Meanwhile, the change in diet frees over 90% of the fossil fuel previously used to produce food. With this liberation of water energy and fossil fuel energy, our reliance on oil imports declines, as does the rationale for building nuclear power plants.

As expenditures for food and medical care drop, personal savings rise—and with them the supply of lendable funds. This lowers the interest rates, as does also the drop in oil imports which eases the pressure on the national debt.

A less obvious effect of our meat-free diet, but perhaps more telling on the deep psychological level, is the release that it brings from the burden and guilt of cruelty inflected on other species. Only a few of us had been able to face directly the obscene conditions we inflicted on animals in our farm factories and modern slaughter houses; but most of us knew on some level that they entailed a suffering that was too much to "stomach."

We can appreciate now what it did to us to eat animals kept long in pain and terror. Because the mass methods employed to raise and kill animals for our tables were relatively new, we did not fully realize the deprivation and torture they entailed. Only a few of us guessed that the glandular responses of the cattle and pigs and chickens pumped adrenalin into their bodies and that we ate with their flesh the rage of the chickens, the terror of the pigs and cattle. It is good for our bodies, our relationships and our politics to have stopped ingesting fear and anger. Acting now with more respect for other beings, we find we have more respect for ourselves.

As I picked my way over the shale and driftwood, I thought to myself, "This scenario is wildly, absurdly utopian. It is also clearly the way we are meant to live, built to live." And I wondered what the means could be that could alter our taste for animal food products and increase our appetite and appreciation for the foods that really are good for us. Then I stopped short, realizing with a laugh that the means is here at hand. I had just read it. It is this very book!

One might argue that information alone is insufficient to alter patterns of behavior. But information of this kind weds itself with both compassion and self-interest. Fifteen years ago such considerations were enough to prompt our whole family to stop eating red meat. Our concerns then were world hunger concerns: a pound of beef costs ten pounds of grain. That change did not strike us as any kind of sacrifice; as a matter of fact, we felt better physically and found our food costs dropping substantially. Now I see how reading John Robbins' book has changed our eating habits again for the better. Like many of our friends, we who had once relished barbecues and roast beef, bacon and eggs, and a chicken-every-Sunday lifestyle, we are changing our eating habits without any trauma or fanfare.

Still, I did not know how much was at stake until I read *Diet for a New America*. For this book reveals the causal links between our animal food habits and the current epidemics of cancer, heart diseases and many other modern health disorders. It reveals as well the role these habits play in the present ecological crisis—in the depletion of our water, topsoil and forests. It shows how the production of animal foods puts toxins into our environment and how our consumption of these foods increases in turn our susceptibility to these toxins. Eating high on the food chain can be seen now as a kind of vicious circle, in which the chemicals we inflict on the environment and other life forms mount exponentially, and in which we ourselves as consumers become progressively more vulnerable to them.

It was clearly not an easy book to write, as John Robbins acknowledges. For he uncovers not only a massive horror in what we as a society are doing to other beings and to ourselves; he uncovers massive deception as well. The information he gives us about what he calls the Great American Food Machine amounts to a powerful indictment of the meat and dairy industries, both in regard to their cruel and dangerous methods of food production and in regard to the falsehoods they purvey. Through their advertising and especially through the "educational" materials they distribute and get taught through our public schools, these industries persuade us of dietary requirements that are inaccurate and promote dietary habits that shorten our lives. In his exposé of their corrupt and corrupting practices, John Robbins stands in the fine American tradition of courageous whistle-blowers, like Ralph Nader and Rachel Carson. In this case, it is both ironic and strangely fitting that the message comes from—or through—the scion of America's largest ice cream company.

A major contribution of a *Diet for a New America* is the welcome news it brings that we need far less protein than we thought we did. Many of us who turned from meat protein in an effort to live more lightly on the earth, believed we should compensate by eating an equal amount of dairy and vegetable protein and by combining grains and legumes to produce it. Frances Moore Lappe, in the first edition of her milestone book *Diet for a Small Planet*, showed us how to do that. Robbins' book is an equally significant milestone, for it shows convincingly that our actual protein requirements are far lower than previously assumed. Using a plethora of recent medical studies, including research and revisions by Lappe herself, *Diet for a New America* debunks what it calls the protein myth, shows we can not only survive on less protein, but live healthier lives. The incidence of osteoporosis, to take an example, declines with lowered protein consumption.

I am grateful that this book is not a sermon. It is too important for that—too important for our health as individuals, as families, as a society and as a planet. John Robbins does not scold or moralize; he takes us on a journey with him, sharing his love for life and his reverence for all life forms, ours included. While he shares as well his surprise and pain at what he discovers in the Great American Food Machine, he wisely lets us draw our own conclusions about how we want to live.

The title is appropriate. There *is* a new America taking birth in our time. I encounter it everywhere I go in this land, in cities and small towns, in churches and schools, where folks are fed up with violence and disease and alienation, where they are creating new forms, new lifestyles, determined to live in ways that lend meaning and sanity to their lives. This new America takes seriously the values of individual dignity, freedom and justice, that were heralded at the birth of our nation. It wants to share these values with all beings—knows it *must* share them in order to survive. It is fed up with consuming over half the world's resources; it is sick of being sick. That is why, I suspect, the fantasy that occurred to me on the beach may not be so unrealistic.

JOANNA MACY

INTRODUCTION

WAS BORN in the heart of the Great American Food Machine. From childhood on it was expected that I would someday take over and run what has become the world's largest ice cream company—Baskin-Robbins. Year after year I was groomed and prepared for the task, given an opportunity to live the Great American Dream on a scale very few people can ever hope to attain. The ice cream cone shaped swimming pool in the backyard of the house in which I lived was a symbol of the success awaiting me.

But when the time came to decide, I said thank you very much, I appreciate the kind offer, but "No!" I had to say no, because something else was calling me, and no matter how hard I tried, I could not ignore it.

There is a sweeter and deeper American dream than the one I turned down. It is the dream of a success in which all beings share because it is founded on a reverence for life. A dream of a society at peace with its conscience because it respects and lives in harmony with all life forms. A dream of a people living in accord with the laws of Creation, cherishing and caring for the natural environment, conserving nature instead of destroying it. A dream of a society that is truly healthy, practicing a wise and compassionate stewardship of a balanced ecosystem.

This is not my dream alone. It is really the dream of all human beings who feel the plight of the earth as their own, and sense our obligation to respect and protect the world in which we live. To some degree, all of us share in this dream. Yet few of us are satisfied that we are doing all that is needed to make it happen.

Almost none of us is aware of just how powerfully our eating habits effect the possibility of this dream becoming a reality. We do not realize that one way or the other, how we eat has a tremendous impact. *Diet For A New America* is the first book to show in full detail the nature of this impact, not only on our own health, but in addition on the vigor of our society, the health of our world, and the well-being of its creatures. As it turns out, we have cause to be grateful, for *what's best for us personally is also best for the other life forms and for the life support systems on which we all depend.*

The more I have uncovered about the dark side of the Great American Food Machine, the more appropriate it has felt to have declined the opportunity to be part of it. And the more urgent it has seemed that people be made aware of the profound and far-reaching consequences of their eating habits.

Diet For A New America exposes the explosive truths behind the food on America's plates. These are truths the purveyors of the Great American Food Machine don't want you to know, for in many cases they are not pretty truths. But if exposing them makes America healthier, the world a kinder and more life-sustaining place, then so be it.

Increasingly in the last few decades, the animals raised for meat, dairy products and eggs in the United States have been subjected to ever more deplorable conditions. Merely to keep the poor creatures alive under these circumstances, even more chemicals have had to be used, and increasingly, hormones, pesticides, antibiotics and countless other chemicals and drugs end up in foods derived from animals. The worst drug pushers don't work city streets— they operate today's "factory farms."

But that's just the half of it. The suffering these animals undergo has become so extreme that to partake of food from these creatures is to partake unknowingly of the abject misery that has been their lives. Millions upon millions of Americans are merrily eating away, unaware of the pain and disease they are taking into their bodies with every bite. We are ingesting nightmares for breakfast, lunch and dinner.

Diet For A New America reveals the effects on your health, on your consciousness, and on the quality of life on earth that comes from eating the products of an obscenely inhumane system of food production. You don't have to forego animal products to derive great benefit from this book. You don't have to be a vegetarian to be concerned about your health, and to want your life to be a statement of compassion. *It's not the killing of the animals that is the chief issue here, but rather the unspeakable quality of the lives they are forced to live.*

The purveyors of the Great American Food Machine don't want you to know how the animals have lived whose flesh, milk and eggs end up in your body. They also don't want you to know the health consequences of consuming the products of such a system, nor do they want you to know its environmental impact. Because they know only too well that if word got out the resultant public outcry would shake the foundations of their industry.

But I want you to know. I'm letting the cat out of the bag. I don't care about their profits. I care about your health, your well-being, and the welfare of our planet and all its creatures.

Eating should be a pleasure. It should be a celebration and a communion with life. The information in this book will provide you access to a whole new sense of pleasure in eating—a pleasure all the deeper for being at no one's expense, a pleasure all the more wonderful for being productive of radiant health.

Exciting things have been learned in the last few decades regarding health and food choices. There have at last been enormous breakthroughs in the science of human nutrition, and for the first time now we are receiving irrefutable scientific evidence of how different eating patterns affect health. We've always known that it was best to eat a "balanced diet," but now we are finding out just what a balanced diet really is, and it's not at all what we had thought. Thousands of impeccably conducted modern research studies now reveal that the traditional assumptions regarding our need for meats, dairy products and eggs have been in error. *In fact it is an excess of these very foods, which had once been thought to be the foundations of good eating habits, that is responsible for the epidemics of heart disease, cancer, osteoporosis, and many other diseases of our time.*

Diet For A New America is the first book to reveal the latest findings of nutritional research in a language anyone can understand, and at the same time document these findings so you can rest assured of their legitimacy. It takes into account the marvelous and undeniable fact that you are a unique person, with your own special tastes, needs, and biochemical individuality. It does not sell you short by presenting rigid rules you have to follow obsessively. On the contrary, the goal is for you to be truly healthy and happy in every dimension of your being, and to be free from any kind of compulsion. *Diet For A New America* contains no dogmatic list of shoulds and shouldn'ts, but instead gives you information that will help you select and enjoy foods that day by day will make you healthier and happier. It shows you how to protect yourself against heart attacks, cancer, osteoporosis, diabetes, strokes, and the other scourges of our time. It shows you how to keep your body free from cholesterol, saturated fat, artificial hormones, antibiotic-resistant bacteria, pesticides, and the countless other disease-producing agents found all too often in many of today's foods. It shows you how you can enjoy eating food that leaves your mind and heart clear and unpolluted.

As Americans we are indeed privileged to have the option of selecting the optimum diet. But for most of the world, the struggle is a far different one; it is survival itself. *Diet For A New America* shows you how your food choices can be of tremendous benefit, not only to your own life, but to the less fortunate of the world as well. No self-deprivation is called for, but simply the understanding that the healthiest, tastiest, and most nourishing way to eat is also the most economical, most compassionate, and least polluting. Heeding this message is without doubt one of the most practical, economical and potent things you can do today to heal, not only your own life, but also the ecosystem on which all life depends. You benefit, the rest of humankind benefits, the animals benefit, and so do the forests and the rivers and the soil and the air and the oceans.

There is enormous suffering today that stems from people feeling isolated and alienated from nature. *Diet For A New America* is a statement of our inter-existence with all forms of life, and provides a means to experience the profound healing powers of our inter-connectedness.

You'll learn how to care for your health and to improve the quality of your life. *You'll see that the very eating habits that can do so much to give you strength and health are exactly the same ones that can significantly reduce the needless suffering in the world, and do much to preserve our ecosystem.* And you'll discover the profound liberation that comes from bringing your eating habits into harmony with life's deepest ecological basis. You will become increasingly sensitive, and increasingly able to live and act as an agent of world spiritual awakening.

Few of us are aware that the act of eating can be a powerful statement of commitment to our own well-being, and at the very same time to the creation of a healthier habitat. In *Diet For A New America* you will learn how your spoon and fork can be tools with which to enjoy life to the fullest, while making it possible that life, itself, might continue. In fact, you will discover that your health, happiness, and the future of life on earth are rarely so much in your own hands as when you sit down to eat.

When I declined to be a top cog in the Great American Food Machine, and turned down the opportunity to live the American Dream, it was because I knew there was a deeper dream. I did it because I knew that with all the reasons that each of us has to despair and become cynical, there still beats in our common heart our deepest prayer for a better life and a more loving world. The book you hold in your hands is a key that will enable you to be an instrument of this prayer.

John Robbins

Summer, 1987

. . . .

The lives of the animals raised for food in the United States today stand in glaring contradiction to our hopes for a better way of life. In order to understand the full significance of what is being done to these animals, it will be helpful to understand what kind of creatures animals really are. This, then, is where our story begins—with a look at the nature of the creatures we call animals, and at our attitudes towards them. The astounding truth may surprise you as much as it has surprised me . . .

PART

ONE

*"Nothing is more powerful than an individual
acting out of his conscience,
thus helping to bring the collective conscience to life."*

(NORMAN COUSINS)

ALL GOD'S CRITTERS HAVE A PLACE IN THE CHOIR

*"I care not much for a man's religion whose
dog or cat are not the better for it."*

(ABRAHAM LINCOLN)

YOU WILL NOT find very many monuments to dogs in this
world. But in Edinburgh, Scotland, in a public area known as
Greyfriar Square, there stands a statue, erected by the local
citizens, in honor of a little terrier named Bobby.

Why did the townspeople erect this statue? Because this little dog
taught them a lesson in the years he lived with them—a most important lesson. Bobby the Scottish terrier had no owner. And as often
happens to smalltown dogs with no master, he was kicked around by
just about everybody, and had to scrounge through garbage to get
anything to eat. Not what you would call an ideal life, even for a dog.

But it happened that there was in the village a dying old man,
named Jock. In his last days, the old man noticed the plight of the
sorry little dog. There wasn't much he could do, but he did buy the
little fellow a meal one evening at the local restaurant. Nothing fancy,
just some scraps. But it would be hard for anyone to over-estimate the
extent of little Bobby's gratitude.

Shortly thereafter, Jock died. When the mourners carried his body
to the grave, the terrier followed them. The gravediggers ordered him

away, and when he refused to leave they kicked him and threw rocks at
him. But still the dog stood his ground, and would not leave no matter
what they did. From then on, for no less than fourteen years, little
Bobby honored the memory of the man who had been kind to him.
Day and night, through harsh winter storms and hot summer days, he
stood by the grave. The only time he ever left the gravesite was for a
brief trip each afternoon back to the restaurant in which he had met
Jock, in hopes of scavenging something to eat. Whatever he got he
would solemnly carry back to the grave, and eat there. The first winter
Bobby had almost no shelter, huddling underneath tombstones when
the snow was deep. By the next winter, the townspeople were so
touched by his brave and lonely vigil that they erected a small shelter
for him. And fourteen years later, when little Bobby died, they buried
him where he lay—alongside the man whose last gesture of kindness he
had honored with such devotion.[1]

THE MOST SELFLESS ANIMAL IN THE WORLD

If the little Scottish terrier whose monument still stands in Edinburgh
is not the most selfless animal who ever lived, a dolphin named Pelorus
Jack might well be. For many years, this dolphin guided ships through
French Pass, a channel through the D'Urville Islands off New
Zealand. This dangerous channel is so full of rocks, and has such
extremely strong currents, that it has been the site of literally hundreds
of shipwrecks. But none occurred when Pelorus Jack was at work.
There is no telling how many lives he saved.

He was first seen by human beings when he appeared in front of a
schooner from Boston named "Brindle," just as the ship was approaching French Pass. When the members of the crew saw the dolphin bobbing up and down in front of the ship, they wanted to kill
him—but, fortunately, the captain's wife was able to talk them out of it.
To their amazement, the dolphin then proceeded to guide the ship
through the narrow channel. And for years thereafter, he safely guided
almost every ship that came by. So regular and reliable was the dolphin
that when ships reached the entrance to French Pass they would look
for him, and if he was not visible, they would wait for him to appear to
guide them safely through the treacherous rocks and currents.

On one sad occasion, a drunken passenger aboard a ship named the "Penguin" took out a gun and shot at Pelorus Jack. The crew was furious, and when they saw Jack swim away with blood pouring from his body they came very close to lynching the passenger. The "Penguin" had to negotiate the channel without Pelorus Jack's help, as did the other ships that came through in the next few weeks. But one day the dolphin reappeared, apparently recovered from his wound. He had evidently forgiven the human species, because he once again proceeded to guide ship after ship through the channel. When the "Penguin" showed up again, however, the dolphin immediately disappeared.

For a number of years thereafter, Pelorus Jack continued to escort ships through French Pass—but never the "Penguin," and the crew of that ship never saw the dolphin again. Ironically, the "Penguin" was later wrecked, and a large number of passengers and crew were drowned, as it sailed—unguided—through French Pass.[2]

WHO IS THE ANIMAL

A San Francisco science fair recently awarded a prize to a junior high school student whose science project consisted of cutting the head off a live frog with a pair of scissors, to find out whether frogs swim better with or without their brains.

Of course, this is not the only case of frogs being treated cruelly in our schools. They are often dissected by children ostensibly learning "how life works." But what did this youngster learn through his experiment? I think he learned that it is all right to treat other living things as if they have no feelings, as if they are nothing but machines. I think he learned disrespect for life. And I wouldn't call that a good thing.

The science fair judges, however, obviously disagree with me, for they commended the boy on his contributions to the forward march of science, predicted great things for his future, and rewarded him for scientifically proving that: "Frogs will not swim with brain missing unless harassed. A frog swims better with head on."[3]

The attitude we develop towards animals as children tends to stay with us through the rest of our lives. And it continues to influence our experience, not only of animals, but of other people, ourselves, and life itself. There is a great deal of evidence from all over the world indicating that people who have, as children, learned to care for animals, grow up more capable of caring for themselves, and for other people. By the same token, people who later become criminals have very often abused animals as children. We find high statistical correlations in every country and culture where research has been done.

The way we treat animals is indicative of the way we treat our fellow humans. One Soviet study, published in *Ogonyok*, found that over 87% of a group of violent criminals had, as children, burned, hanged, or stabbed domestic animals.[4] In our own country, a major study by Dr. Stephen Kellert of Yale University found that children who abuse animals have a much higher likelihood of becoming violent criminals.[5]

Studies of inmates in a number of U.S. prisons reveal that almost none of the convicts had a pet as a child. None of them had this opportunity to learn to respect and care for another creature's life, and to feel valuable in so doing.

But these attitudes can be reversed, even in criminals. Heartwarming research has been done in which convicts nearing their release dates were allowed to have pet cats in their cells with them. The result? "Of the men who loved and cared for their cats, not a single one later failed as a free man to adjust to society."[6] This in a penal system where over 70% of released convicts are expected to return to jail.

The attitudes towards animals shown by the youngster at the science fair, and by the Soviet criminals when they were youths, are not at all unusual. We've all grown up in a system that condones such cruelty. Our public stance is basically that animals are ours to treat any way we wish, and that kindness to animals and sensitivity to them as fellow beings is an option some may choose if they want to, but it is no more incumbent upon us than being nice to plastic dolls.

This attitude towards animals has been given voice, even by modern religious leaders, one of whom said that when animals are being slaughtered:

"Their cries should not arouse unreasonable compassion any more than to red-hot metals undergoing the blows of a hammer, seeds

*spoiling underground, branches crackling when they are pruned,
grain that is surrendered to the harvester, wheat being ground by
the milling machine."*[7]

For this religious leader, animals are not creatures who merit any sort
of empathy. They are merely machines, bundles of reflexes and instincts, mechanical things with no feelings to speak of, objects which
we can treat without qualm in any way whatever. This is a far cry from
the attitude of Albert Schweitzer, who believed that . . .

> *"Any religion which is not based on a respect for life is not a true
> religion . . .*[8] *Until he extends his circle of compassion to all living
> things, man will not himself find peace."*[9]

Toward the end of his long life, Schweitzer was awarded the Nobel
Peace Prize, for dedicating his whole life to teaching that:

> *"We must never permit the voice of humanity within us to be
> silenced. It is man's sympathy with all creatures that first makes
> him truly a man."*[10]

DOLPHINS TO THE RESCUE

The official position of the Catholic Church has long been that animals don't have souls. During a Church council in the Middle Ages a
vote was taken on whether women and animals have souls. Women
squeaked by. Animals lost.

One thing is sure. Yvonne Vladislavich would give you quite an
argument if you tried to tell her animals don't have souls. In June,
1971, Yvonne was aboard a yacht that exploded and sank in the Indian
Ocean. Utterly terrified, she was thrown into shark-infested waters.
Then she saw three dolphins approach her. One of them proceeded to
buoy her up, while the other two swam in circles around her and
guarded her from the sharks. The dolphins continued to take care of
Yvonne, and protect her, until she finally drifted to a marker in the sea
and climbed up onto it. When she was rescued from this marker, it was
determined that the dolphins had stayed with her, kept her afloat, and
protected her across more than 200 miles of open sea.[11]

And there's more. On May 28, 1978, four fishermen became lost in a fog off the coast of Dassen Island, South Africa. They knew there were dangerous rocks in the vicinity, and they feared running into them because the fog had become so thick they couldn't see where they were going. Then they became aware of a group of dolphins nudging and pushing the boat, and forcing them to change course. Suddenly, through the fog, they saw sharp rocks protruding through the water. The rocks only became visible as they floated by them, and the fishermen realized at once that the dolphins had saved their lives. Meanwhile, the dolphins continued to push the boat along a course known only to them, until it reached calm waters. Then they swam away, evidently feeling their job was done. When the fog lifted, the men were flabbergasted to find themselves in the very bay from which they had originally set out early that morning.[12]

MAN'S BEST FRIEND AT HIS BEST
Human contact with dolphins is limited. In recent years, the animal with whom most of us have had the greatest contact is the dog. One doesn't have to be a "dog-lover" to recognize that these beings have provided enormous amounts of companionship, devotion and loyalty to people over the years.

Television shows like "Lassie" and "Rin Tin Tin" were not wholly contrived fantasies. They were dramatic representations of the loyalty, devotion, and intelligence of dogs. There are actually thousands of fully-documented and independently verified incidents that make the adventures of Lassie and Rin Tin Tin pale by comparison.

One day in Coeur d'Alene, Idaho, in 1955, a man named Ken Wilson was trying to teach a horse to accept a saddle in his corral. Ken wasn't at all concerned about his three-year-old son, Stevie, who he thought was playing at a neighbor's. But what he didn't know was that little Stevie had wandered off alone, fallen into a pond, and sunk to the bottom. The boy's dog, Taffy, however, saw the disaster and immediately raced to the corral, barking uproariously, and demanding Mr. Wilson's attention. When the man ignored him, Taffy made a big show of charging into the pond, all the while continuing to bark at the top of his lungs. Then he raced back and nipped at the horse's legs. Finally

Mr. Wilson realized the dog was trying to tell him something, and dismounted. Immediately, Taffy bolted to the pond, barking for the bewildered man to follow him. When Wilson got to the pond, he saw his little son's red jacket floating on the surface of the water. Finally realizing what had happened, he instantly dove headlong into the four-foot-deep water, found his unconscious son, and lifted him from the bottom. It was six hours before Stevie regained consciousness. But when he did, the first thing he saw was his little dog Taffy, sitting prayerfully beside his bed.[13]

Taffy is not the only dog that has saved the lives of children. There are thousands of such cases, fully documented and verified.

One such child was two-year-old Randy Saleh, of Euless, Texas. Little Randy wandered away from home one day. When his parents noticed his absence and couldn't find him anywhere, they called the police. But even a two-hour police search did not locate young Randy. The parents were becoming extremely alarmed, and when they noticed that the boy's dog, a St. Bernard named Ringo, was also missing, they found themselves praying that the big dog was with their little son, and was somehow protecting him.

Meanwhile, a man named Harley Jones had to stop his car for a traffic jam on a highway about three quarters of a mile from Randy's home. Getting out of his car, he asked other stopped motorists if they knew what was the problem. They told him the trouble was "caused by a mad dog in the road ahead." Curious, Jones walked toward the head of the line of stopped cars to see for himself what was going on. What he saw was a St. Bernard, stationed resolutely in the center of the highway, barking wildly, and letting no car move by in either direction. Jones saw the dog was protecting a little boy who was merrily playing in the center of the heavily-traveled thoroughfare. The dog would stop any car that dared attempt to drive through the area, and then would immediately rush back to the little boy, and nudge him toward the side of the road. But the little fellow, thinking the whole thing was just a game, would return to the center of the highway.

Jones spoke soothingly to the St. Bernard, and managed to calm him down. But the dog would not let a single car move by until little Randy was safely off the road.[14]

I think you'd have a hard time convincing little Randy's parents that animals are just mechanical contraptions.

Now, if you are like me, you may get a little choked up when you learn of these incidents. These are not just cases of dogs waking up their masters because they are panicking in the midst of a fire, and then later getting credit. These are not the work of machines without feeling, driven only by instincts and reflexes. They are demonstrations of courage and devotion and selfless love. They are intelligent and brave responses to emergencies.

UNLIKELY HEROES

It is not only dogs and dolphins who have shown their reverence and devotion to human life by going to enormous lengths to save it. The animal kingdom, it turns out, is full of remarkable samaritans.

In 1975, a desperate shipwreck victim off the coast of Manila was stupefied to see a giant sea turtle swimming towards her, seemingly offering its aid. The floundering woman climbed aboard the turtle, which then did something turtles supposedly "never do." Sea turtles spend most of their time underwater, but this one must have somehow known the poor woman needed constant support to survive, and must also have wanted very much to take care of her. It proceeded to stay at the surface for two full days, going without food itself, so it could continue to carry her and keep her alive. When human rescuers finally appeared: "Eyewitnesses thought the woman was floating on an oil drum until she was safely on board—whereupon the 'oil drum' circled the area twice and disappeared."[15]

To be taken for an oil drum might not have surprised the turtle all that much. You see, for many years, turtles were not legally recognized as animals in the U.S. One of the earliest crusaders for animal protection, Henry Bergh, found this out when he tried to stop the torments visited upon green turtles. These great animals, which have been known to live for hundreds of years, and grow to 600 pounds or more, are sought after as a status source of soup and steak for the wealthy, with the children being eaten when they weigh only about 50 pounds. Bergh found that the turtles were transported by ships from the tropics to the Fulton Fish Market in New York. En route, the turtles did not exactly travel first class. They lay on their backs for several weeks, out of the water, with nothing to eat or drink, like so much upside-down luggage. They were held in place by ropes strung through holes punched in their flippers.[16]

Bergh did everything he could to halt this activity, but when he brought the perpetrators to court, the judge acquitted them on the grounds that a turtle was "not an animal within the meaning of the law."[17] Accordingly, ruled the judge, even the barest minimum of protection against cruelty that was afforded animals by the law at that time could not be applied to turtles.[18]

Most of us, like that judge, are conditioned by a culture that thinks of animals as mere machinery, and could never imagine that a sea turtle would be capable of saving a human life. Nor would that same type of thinking allow us to believe that a canary, however sweet its song and pretty its feathers, could be much more than a decorative and bright adornment to a house. But the residents of Hermitage, Tennessee, know better.

In 1950, an elderly woman lived in Hermitage, who was known to everyone around simply as Aunt Tess. The old lady lived alone with only her cat and a canary named Bibs. Aunt Tess's niece and her husband lived a few hundred yards away from her house, and they were concerned lest something happen to the aging woman without anyone knowing.

One night they were awakened by what seemed like a tapping on the window. It wasn't loud, and they tried to ignore it, but the tapping continued.

Finally, the niece got out of bed and went to the window to investigate. She drew back the curtains, and there, to her amazement, beating frantically against the window pane, was Aunt Tess's canary, Bibs. The little bird had never before been outside the aunt's house, but she had somehow managed not only to get out, but then to find her way several hundred yards to the niece's window. The task took all the little bird had, however. Before the niece's eyes, Bibs literally dropped dead from exhaustion on the windowsill. The niece and her husband immediately rushed over to Aunt Tess's house and there found the old lady lying unconscious and bleeding on the floor. She had suffered a bad fall, and may well have died had not help arrived when it did. The canary had given its own life to save that of Aunt Tess.[19]

The more I have learned about animals, the more I have realized how conditioned I have been in my attitudes towards them. I never would have imagined a bird capable of this kind of thing. Nor would I have thought a pig likely to be a lifesaver. But I would have been wrong.

A couple of years ago United Press International carried a photograph and story that was picked up and printed in many of the country's major newspapers. The photo was of Carol Burk, her 11-year-old son Anthony Melton, and a pig. What made the story newsworthy was that mother and son had gone swimming in a Houston lake. The boy inadvertently strayed too far from shore, panicked, and began to sink. The boy's pet pig, Priscilla, evidently felt his distress because she rushed into the water and began to swim towards him. While Anthony's anguished mother watched helplessly, the boy managed to stay afloat until the pig reached him. Then he caught hold of her leash. Anthony's mother watched awe-struck as Priscilla the pig proceeded to tow her son safely to shore.

THE VALUE OF LIFE ITSELF

Human-centered animal that I am, I find it easiest to appreciate the heroism of animals who save human lives, who rescue people. But I've come to be impressed, too, by the numerous accounts of animals inexplicably going out of their way to save the lives of other animals.

Now, the official government-run Soviet News Agency TASS does not ordinarily carry "human interest" stories. But in September, 1977, TASS reported a remarkable incident that occurred in the Black Sea. A Russian fishing boat found itself being circled by a small group of dolphins. The animals seemed to want something, and kept circling, until the sailors decided to raise anchor. Immediately, the dolphins sped off, as if they had been waiting for the anchor to be lifted, and wanted to be followed. The puzzled sailors decided to follow along to see what would happen, and were lead to a buoy near which they saw a young dolphin trapped in a fishing net. Understanding now why the dolphins had come to them, the men released the trapped dolphin.

The dolphins then proceeded to guide the boat back to the exact spot where it had been originally anchored.[20]

In this case, dolphins teamed up with human beings to save the life of one of their own kind. But there are many cases, perhaps even more remarkable, in which dolphins and human beings have collaborated to save the lives of other species, such as whales.

On September 30, 1978, about 50 pilot whales became beached just north of Auckland, New Zealand. Government officials tried in every way to lure the great whales out to sea, because if they remained where they were they would all certainly die. Nothing worked. Then the officials got the idea of guiding a passing group of dolphins into the harbor. This they did, and when the dolphins saw the whales they seemed instantly to understand the whole situation. Wasting no time, the dolphins immediately took charge, and literally herded the whales back to the open sea, thereby saving their lives.[21]

Of all the accounts I have on record of dolphin heroism, perhaps the most amazing comes, once again, from TASS. Their report tells of sailors on board the fishing vessel "Neverskoil," which was sailing off the coast of Kamchatka on August 14, 1978. The sailors heard a sea lion bellowing for help, and saw that the creature was surrounded by a number of killer whales. But before the whales could devour the sea lion, a group of dolphins appeared, and the whales backed off. The sailors watched as the dolphins then swam away, and they thought this high drama of the seas was over. But the whales made another run at the beleaguered sea lion, who again began bellowing in fear. I can't help but think that what the sailors saw next must have astounded even these hardened veterans of the sea. The dolphins, hearing the distressed cries of the sea lion, realized that the killer whales were again honing in on the creature. They rushed back to the scene, leapt over the heads of the whales, and formed a ring around the sea lion, protecting it. They did not leave until the killer whales were well out of sight.[22]

There are reports of dolphins coming to the aid of whales giving birth. When sharks are menacingly near, the dolphins take up positions around a mother whale and her female "attendants," forming a ring around the helpless mother during her labor and delivery. Should the sharks attack, the dolphins bump them away with their bottle-nosed beaks.

There are so many cases of dolphins saving lives—both human and non-human—that we should really think of them as the "Life-guards of the Seas." We should. But we don't. Instead, we often treat them with utter contempt.

One type of dolphin, called the Dall Porpoise, often swims in the water above salmon and tuna fish schools. Current salmon and tuna fishing methods use huge nets which trap the salmon and tuna—and the dolphins. In the last ten years, according to official figures, 1,649,189 were killed in the course of tuna fishing. The Marine Mammal Protection Act of 1972 required fishermen to reduce their porpoise kill gradually to zero. However, in September 1981, President Reagan's Administration convinced Congress to exempt the U.S. commercial tuna fleet, resulting in the continued use of purse-seine nets which trap and kill thousands of dolphin along with the tuna. Thus fifty dolphins will be killed in the time it takes you to read this chapter. Two have been killed while you've been reading this page, and this rate of massacre goes on 24 hours a day, 365 days a year. The huge corporations which own the fishing fleets tell the public they have modified the nets to permit the porpoises to escape. But they don't tell the public that many of the animals are netted and released, netted and released, until they are mangled and dead. The Reagan Administration has also allowed the Japanese to kill porpoises while fishing for salmon in the U.S. waters of the North Pacific. Over a million dolphins have died in their huge nets, which also trap and kill seals and birds. As a result, organizations like "Friends of Animals, Inc." have called for a boycott of all tuna and salmon products.

The more I've learned, the harder it has become to avoid the conclusion that animals are capable of a respect and reverence for life that cuts across species boundaries. One veterinarian reports:

"I have six cases on record of pet dogs and cats becoming depressed and calling mournfully when a companion animal in the same house has been taken away to be put to sleep because of some incurable disease. In all cases, at about the same time that the

companion pet was being destroyed, the surviving animal showed a
sudden and obvious change in behavior. In one case, the owner did
not know that the vet had put the other pet to sleep until he called
an hour later, and for an hour before, her cat had been calling
frantically and showing distress." [23]

I find it difficult to dismiss these cases and attribute them merely to
instinct. They speak to me rather of a thread binding all creatures in
the great web of life.

A GUIDE-DUCK FOR THE BLIND

One of the most marvelous examples of animals caring for each other is
recalled by Cleveland Amory in his lovely little book, *Animail*. He tells
of a scientist named Dr. Arthur Peterson, who lives in DeBary, Florida. A few years ago, Dr. Peterson noticed some odd activity by ducks
on a lake on his property. Becoming extremely fascinated with what he
saw, Dr. Peterson began to study the ducks, and soon realized that a
male duck (whom he called for the sake of clarity "John-Duck") was
uncannily and persistently attentive to a certain female duck (whom
Dr. Peterson called "Mary-Duck"). It was not mating season, so there
was no apparent explanation for this behavior, but he was terribly
curious, and kept observing the ducks, looking for clues. One day he
noticed that John-Duck had left Mary-Duck alone for a minute, and he
quickly approached her, slipped a net over her, and examined her. To
his astonishment, Dr. Peterson found that Mary-Duck was completely
blind.

Touched by the implications of his discovery, Dr. Peterson released the unseeing Mary-Duck. Moments later, John-Duck reappeared, and went immediately over to her. Then this "seeing-eye
duck" gave a loud series of reassuring quacks, and guided her off. [24]

THE TRAPPER AND THE BEAVER CUBS

Animals with whom humans have little contact also have the potential
for kindness and friendship. One man who came to understand something of the spirit of such animals was the Englishman Archie Belanie,
who later became known as "Grey Owl" when he turned his back on

his past and totally adopted American Indian ways.[25] A prodigiously successful trapper, he fell in love with an Iroquois woman named Anahareo. One day the two of them came upon a female beaver who had been killed in one of Grey Owl's traps. They were about to leave with the fur when two small heads appeared above the water. At Anahareo's urging, Grey Owl rescued the little beavers, whose mother had been killed in his trap, and took them home. Getting to know these two little beaver kittens was such a powerful experience for the great trapper that he never trapped animals again. He wrote movingly of:

> *". . . their almost childlike intimacies and murmurings of affection, their rollicking good fellowship with not only each other but ourselves, their keen awareness, their air of knowing what it was all about. They seemed like little folk from some other planet, whose language we could not quite understand. To kill such creatures seemed monstrous. I would do no more of it."* [26]

YOU REAP WHAT YOU SOW

All animals—including those we have been taught to fear—can respond to love and give it. Nowhere has this been proven more profoundly than by Ralph Helfer and his wife Toni, two of Hollywood's foremost wild animal trainers. Helfer operates an animal park and training center in Buena Vista, California, where he handles and trains the fiercest of animals. Conventional wisdom has it that training these wild animals for show business requires instilling fear in the creatures, and breaking their wills. But Helfer is successful with a radically different approach. He says the idea first came to him in a hospital bed:

> *"Violence begets violence, I mused, as I lay in my hospital bed 25 years ago after being mauled by a 500-pound lion. The big cat had been 'fear-trained,' with whips, chairs, and screams, as animals in captivity traditionally are; and though he performed his tricks well enough, he had no love for humans. Just as a battered child grows up to be a child abuser, a battered animal awaits its chance to do unto others as has been done unto him. I had been done unto royally by that lion, and I had plenty of time during a long*

convalescence to figure out why. That lion had attacked me, as so many other animals have attacked humans over the centuries, not because he was 'wild,' but because he was unloved. Your dog or cat is no different, nor is your horse or fish or pig or bird.

"The idea of affection-training was born in that hospital bed. Animals respond to their lives emotionally, I reasoned. If an animal could be trained by addressing its negative emotions (with threats and punishment), he could probably also be trained by appealing to his positive emotions. Surely the results would be even better with love than with pain, for the animal would be motivated to cooperate. Where pain might get the horse to water, love could induce him to drink.

"Since that time, I've proved my theory with almost every animal known to man. I've traveled from the jungles of Africa to the forests of India, working with everything from hippopotami to tarantulas." [27]

When I first heard of training wild animals through affection, I was skeptical. But Helfer's success record, "with everything from hippopotami to tarantulas," is hard to discount. His animals have been used in many television shows, movies, and commercials. There is one thing, however, that affection-training cannot accomplish.

There are some circus "tricks" which animals can be forced to perform through threats and fear, but which they cannot be coaxed to perform through positive means. The reason for this is simple: the tricks we see in circus rings are often in violation of the anatomical structure and deepest instincts of the animals. Horses dancing on their hind feet, bears roller-skating, dogs walking on their back legs and pushing prams, cats firing off cannons, tigers jumping through burning hoops. These are displays, not of the magnificent natural capacities of the animals, but of their degrading obedience to the dominance of their trainers, a dominance achieved in the ugliest of ways. The quickest and least expensive method of breaking the spirits of the animals held prisoner by the circus trainers is by using whips, electric shocks, sharp hooks, loud noises, and starvation. The training is done in seclusion, and if local SPCA's get too nosey about what is being done to the animals to force their compliance, the animals are moved to foreign countries where there are no restrictions on animal treatment.

One elephant, trained to dance and to play "Yes, Sir, That's My Baby" on the harmonica, was described recently as being probably the meanest elephant in the United States. I wouldn't be at all surprised if he had good reason.

THE EASIEST WAY TO BE WRONG AGAIN

The conventional assumption of our culture is still that animals do not have any of the higher feelings of which we are capable, such as compassion and love and reverence for life. It can be difficult for us to see how tainted we might be by the culturally sanctioned misunderstanding that animals are only mechanical bundles of instincts and reflexes, with no hearts or souls. Few of us have had the opportunity to learn to respect them for what they are—creatures of marvelous complexity, beauty, and mystery.

The idea of animals as machines without feeling has held sway in the collective psyche for so long that it has acquired a momentum of its own. We have gotten stuck in a very deep mental rut, a habit, from which it is not easy to uproot ourselves.

And habit, as Laurence Peter put it, is often "simply the easiest way to be wrong again."

We have seen this mental habit given credence by the church and philosophical expression through thinkers such as Descartes. To him, the body and soul were completely separate; thinking and feeling were attributes of the soul, not the body; and the body itself was simply a machine.[28] Since animals could not speak, it followed for Descartes that they had no soul, and so could not feel. According to Descartes' point of view, which still permeates the psychic atmosphere of our times, all the non-human animals, from the ants up to what he called the "ape-machines," have no capacity for ideas, freedom of action, choice, knowledge of any kind, or feeling. They are merely robots, driven by instincts. He likened animals to watches and clocks, with wheels, springs, gears and weights. Marvelously contrived though they might be, they are, said Descartes, "mere automatons."[29]

Descartes would sometimes kick his dog, just to "hear the machine creak."

DO ANIMALS SUFFER?

I'm sorry to say that the point of view that animals are only machines, and thus incapable of suffering, is still very much with us today. It is part of our cultural heritage, and I am still frequently amazed as I discover how conditioned I am by it. In the culture-at-large, it is so taken for granted that it is rarely questioned.

I don't know if the gentlemen of Kewaskum, Wisconsin are still enjoying their annual Kiwanis turkey shoots. But I know that as of 1971 they had not felt any compunction about their annual "fun and games." What, you may wonder, could be amiss in the "sport" from which the Kiwanis Club members derived so much amusement? Well, turkeys, those great birds who so astounded the Pilgrims when they first arrived in this land, may not be the smartest of God's creatures, but with a dignity all their own they have long been a symbol of the New World for many Europeans seeking freedom. Dignity notwithstanding, at the annual Kiwanis festival they were tied into stalls by the legs in such a way that their heads were exposed as a target for the participants in the "gala" event. The birds couldn't do anything to free themselves and they were shot at again and again by the drunken celebrants. In fact, they were tied in such a way as to guarantee that if they broke their wings or legs in their struggle to save their lives, as they often did, their heads would nevertheless be kept jiggling and exposed to the aim and merriment of the "brave" hunters.[31]

Champions of the idea that other animals don't feel pain as we do say that animals operate entirely from instinct. Thus the Kiwanis marksmen felt no more pangs of conscience than they would if the turkeys whose heads they gaily shot off were made of cardboard. They probably honestly believed turkeys don't suffer.

But a reliance on instincts is very different from a lack of ability to feel pain. The capacity to feel pain has an obvious survival value to any species, enabling it to avoid sources of injury. It is with our senses and nervous systems that we feel pain, not with our capacity for abstract thought. The nervous systems of non-human animals are finely tuned to their environments. Their senses, in many cases, are vastly more sensitive and refined than our own. Physiologically, there is no basis at all for saying that animals don't feel pain. In fact, in *The Spectrum of Pain*, Richard Serjeant writes:

> *"Every particle of factual evidence supports the contention that the higher mammalian vertebrates experience pain sensations at least as acute as our own. Apart from the complexity of the cerebral cortex (which does not directly feel pain) their nervous systems are almost identical to ours and their reactions to pain remarkably similar . . ."*[32]

The senses of animals often make ours look pathetic in comparison. For example, the cells essential for smelling are ethmoidal cells. We have about 5 million of these in our noses. A German shepherd, by way of contrast, has about 200 million. And when it comes to hearing, once again we pale in comparison. The German shepherd can hear sounds clearly at 200 yards which we cannot detect at a mere 20. Even the much maligned shark has enormously sensitive hearing. An Australian named Theo Brown has taken advantage of this fact to develop a musical shark repellent. He conceived the idea when he discovered that if he played fox trots or waltzes the sharks were attracted from great distances, but if he played rock music they left at once.[33]

WE ALL NEED LOVE

Proponents of the attitude that animals are "ours to use," while sometimes acknowledging that animals may experience pain at a physical level, assert that they are not capable of suffering as we know it because their pain has no meaning to them. It is, say these "experts," just sensation. Accordingly, animals can't suffer as we can because their sensations of pain have no emotional meaning for them.

I don't agree. There are many kinds of emotional suffering which we human beings have the ability to experience and all are connected, in one way or another, to our capacity to feel with other beings. And animals have that capacity.

There is a relationship between the capacity of a being to love, and its capacity to suffer, regardless of its species. If a being, of whatever species, has the capacity to give and receive love, then certainly it will suffer if that capacity is thwarted. This is one of the reasons all the wisdom traditions of the world teach us that a sure way to make yourself miserable is not to express your love.

We need both to receive and to give love. Love is food for our souls, and without it we suffer greatly, just as we suffer physically if we starve. Have you ever watched an infant carefully, while it is being stroked and petted? We all know babies love and thrive on this kind of attention, but have you ever looked closely at the physiological changes they undergo? There is a distinct and well defined pattern in their young nervous systems. The heart rate slows down, muscles relax, peristaltic waves increase, and digestive juices flow. Among other things, these changes allow for the formation of the crucial mother-child bonding. And so if the little one is not petted and stroked, and thus does not undergo these physiological changes, the bonding will not occur.

One of the results of this is that the little human baby will have a hard time establishing social bonds in its later life. Another result when an infant is deprived of touching is that it literally shrivels. Because its digestive juices are not fully activated, it fails to receive proper nourishment and so its physical growth is retarded. The little one will do the best it can to survive under the circumstances, and this may mean developing what we call neurotic, or in extreme cases, psychotic symptoms, in the attempt somehow to compensate for the missing mother-love. If the deprivation is sufficiently severe, the infant will habitually repeat the gestures of its compensation for the rest of its life.

Now, it may surprise people who think animals are objects, but every single word you have just read about human infants, about their physiological and emotional responses to stroking and petting, and about the consequences if they are deprived of this attention, is true not only for human babies. It is also true, in every detail, for puppies, kittens, baby monkeys, and a large number of other mammals.[34]

Dr. Harry Harlow, at the University of Wisconsin, has done extensive studies on the influence of love and affection in the lives of sub-human primates. In one appalling experiment, monkeys were deprived of their mothers. The result?

"They have shown many signs of extreme neuroticism and even psychosis. Most of them spend their time sitting passively staring out into space, not interested in other monkeys or anything else.

> *Some of them tensely wind themselves into tortured positions,*
> *and others tear at their flesh with their teeth . . . These are all*
> *symptoms found in human adults confined in institutions for the*
> *insane.*"

Mother dolphins nurse their young for 18 months, and the mother-child bond is deep and enduring. Dolphins four to six years old have been known to seek out their mothers from a group when they become sleepy or frightened. So devoted are these animals to the welfare of one another that they will not abandon or desert a fellow dolphin who seems to be injured or distressed even if it costs them their life. When infant dolphins are caught in tuna nets, their mothers will go to extraordinary lengths to join their doomed young. Once in the nets, they will huddle together with their offspring, singing to them. The tuna industry takes note of this only to acknowledge that the majority of dolphins killed in their nets are females and infants.[35]

It's not only dolphins. Even hard-nosed scientists who have studied wolves have been consistently amazed at the exceptional degree of what can only be called love and affection they show for each other. Gordon Haber, who has studied wolves for decades and is recognized as one of the world's leading wolf experts, notes that one of the outstanding features of these animals is their profound devotion and caring for one another. For example, he saw a wounded wolf in Alaska, its shoulder shattered and bleeding from being kicked by a caribou, limp into an abandoned cabin and lie down, seemingly to die alone as animals often do. But each night another wolf crept into the cabin and fed its crippled friend by bringing it chunks of meat. He continued to care for the wounded wolf until it recovered.[36]

And it is not only in the parent-child relationship that animal love is evident. Many animals, including beavers, geese, eagles, wolves, hawks, penguins, lynxes and mountain lions, mate monogamously for life, and are utterly devoted to their mates in a way that most married humans—who have pledged to care for each other "until death do us part"—could never imagine. Animals can suffer precisely because they have the ability to give and receive love, and a need to do so.

INTELLIGENCE

Still the blindness continues. Those who say that animals can't suffer in any meaningful way often claim that any pain sensations the animals might feel would have no meaning because they are too stupid to know that they hurt. However, it seems to me remarkably limited for us to assume that because an animal does not display intelligence as we know it, it is therefore stupid.

"It is just like man's vanity and impertinence to call an animal dumb because it is dumb to his dull perceptions."

(MARK TWAIN)

Even among our own species, we often don't recognize forms of intelligence which are perhaps a little different from the norm. Albert Einstein's parents were sure he was retarded because he spoke haltingly until the age of nine, and even after that would respond to questions only after a long period of deliberation. He performed so badly in his high school courses, except mathematics, that a teacher told him to drop out, saying, "You will never amount to anything, Einstein."[37] Charles Darwin did so poorly in school that his father told him, "You will be a disgrace to yourself and all your family."[38] Thomas Edison was called "dunce" by his father, "addled" by his high school teacher, and was told by his headmaster that he "would never make a success of anything."[39] Henry Ford barely made it through school with the minimum grasp of reading and writing.[40] Sir Isaac Newton was so poor in school that he was allowed to continue only because he was a complete flop at running the family farm.[41] Pablo Picasso was pulled out of school at the age of ten because he was doing so badly. His father hired a tutor to prepare him to go back to school, but the tutor gave up on the hopeless pupil.[42] Giacomo Puccini, the Italian opera composer, was so poor at everything as a child, including music, that his first music teacher gave up in despair, concluding the boy had no talent.[43]

If we can be so far amiss in recognizing types of intelligence which are a bit different from the normal, and yet belong to members of our own species who are destined to make great contributions, it seems likely we might fail to recognize some forms of intelligence which belong to beings of other species.

Researchers have done exhaustive studies of animal and human brains. Most of these studies have been motivated by a desire to find a biological basis for the belief that there is a profound difference between human and animal forms of intelligence.

No cut and dried dividing line has emerged. Comparing the "structure and function of the human brain with the brains of other animals," scientists have found that humans and other animals:

> ". . . *differ in fewer ways than we may think; surprisingly, the similarities are greater than the differences . . . A striking similarity between the human and non-human mammalian brain is seen in the electrical activity patterns of electroencephalograph (EEG) readings. A dog, for example, has the same states of activity as man, its EEG patterns being almost identical in wakefulness, quiet sleep, dreaming, and daydreaming. As for the chemistry of the central nervous and endocrine systems, we know that there is no difference in kind between human and other animals. The biochemistry of physiological and emotional states (of stress and anxiety, for example) differ little between mice and men."* [44]

INCREDIBLE JOURNEYS

There are so many instances in which animals have demonstrated profound intelligence that, frankly, I wonder sometimes about the intelligence of the people who insist that animals are dumb. Everyone has heard tales of dogs traveling great distances across unknown terrain to rejoin their people. What you might not know, however, is that many of these stories are documented, verified, and, incredible as they seem, literally true.

For example, Mr. and Mrs. Robert Martin moved from Des Moines to Denver. But their German shepherd, Max, evidently preferred Des Moines, because he went back on his own, a distance of 750 snow covered miles. [45]

Another German shepherd, living in Italy, missed his human companion, who had recently moved from Brindisi to Milan and left the animal behind. It took the dog four months to cover the 745 miles, but he managed to do it and found his person to boot.[46]

Even more remarkable is a shorter journey of "only" 200 miles, described by Sheila Burnford in her book *The Incredible Journey*. Three animals—an old English bull terrier, a young Labrador retriever, and believe it or not, a Siamese cat—stayed together, took care of each other, and found their way across 200 miles of rugged Canadian wilderness in Northwestern Ontario.[47]

I would never have thought a cat capable of such a feat. But I was wrong. There are actually many documented and verified accounts of cats traveling great distances to be with their people. The longest I know of is also one of the best authenticated. It concerns a New York veterinarian who moved to a new job and house in California, and had to leave his cat behind, expecting to send for him later. But the cat disappeared prematurely, so the doctor understandably assumed he had seen the last of his cat. Five months later, however, the cat "calmly walked into the (new) house, and jumped onto its favorite armchair." As you might imagine, the vet was startled. For a moment, he was so shocked he just stood there, gaping. Was this his cat? Then he remembered that his cat had once been in a bad fight, in which its tail had been bitten. The injury had left a distinct growth on the fourth vertebra of the cat's tail. Remembering this, the vet walked over to the cat, and felt it's tail. Sure enough, there, on the fourth vertebra, was the telltale growth![48]

We may surely be justified in considering the possibility that animals have access to a kind of intelligence beyond our comprehension. It is hard to attribute such accomplishments to mere instinct.

AN ELEPHANT WITH A SWEET TOOTH

If the only time you've seen an elephant is in a zoo, you've only seen the most devastated and abused specimens of this grand species. But even captive elephants are capable of sophisticated reasoning. One five-ton lady elephant, known as Bertha, was kept for years in the Nugget Casino in Las Vegas. She used to wake up her handler, Jenda Smaha, when it was time for a show by brushing her eyelashes against his cheek! Also, she had a clever way of getting at the sweets Jenda used in the show, but kept stored between times in a cabinet in Bertha's house. Of course, Bertha was an enormously powerful animal, and could easily have smashed the cabinet to smithereens, and nabbed the goodies. But that, evidently, would have been too gross a strategy for a being of her subtlety. Instead, when a stranger would wander into the elephant house, Bertha would grab his arm with her trunk. You can imagine how this would startle just about anybody, so Bertha, sensitive as she was to others' feelings, was just as gentle about it as she could be. But if her captive tried to pull away, she'd tighten her grip enough to let him know who was boss. Thus ensnared, the stranger would be guided to the cabinet where the sweets were stored. Then Bertha would place the person's hand on the handle, and hope the human had enough intelligence to deduce what was wanted of him.

On one occasion, however, the cabinet was unexpectedly locked, and the poor woman in Bertha's grasp didn't know what to do. When Bertha let go of her, she made a beeline for the door, trying to get out of there as fast as possible, but trying at the same time not to move so quickly as to panic the "dumb beast." Just before she could reach the door, however, there came a tap on her shoulder. Astonished, she turned around, and found herself staring at the great elephant. In her trunk, the elephant held the key to the cabinet, which she now dropped carefully into the woman's hand.[49]

Almost always, what is taken for rank stupidity on the part of animals turns out to be, instead, a lack of understanding on our human part. Ostriches, for example, are famed for stupidly sticking their heads in the sand when they want not to be seen. The truth of the matter, though, is that ostriches do not put their heads in the sand at all. When they sit on their massive eggs, their long necks and prominent heads make them a conspicuous and vulnerable target, visible to their enemies for miles. And so they have developed an ingenious and effective method of camouflaging themselves when they sense danger, but must remain on their eggs. By stretching their necks down and along the sand, they not only become less conspicuous, but also, from a distance, look very much like a small hill of sand.

The more I learn about animals, the more they astound me. There are birds who fly halfway around the globe, and yet return precisely to the same spot year after year. There are dolphin midwives who usher the newborn dolphins up for their first breath of air, while other dolphin midwives stay with the new mother and care for her. There are whales who communicate with each other through sound patterns of such wondrous beauty that some feel they have more intricacy than even a Beethoven symphony. But sometimes it seems as if we humans will recognize their forms of intelligence as worthy of our respect only if they discuss matters with us, in English and over tea.

FRESH FROM THE LAP OF GOD

There is always something adorable to me about a new born fawn, or a freshly-hatched duckling, or a new born calf, or, in fact, a new born animal of any kind, including human new borns. They shine, there is a lustre about them, a shimmering statement of the freshness they bring to life. To me, the fact that new born human infants and new born animal babies of all kinds glow with this ineffable sweetness testifies to our common source. They are born as we are—fresh from the lap of God, wanting to express their qualities in the service of the divine spark within them. They are born, as we are, thirsting for life. They are born, as we are, wanting to be all they are, and become all they can become.

They want to play their part in the universe, live the lives they were born to live. In many ways they remain like babies as they age, even if they grow as big as an elephant, for their lives are always intense with immediacy, rich with emotional and sensory experience.

Animals are part of our world, part of our existence. They give us reasons to celebrate life. They are part of us.

Sometimes they bring us challenges, sometimes they bring us the opportunity to help them, sometimes they bring us companionship. Often, they bring us play, beauty, and laughter, as they go about their business of being themselves. What we would miss if they were not here!

"If the stars should appear one night in a thousand, how men would believe and adore!"

So said Ralph Waldo Emerson. Can you imagine how we would feel if such were the fate of animals?

WHAT THE CHILDREN KNOW
Sometimes children understand these things better than we do. A young Girl Scout named Karyl Carter wrote a simple report that says it all so well.

"A beaver who swam, dove and somersaulted among canoeing Girl Scouts—that's what you would have seen at Camp Sacajawea Girl Scout Camp in Nefield, New Jersey, this summer.

"It was a late morning discovery. Girls from Holly Shores Girl Scout Council were taking canoeing lessons in Sacy's Lake when a large stump started to move and perform numerous swimming feats. Hearing laughter, squeals and screams, the waterfront director canoed out to the girls, identified the stump as a real beaver, and yelled to those on the beach, 'Go get the rest of the camp . . . they've never seen anything like this before.' In no time flat, the entire camp lined the lakefront, playing audience to a most talented but different kind of swimmer.

"The waterfront director, who was wary but excited, told the canoers, 'Just keep canoeing, don't pet the beaver, but enjoy the experience.' Meanwhile, a beach bystander ran to the camp office and called Hope Buyukmihci, naturalist and author, at Unexpected Wildlife Refuge, three miles away. 'Are you missing a beaver . . . a very friendly one?' The answer was yes. The beaver was Chopper, an orphan Ms. Buyukmihci had raised from infancy, and he was now over a year old and beginning to make it on his own in the wild.

"Minutes later, Hope drove in to Camp Sacy to con Chopper back home. But the next day Chopper was back in Sacy's lake, entertaining campers with his swimabatics. 'Maybe he's building a dam. Maybe he's going to raise a family,' said some of his young admirers.

"All of us were excited over these prospects. We told Hope about Chopper's whereabouts. She said he could stay and was happy that Chopper was on his own.

"Every day the staff members kept Hope informed of Chopper's activities. 'He may try to climb into your boats,' she

said, 'but he's just playing. He'll dive off immediately. And he
might just swim along or wrestle with you if you're in the water!'

"For the next three days, campers, leaders and staff members
observed, petted, fed and just plain enjoyed Chopper. The Girl
Scouts also learned about the looks, diet, habits and temperament of
a beaver who is accustomed to the world of people.

"During these beaver days, the atmosphere in the camp
drastically changed. There was a profound awareness that there
really was something alive and friendly out there in the woods and
waters.

"One afternoon the camp director decided to take some pictures
of Chopper. He found him swimming in a swampy area near the
Comanche campsite. An animal enthusiast, the director walked
right into the swamp, click-clicked the camera, and was then
promptly but playfully grabbed around the leg by Chopper. The
following day was hectic, with camp closing and campers leaving. It
wasn't until late Saturday afternoon that a few remaining staff
members decided to walk down to the lake to say goodbye to
Chopper.

"As we approached the lakefront, there were other last-minute
beaver admirers standing on the dock. They screamed—'Come
quickly!!!' We ran, only to find Chopper lying on the edge of the
dock, dead.

"These people, many of whom were young campers, had just
witnessed an unidentified fisherman maliciously beat Chopper to
death.

It seemed Chopper was disturbing this trespassing man's sport.
The fisherman, who was rowing away, shouted to us, 'That thing
tried to climb into my boat, so I hit it with my fishing pole. Then
it started to hiss at me. I had to hit it with my oar.'

"We wrapped Chopper up in a beach towel.

"We cried . . .'[50]

MY DREAM

I have a dream. I see humankind understanding that the spirit which
sings in our hearts sings as well in the hearts of the other animals. I see

us realizing that there are many kinds of intelligence, many kinds of souls, many kinds of suffering and striving. I see us knowing that all creatures are endowed with the same will-to-live which we possess. I see us respecting theirs, as we would like our own to be respected were we in the less powerful position and they dominant upon the earth.

I see us grateful for these extraordinary companions.

I see our lives rich with animals. I see us with many animal friends. I see our cities sprinkled with wild places, shorelines, parks, ravines and creek-canyons, where wild creatures can live. I see all life forms working together in harmony, cultivating the full potential of the planet.

I see us appreciating the different needs, different kinds of intelligence, and different responsibilities of the various animals. I see us sensing the unique ways in which they feel, they think, they suffer, and they love.

I see us learning to treat with respect those who are, in the greater scheme of things, but our younger brothers and sisters. I see us realizing they, too, are expressions, in their individual ways, of the universal life-force. I see us acting from the knowledge that it is the same God-Force that gives us all breath.

I see us realizing that all God's critters have a place in the choir.

BRAVE NEW CHICKEN

"Teaching a child not to step on a caterpillar is as valuable to the child as it is to the caterpillar."

(BRADLEY MILLER)

"The greatness of a nation can be judged by the way its animals are treated."

(GANDHI)

LIKE MOST PEOPLE, I would like to minimize the unnecessary suffering in the world. I want to eliminate needless violence and pain and I give my support, wherever I can, to a positive approach to this goal. But like most people I never gave much of a thought to the impact my way of eating had on the world. Sure, I knew animals were killed for meat, but isn't that the way of nature? Isn't that the way of life's food chains?

But I've learned that the animals used for food in the United States today are not just killed; something else happens to them. And finding out about it has changed me forever.

The more I've learned, the more I've felt that if people knew what really goes on they would make major changes in their food choices. Major changes that would go a very long way, not only towards improving their own health, but towards reducing the suffering in the world as well.

Let's start with chickens. In order to understand what happens to these animals, it helps to have a feeling for what kind of beings they are. Unfortunately, most of us have rather stereotyped visions of them.

The word "chicken" is often used as a synonym for "coward." But that is a human moniker. Chickens, while high-strung and quick to startle, are anything but gutless, timid creatures. Roosters are renowned for their pride, ferocity, and the adamant assertion of their power. Many cultures have exploited this fact in the so-called "sport" of cock fighting. And throughout the world a wide variety of cultures have acknowledged the potent spirit of the cock by using his name as a synonym for the male penis.[1] In languages all over the world the word for the male chicken is also used to signify human male sexual potency.[2]

Female hens are likewise not the craven creatures we've been conditioned to think they are. They can be absolutely fierce in defending their little ones, even against terrible odds and much larger predatory birds. A scientist who studied chickens for years, E. L. Watson, watched a mother hen defend her little chicks against the awesome attack of the dreaded raven.

> *"I have known one little old hen who reared chicks on the far western coast of Scotland near cliffs where ravens built their nests. On ordinary occasions, ravens are the terror of domesticated fowls, that fly to shelter at the first sight of the black wings. They dare not face beaks so much stronger than their own. (But) this little mother of a brood of ten would stand her ground with her hackles up, eyes glaring defiance. Such was her courage that she lost but one of her brood when two ravens came against her."*[3]

Chickens are not the fearful creatures we have been conditioned to think. And the generally-agreed-upon idea that they are stupid is equally ungrounded in fact.

Now, I'm not saying that chickens are the most brilliant of animals. But I do know that our understanding of what constitutes intelligence is utterly relative. If an aborigine drafted an I. Q. test, for example, all of Western civilization would probably flunk. We have a very convenient and self-serving way of defining intelligence. If an animal does something, we call it instinct. If we do the same thing for the same reason, we call it intelligence.

Personally, I wouldn't be too quick to try to define the intelligence of chickens. I'd be afraid of judging them by standards that are irrelevant to them. For the more I've learned about the kinds of creatures they are and what they have been known to do, the more I've been impressed by their unique kind of intelligence.

One naturalist gave a chicken-hen 21 guinea-fowl eggs he had found, just to see what would happen. These small, hard-shelled eggs are a far cry from a chicken's eggs. But the hen took the task to heart, and somehow managed to tend to all 21 of the eggs without a sign of protest. As a product of our conditioned conventional notions about chickens, I originally thought she did this simply because she was too stupid to notice they weren't her own eggs. When the chicks hatched, she didn't seem at all perturbed by the fact that they weren't chickens. Their small partridge-like appearance and unfamiliar ways evidently presented no problem to her. Again, I thought she was simply too stupid to notice they were not chickens. But I was wrong. She was far more tuned in to reality than I knew. After a few days brooding the little guinea fowl, she took them away out into the cover of some bushes. Instead of asking them to feed on the ordinary mash that was given the chickens, she scratched in some ants' nests for the white pupae. Chickens don't eat such food, but guinea fowl do! The little ones took to it with instinctive relish.[4]

How could she have known? What form of intelligence was she displaying? Was she perhaps sufficiently tuned in to have received some sort of message from their collective psyche? That's more than man can do!

On another occasion, a naturalist gave a chicken-hen some duck eggs. She tended them and hatched them as if they were her own, yet wasn't fazed at all when ducklings emerged from her labors instead of chicks. Utterly nonplussed by the situation, she proceeded to do something neither she nor any other chicken in the area had ever done before. She walked up on a plank bridging a stream. Then, clucking, she invited the little ducklings into the water.[5]

It is a mystery to me how these mother hens knew what to do for the babies they hatched who were of another species. But somehow they did. It appears that when we speak of being "taken under someone's wing" we are correctly referring to a remarkably caring and sensitive kind of nurturing.

Living as divorced from nature as most of us unfortunately do, we may not have much personal experience with chickens anymore, and so may not know what wonderful mothers they are. But throughout recorded history the hen has been a supreme symbol of the best kind of mothering. In fact, the Romans thought so much of the maternal qualities of the hen that they frequently used the phrase "son-of-a-hen" to mean a fortunate and well-cared-for man.[6]

NAKED AMIDST THE RUINS

Although the experiences and memories most of us have of chickens are colored by ill-founded biases, it is hard to forget the feeling of seeing freshly-hatched baby chicks, their little yellow heads pushing out from under their mother hen's feathers, their tiny yellow beaks just beginning to peck about. To many of us, freshly-hatched baby chicks are the very picture of innocence and adorability. Yet perhaps they also speak of something deeper, something inspirational. In pecking their way out of the egg, they can seem as well to symbolize our ongoing need to outgrow old limitations, our deep need to push against and expand beyond boundaries which have served a needed purpose, but which now must be left behind. In this, the little ones stand for the very opposite of the gutlessness we have been conditioned to think of as "chicken." They stand for courage. They peck their way out, not knowing what will await them. And when they emerge, they stand naked and new amidst the ruins of a past to which they can never return, having undertaken an irreversible journey into the unknown, simply because it is their destiny to do so.

Somehow these little chicks remind me of the bravery of the human spirit, and as well, of our situation as a species. Are we not also driven by an evolutionary imperative, by the call of our own growth and potential for expansion? Are we not, as a race, standing now amidst the slime and eggshells of our primeval past, not knowing what will become of us, yet already dreaming of the stars?

One thing's for sure. Chickens are far more sensitive than most of us give them credit for. A study at Virginia Polytechnic Institute found that chickens flourished when treated with affection. Researchers there spoke and sang gently to a group of baby chicks. As a result the chickens were friendlier, and put on more weight for the amount of feed consumed than did chickens who were ignored. The well treated birds were also more resistant to infection than the other chickens.[7]

WELCOME TO CHICKEN HEAVEN

The raising of chickens in the United States today is not, however, a process which overflows with compassion for these animals. Nor is it anything like the barnyard operation that comes to most of our minds when we imagine the lives of chickens. Fundamental changes have taken place in the past 30 years. Formerly, chickens were free-range birds, scratching and rooting around in the soil for grubs, earthworms, grass and larvae. They knew the sun and the wind and the stars, and the rooster crowing at the break of day was only one of many signs that showed they were deeply attuned to the natural cycles of light and dark.

But today this has all changed. The raising of chickens in the United States has become completely industrialized. We no longer live in the day of the barnyard chicken. We live now, I'm sorry to say, in the day of the assembly-line chicken.

There is a story behind today's poultry and eggs which we would never know from the clean little packages for sale in brightly lit modern supermarkets. It all looks so neat, comfortable and dependable, so carefully wrapped and labeled. As I stand in a tastefully decorated supermarket, serenaded by piped-in music, looking at egg cartons and poultry packages with happy drawings of smiling chickens, I find it hard indeed to imagine anything could be amiss. Every attempt is made to assure us that the chickens of today couldn't be happier or better cared for, and that no expense is spared in bringing us quality eggs and produce. Advertisements for Perdue, Inc., one of the nation's largest producers of chickens for meat, are typical. In them, the company president, Frank Perdue, tells us that his chickens live in "a house that's just chicken heaven."[8]

But it turns out there's not a great deal of truth in describing contemporary chicken accommodations as "chicken heaven."

To begin with, today's chicken farms are not really "farms" anymore, but should more accurately be called "chicken factories." Factories, because the chickens live their whole lives inside buildings entirely devoid of natural light. The day of the barnyard is long gone. There are no barns and no yards in today's mechanized world of poultry production, only assembly lines, conveyer belts, and fluorescent lights. Factories, because these proud and sensitive creatures are treated strictly as merchandise, with utter contempt for their spirits, with not a trace of feeling or compassion for the fact that they are living, breathing animals. Factories, because the chickens are systematically deprived of every conceivable expression of their natural urges.

Today's chicken factories are not farming as most of us conceive it. They are living expressions of the attitude that animals are things, raw materials to be consumed however we might wish.

I wish I were exaggerating. I wish I were describing isolated cases of negligent management. But I'm not. I'm describing the standard operating procedures of the egg and poultry industries today. I'm describing the operations that produce 98% of our eggs and poultry. I'm describing techniques and practices that are outlined and discussed every day of the week in trade journals such as *Poultry World, Poultry Tribune, Poultry Digest, Farmer and Stockbreeder,* and *Farm Journal.*

In the assembly-line world of today's chicken factories, chickens aren't called "chickens" anymore. If they have been bred for their flesh, they are called "broilers." If they have been bred for their eggs, they are called "layers." Now, not calling animals by their animal names, but giving them new names according the their food value to humans may not seem like a big deal in itself, but it is part of a process which deeply conditions us all into forgetting the spirit of the animals as living beings with their own dignity. In fact, the industry makes a deliberate point of not seeing the animals as animals.

"The modern layer is, after all, only a very efficient converting machine, changing the raw material—feedstuffs—into the finished product—the egg—less, of course, maintenance requirements."

(*FARMER AND STOCKBREEDER*[9])

HAPPY BIRTHDAY FACTORY STYLE

Male chicks, of course, have little use in the manufacture of eggs. So what do you think happens to the males? How are the little fellows greeted when, having pecked their way out of their shells, expecting to be met by the warmth of a waiting mother hen, they look around and seek to begin their lives on earth?

> *"They are, literally, thrown away. We watched at one hatchery as 'chicken-pullers' weeded males from each tray and dropped them into heavy-duty plastic bags. Our guide explained: 'We put them in a bag and let them suffocate.' "* [10]

It's not a picture to bring joy to a mother's heart, but over half-a-million little baby chicks are "disposed of" in this fashion every day of the year in the United States. In the seconds it takes you to read this paragraph, over 2,000 newborn male chicks will be thrown by human hands into garbage bags to smother among their brothers, without the slightest acknowledgment that they are alive.

And they are, perhaps, the lucky ones. Because for those chicks allowed to live, the "life" that follows is truly a nightmare.

In today's modern factories, chickens, exquisitely sensitive to the earth's natural rhythms of light and dark, never see or feel the light of the sun. Broiler chicks arrive at the producers via conveyer belt, in batches of tens of thousands. Fresh from the incubators and mechanized hatcheries, only a few hours old, the fluffy yellow babies peep constantly in frail little voices for their missing mothers. But they will never know the sound of their mother's voice, nor the warmth of her body, nor the comfort of her protection. There will be no scratching in the dust for tasty bugs, no strutting and preening, no crowing to announce the dawn.

These little chicks come equipped with a God-given life expectancy of 15 to 20 years. But under the conditions of modern factory farming, modern "broilers" might make it to the ripe old age of two months. In comparison, the "layers" are veritable Methuselahs—the longest lived amongst them might possibly live as long as two years.

The more I've learned about these factories, the more ironic it has seemed to call them "chicken heavens." Consisting of windowless warehouses, with tiers of cages stacked on top of each other from floor to ceiling, like shipping crates, the environment has been systematically designed to maximize the profits of the agribusiness corporations that own the sheds and the birds. It has not been designed with any concern whatever for the chickens' natural urges, minimum comfort, or even their health.

Inside the windowless warehouse, every aspect of the birds' environment is totally controlled, in order to make them grow as fast as possible, or produce as many eggs as possible, at the least possible cost to the company that owns the operation. Incidentally, the companies that own our nation's chicken factories are not generally agricultural enterprises, as you might have imagined. As Peter Singer has shown in his excellent *Animal Liberation*, they are companies like Textron, Inc., a manufacturer of pencils and helicopters. These companies go into the business simply because it looks like a profitable venture.[11] Accordingly, they apply to chickens the business practices that work with pencils and helicopters, thus treating these breathing, passionate animals with the same consideration they use for pencils.

THE SOCIAL LIFE OF HENS
The renowned English ethologist, Desmond Morris, author of *The Naked Ape*, has written about today's methods of raising hens in cages (also called "batteries").

> *"Anyone who has studied the social life of birds carefully will know that theirs is a subtle and complex world, where food and water are only a small part of their behavioral needs. The brain of each bird is programmed with a complicated set of drives and responses which set it on the path to a life full of special territorial, nesting, roosting, grooming, parental, aggressive and sexual activities, in addition to the feeding behavior. All of these activities are totally denied the battery hens."[12]*

Chickens are by nature highly social animals. In any kind of natural setting, be it a farmyard or the wild, they develop a social hierarchy, often known as a "pecking order." Every bird yields, at the food trough and elsewhere, to those above it in rank, and takes precedence over those below.

The social order is extremely important to these birds. According to studies published in *The New Scientist*, chickens can maintain a stable pecking order, with each bird knowing all the others individually, and aware of its place among them, in flocks with up to 90 chickens.[13] Beyond 90 birds, however, things can get out of hand. Of course, in any kind of natural setting, flocks would never get nearly that large. But in today's "chicken heavens," flocks tend to be larger than the 90 bird limit.

How much larger? *Poultry Digest* reports that the flock size in a typical egg factory is 80,000 birds per warehouse![14]

JUST LIKE A MOTHER HEN

In such a situation the birds are completely unable to satisfy one of the most basic and intense priorities of their nature, which is to develop a sense of social order and their place within it.

The results aren't very pretty. Unable to establish any kind of social identity for themselves, the cooped-up animals fight constantly with each other. They are driven berserk by the lack of space and the complete frustration of their primal need for a social order. In their frustration they peck viciously at each other's feathers, frequently try to kill one another and even try to eat each other alive. The industry takes note of these developments, but only in terms of its effect on profits.

> *"Feather-pecking and cannibalism easily become serious vices among birds kept under intensive conditions. They mean lower productivity and lost profits."*
>
> *(THE FARMING EXPRESS)*[15]

Any behavior among chickens which threatens profits is known in the trade as a "vice," a term that truly gives me pause. Where is the virtue in keeping birds in these conditions?

Since the animals insist on behaving like the proud and sensitive creatures they are, and trying even under these bizarre conditions to express their natural urges, the experts who manage today's factory farms have to respond. They have to do something, because if very many of the birds kill each other money is lost, and that is the one thing they can't let happen. They know that the birds' berserk behavior arises out of the unnatural ways in which the birds are kept. So what do the factory managers do? Make the conditions even more unnatural, of course.

The preferred method in the industry today is to cut off part of the chickens' beaks, a process known as "de-beaking."[16] This does nothing to reduce the conditions which drive the chickens so mad that they attack each other viciously. But it renders them incapable of doing much harm to company profits.

The people who run today's poultry factories are not concerned that the process of cutting off part of the chickens' beaks requires cutting through highly sensitive soft tissue, similar to the tender sensitive flesh under human fingernails and causes the animals severe pain. Nor do they mind the fact that they are crippling the animals, and cutting off the animals' most important member. Today's poultry producers are highly satisfied with de-beaking. Employed almost universally in the industry today,[17] this practice helps the producers to keep the chickens alive under the stressful, inhumane and overcrowded conditions which are the cause of the animals unnatural aggression and cannibalism in the first place.

Even from a strictly dollars-and-cents viewpoint, however, there are a few drawbacks to the procedure. As one farm publication noted:

> *"Sometimes the irregular growth of beaks on a de-beaked bird makes it difficult or impossible to drink where a normal bird would have no trouble."* [18]

The factory experts are not pleased with the tendency of ungrateful young de-beaked birds either to die of thirst because they are unable to drink from nipple-type watering devices or else to starve to death within inches of their food supply because they can't manage to eat. Nor are they happy with the birds who survive but can't gain weight according to schedule because they have trouble eating. This is not something they want to see, because chicken flesh is sold by the pound.

Not ones to be defeated by the deaths and disabilities of de-beaked birds, however, today's producers have sought to counter such losses and increase profits, through advertising. They simply tell the public that their chickens "couldn't be happier." One huge broiler producer, Paramount Chickens, has aired TV commercials in which a smiling Pearl Bailey (who probably doesn't know the truth any more than most of us) reassures us that Paramount looks after their chickens "just like a mother hen."[19]

This is a remarkable statement. How many mother hens have been known to cut the beaks off their babies, and force them to live under conditions in which they cannot establish a social identity, and so are driven berserk?

ENLIGHTENED?
You have probably heard the magnificent trumpeting of roosters at daybreak, the passionate, full-throated announcement that dawn has come. The sound with which they welcome the day testifies, not only to their proud and passionate spirits, but also to how sensitive chickens are to light. This is a fact that modern poultrymen know, and do not hesitate to exploit.

In the windowless warehouses we are asked to believe are "chicken heavens," the artificial lighting is manipulated in the most unnatural ways to maximize profits and minimize costs. Broilers are often subjected to bright light 24 hours a day for the first two weeks. Then the lights may be dimmed slightly and go off and on every two hours.[20] At about six weeks of age, the animals have gone so completely crazy from all this that the lights must be turned off completely in an attempt to calm them down. But even then the absence of any outlet whatsoever for the birds' natural energies and drives leads to a great deal of fighting, with the de-beaked birds pecking painfully at each other in the dark, often managing despite the mutilation of their beaks to kill each other. It's at times like this that farm managers will sometimes reveal the depth of their compassion for the animals in their care.

"It's a damn shame when they kill each other. It means we wasted all the feed that went into the damn thing."

(HERBERT REED, POULTRY PRODUCER)[21]

The lighting conditions for young layer hens (called "pullets") are a little different from those provided for broilers, though not exactly what you'd call natural. These youngsters are kept in "grow-out" buildings which are usually kept completely dark except for feeding times.[22] Then, when the young hens reach the age where they can begin to lay eggs, everything suddenly changes. Having lived their entire lives in complete darkness, except for feeding times, the hens now find themselves subjected to harsh and continuous light.

> *"At one farm, a period of 23 hours lighting a day has been tested."* [23]

AGRIBUSINESS LAYS AN EGG

The folks who design what the industry tells us are "chicken heavens" are real virtuosos when it comes to manipulating the environment of the animals for maximum profit. When a layer hen's production begins to slacken, the producers do not just sit back and let her output wane. Not when they have found it possible to bolster her egg production by a procedure known in the trade as "force-moulting."[24] The already panicked and exhausted hen will suddenly find herself plunged into complete darkness. The artificial lighting, which heretofore had been on for upwards of 17 hours a day, is now completely cut off, and at the same time her food and water are removed. After two days of starving without even water in the dark, the bird, still without food or light, is allowed water. Eventually lighting and food will be returned to what passes for "normal." Those hens who survive this ingenious procedure will have been shocked into physiological processes associated, under natural conditions, with the seasonal loss of plumage and growth of fresh feathers. After the forced moulting, those hens who survive the ordeal may be sufficiently productive to be kept around for another two months. Then they join those who did not survive the procedure in the first place in our chicken soup.

Hopefully, the hen will have learned something from the days without food or water, because the farm managers certainly have. During her last 30 hours before slaughter she will again receive no food. A headline in *Poultry Tribune* reminded poultry producers to "Take Feed

Away From Spent Hens."[25] The trade journal brilliantly calculated that food given to hens during the last 30 hours of their lives doesn't have time to turn into flesh. It stays in the digestive system, and so, counsel the experts, is nothing but a waste of feed.

THE PANIC BUTTON

Despite being treated consistently as machinery in today's chicken factories, the chickens still stubbornly refuse to settle down and devote themselves singlemindedly to producing as many eggs as possible and growing as fat as they can, in the shortest possible length of time. Instead, they insist on thinking of themselves as animals, with drives and needs.

But today's chickens are allowed no expression of their natural urges. They cannot walk around, scratch the ground, build a nest, or even stretch their wings. Every instinct is frustrated. The bizarre lighting manipulations allow these light-sensitive creatures no vestige of a natural sleep cycle. They cannot establish a pecking order, or any sense of social identity. They cannot keep out of each other's way, and weaker birds have no escape from the stronger ones, already maddened by the grotesque conditions in which they live.

The result is that these passionate creatures live in a state of perpetual panic. They fly into an uproar at the slightest disturbance, and show every sign of having been driven completely out of their minds. One naturalist noted:

> *"The battery chickens I have observed seem to lose their minds about the time they would normally be weaned by their mothers and off in the weeds chasing grasshoppers on their own account. Yes, literally, the battery becomes a gallinaceous madhouse."* [26]

Another reporter states:

> *"The birds in the laying house are hysterical . . . Birds squawk, cackle and cluck as they scramble over one another for a peck at the automatically controlled grain trough or a drink of water. This is how the hens spend their short life of ceaseless production."* [27]

Another account, this one from a scientist who has spent his whole life observing animal behavior, tells us that today's chickens are prone to:

> ". . . *stampedes. With no apparent cause, a wave of hysteria sweeps over the whole battery; wild, unnatural chirps, jumbled screams, and a fluttering as if every feather on every chicken had become possessed and frantic.*" [28]

In their panic, the birds will sometimes pile on top of each other and some will smother to death. Poultry producers are not by and large what you would call sentimental types, but since smothered birds represent a "waste of feed" this is the type of thing that will definitely spur them into action. Not to be outsmarted, they have found the piling problem can be decreased by crowding the chickens so tightly into wire cages they can hardly move. This way, when they panic, they can't pile on top of each other as readily.

The cages produce a few problems of their own, however, that make the calling of them "chicken heavens" even more deceitful: the caged hens still try to behave as if they were designed by Nature to live on the earth, instead of in wire cages. For instance, their toenails continue to grow. With no solid ground to wear the nails down, they become very long, and can get permanently entangled in the wire. The ex-president of a national poultry organization wrote in the *Poultry Tribune* about the many times when, on removing a batch of hens from a cage:

> ". . . *we have discovered chickens literally grown fast to the cage. It seems the chickens' toes got caught in the wire mesh in some manner and would not loosen. So, in time, the flesh of the toes grew completely around the wire.*" [29]

Needless to say, those birds who get stuck in the back of the cage, where they cannot reach food or water, starve to death.

Once again, however, the minds that created this whole situation have come up with an ingenious solution to prevent such a distressing "waste of feed." The idea is simply to cut off the toes of the little chicks when they are a day or two of age.

In most cages, there is at least one poor bird who has undergone these grotesque conditions and has entirely lost the will to live. These sad creatures no longer resist being shoved aside, pushed underfoot and trampled by the other birds. They are probably the birds who, in a natural flock, would be low on the pecking order. Although they would defer to the others, and not have much status, they would nevertheless play a needed part in the life of the flock. They would mate, have chicks to care for, and live out their lives. In the cages, however, life is not very kind to the little guy. The results are pathetic.

> *". . . these birds can do nothing but huddle in a corner of the cage, usually near the bottom of the sloping floor, where their fellow inmates trample over them as they try to get to the food or water trough."* [30]

SPACE FOR RENT

I have met quite a few people who seem to think that chickens are vegetables. When someone says he or she is a vegetarian, these people reply with something like, "Yes, but you do eat chicken, don't you?" I feel reasonably confident that most of today's poultry producers know their stock well enough to realize that chickens aren't vegetables. But they seem unable to grasp the fact that they are animals, and as such have profound territorial needs.

At the Hainsworth Farm in Mt. Morris, New York, naturalist Roy Bedichèk found four and even five hens squeezed into cages 12 inches by 12 inches.[31] Under these conditions, the birds are unable to lift a single wing. In fact, they are squeezed together so tightly that they have a great deal of difficulty even turning around in place. This is not seen by the factory managers as a bad thing, though. With their bodies in forced contact at all times on all sides with other chickens, they absorb heat from their fellow inmates, so this cuts down on heating costs.

The Hainsworth farm is an extreme example. But the industry norm isn't much better. A surprisingly large percentage of the eggs eaten in Los Angeles come from the 345 acre "Egg City" in Moorpark, California.[32] Here, some 2,200,000 eggs are laid daily by 3 million hens. The hens are housed five to each 16-by-18 cage.[33]

To get a chicken's eye view of these conditions, picture yourself standing in a crowded elevator. The elevator is so crowded, in fact, that your body is in contact on all sides with other bodies. Even to turn around in place would be difficult. And one more thing to keep in mind—this is your life. It is not just a temporary bother, until you get to your floor. This is permanent. Your only release will be at the hands of the executioner.

By the way, in your picture of the elevator, you may have imagined the other people trapped with you as doing the very best they can to hold still, and not make things difficult for you. But what if all the others do not have the ability to understand what is happening? What if they react to the terror of it all with raw instinct, without even a trace of a civilized veneer? What if, like you, they have powerful territorial needs, and the utter frustration of the situation has driven them literally insane, prone to erupt into violence with or without provocation?

Now imagine further that the floor of the elevator is slanted sharply, so gravity tends to push you all in one direction. The ceiling is so short that you and the others can only stand upright towards one side, and the floor is made of a wire mesh that is terribly uncomfortable to everyone's feet. And to complete this approximation of the living conditions in today's factory farms, what if some of the others trapped with you in the elevator have, in their madness, become cannibalistic?

These are the conditions which the industry tells us is a "chicken heaven."

This is the actual living situation of the chickens whose flesh and eggs Americans eat.

BREEDING A "BETTER" CHICKEN

Chicken breeders have been hard at work developing a "better" chicken, which to their way of thinking is the heaviest possible one. (Remember, profit is per pound.) The result is a bird whose skeleton becomes, every year, less able to support his increasingly massive weight. The fleshy bodies of "broilers" today grow so fast that their bones and joints can't keep pace. The trade journal, *Broiler Industry*, reports that the chickens raised for meat today can hardly stand under their weight, so spend most of their time huddling "down on their haunches."[34]

> *"Skeletal disorders are common. Many of these animals crouch or hobble about in pain on flawed feet and legs."* [35]

Problems like these are not considered particularly noteworthy by the industry which tells us they take care of their chickens "just like a mother hen," because lameness effects only the living animal, not the price to be had for his flesh. Animals can be sold for meat whether or not they are crippled.

The same breeders who brought us these grossly top-heavy birds are hard at work to accomplish other grotesque feats of genetic engineering. You may have thought, as I did, that God pretty much knew what He was doing when He designed animals. But the folks at the Animal Research Institute of Agriculture, Canada, have a better idea. The director of the Institute, R. S. Gowe, enlightened me on the subject when he spoke at a conference in Ottawa in December, 1978, on "Livestock Intensive Methods of Production." Said Gowe, proudly:

> *"At the Animal Research Institute, we are trying to breed animals without legs, and chickens without feathers."* [36]

I must admit it took me awhile to comprehend why anyone would want to breed a chicken without feathers. But I finally came to understand why at least six universities in the U. S. and Canada are presently trying to do so.[37] If only chickens didn't have feathers, then the folks who care for them "just like a mother hen" would be spared the bother of plucking them out.

FLIPPED OUT
There are many other ways, besides having feathers, that chickens make themselves difficult to their caretakers. *Poultry Digest* describes the growing problem of "Flip-Over Syndrome." This condition:

". . . is characterized by birds jumping into the air, sometimes emitting a loud squawk, and then falling over dead." [38]

Post-mortem exams show the bird's hearts are full of blood clots, but it is not known whether this is a result or a cause of their deaths. The problem of "Flip-Over Syndrome" has the experts stymied. They don't have any idea what makes the birds suddenly jump into the air and die. I don't know either, but I think it is probably safe to say that the birds are not jumping into the air because they cannot restrain a spontaneous upsurge of joy and delight.

THE FINE CUISINE OF CHICKEN HEAVEN
What do you think the lucky residents of today's chicken heavens dine on before we dine on them? Researchers who wrote an article titled "Poultry Production" in *Scientific American* investigated contemporary chicken cuisine, and they were seriously concerned with its quality:

"The modern fowl thrives (sic) on a diet almost totally foreign to any food it ever found in nature. Its feed is a product of the laboratory." [39]

A poultryman summarized the matter this way:

"Virtually all chickens raised in the United States today are fed a diet laced with antibiotics from their first day to their last. Without antibiotics, the industry could not maintain the intensive farming practices. An awful lot of them die anyway, before we can get our profit out of them. Without antibiotics, why, we'd be back to the backward practices of yesteryear." [40]

Heaven forbid! Why, back then the chickens were deprived of a steady supply of sulfa drugs, hormones, antibiotics and nitrofurans.[41] And what on earth did the poor birds ever do without the arsenicals? Over 90% of today's chickens are fed arsenic compounds.[42]

I had assumed that the diet fed to chickens would be one chosen for its ability to keep the animals healthy. But such, I have found, is not the case. Broilers fetch a price according to their weight, not according to their health, so their diet is selected purely for its ability to maximize their weight as cheaply as possible. Similarly, the diet fed to layers is selected strictly for its ability to stimulate egg production at the lowest possible cost.

As a result, these are not the healthiest animals you could find. According to *Poultry Digest*, an increasing number of today's chickens suffer from "Caged Layer Fatigue." These birds undergo the withdrawal of minerals from their bones and muscles, and eventually are unable to stand.[43]

Caged Layer Fatigue is actually only one of many health problems that flourish among modern chickens, whose diet is not designed with their health in mind. In the classic work on contemporary animal agriculture, *Animal Factories*, Peter Singer and Jim Mason report:

> *"Vitamin deficiencies common in poultry factories . . . result in a variety of conditions, including retarded growth, eye damage, blindness, lethargy, kidney damage, disturbed sexual development, bone and muscle weakness, brain damage, paralysis, internal bleeding, anemia, and deformed beaks and joints. Dietary deficiencies and other factory conditions can cause a variety of bodily deformities. In poultry, fragile bones, slipped tendons, twisted lower legs, and swollen joints are among the symptoms of mineral deficient diets . . . Some poultry diseases can leave birds with malformed backbones, twisted necks, and inflamed joints."*[44]

These poor animals are riddled with disease. In fact, due to the danger of contracting diseases from chickens, the Bureau of Labor has listed the poultry processing industry as one of the most hazardous of all occupations.[45]

Many of the health problems which occur regularly to these sad creatures were unknown only a few years ago. It is common today for caged birds to lose their feathers. It isn't known whether this is from rubbing constantly against the wire, from feather-pecking by other birds, or because of the totally unnatural diet and lack of sunlight. But whatever the cause, the result is that without their feathers the chickens' skin begins to rub directly against the wire.[46] When I first saw these birds I was startled by the sight, and didn't even recognize they were chickens. Their skins are raw and sore and bright red. They look more like a walking wound than a bird.

It is hard to underestimate the health of today's chickens. Driven to a state of hysteria, their raw skins rubbing constantly against the wire cages in which they are packed like living sardines, a staggering percentage of these animals contract cancer. A government report found that over 90% of the chickens from most of the flocks in the country are infected with chicken cancer (leukosis)![47]

You and I may wonder at the level of health in food produced by a system which so totally disregards the health and well-being of its animals. But today's poultry producers are rarely hampered by such considerations. They are a dedicated group, with a steadfast single-mindedness of purpose. Only their purpose is not, as you might have thought, to produce healthy food. As Fred C. Haley, president of a 225,000 hen Georgia poultry firm put it:

"The object of producing eggs is to make money. When we forget this objective, we have forgotten what it is all about." [48]

The money Mr. Haley is talking about is not made by the farmer who spends his day with the animals. It is made by agribusiness oligopolies. The actual chicken farmer amounts to a mere hired hand who virtually works for the huge "integrated chicken processors," and "amalgamated poultry producers." He is the one in daily contact with the birds; he is the one who sees and lives with the animals; and he may very well have feelings about what is being done to them. But if he protests, well, he can always be replaced by someone "better suited" to the job. He is not the one who has devised the production strategies that prevail in the industry today, and though he may have to implement them, he is not the one who profits by them. A study by the director of the Agribusiness Accountability Project, Jim Hightower, showed that in 1974, when chicken prices were running 80 to 90 cents a pound in the supermarket, the chicken farmers themselves were getting just two cents a pound.[49]

Of course, the corporate managers who are making the money love to portray themselves in the public eye as old-fashioned farmers. In one case, a number of the top executives of one of the international cartels that control the nation's poultry production testified before Congress dressed in overalls.

AN ASSEMBLY-LINE CHICKEN IN EVERY POT

We are a nation with an assembly-line chicken in every pot. We do not know that we eat the bodies and eggs of tortured creatures. We do not know they have been inoculated, dosed with hormones and antibiotics, and injected with dyes so that their meat and yolks will appear to be a "healthy-looking" yellow. How far out of touch we have become, not only with animals but with our own taste buds, to be susceptible to being so deceived.

Some people are beginning to suspect, however, that today's poultry products aren't what they should be. The comedian George Burns spoke of the first time he ate scrambled eggs without ketchup.

> *"I never knew they tasted like that. They tasted like the chicken wasn't getting paid."*

Needless to say, with money at stake, the industry isn't taking the matter of tasteless chicken lying down. The trade journal *Broiler Industry* has come up with an idea they think will remedy the situation. It is an idea which exemplifies their whole approach to food production.

> *"We've been accused of selling a chicken with less flavor than the 'old-time' chicken . . . Attempts are being made at overcoming the flavor problem by injection."* [50]

That should take care of everything!

In another issue, *Broiler Industry* saliently proposes:

> *"It should be possible to uncover a material, or materials, that could impart that 'old-fashioned flavor' to chickens."* [51]

And if that doesn't do the trick, don't think for a moment that the agribusiness experts are going to admit defeat. In spite of the universal use of ever more chemicals and drugs in egg production today, one industry leader tersely advises a marketing strategy designed to take care of the problem once and for all. His suggestion?

"Slant egg carton copy along this line: 'Eggs are a health food. A natural human food. No additives, no preservatives.'" [52]

I find the latest developments in poultry production truly disturbing. The huge multinational conglomerates, and those who must compete with them or be forced out of business, in their utter disregard for the suffering of innocent animals, have lost touch with something very basic.

Today's egg and poultry consumers know nothing of this. We have been deliberately kept in the dark about what modern poultry production has become, and have no idea of the relentless and systematic misery in which the chickens live. Every day people eat the flesh and eggs of these poor creatures, utterly unaware what they have suffered.

What are the consequences of eating the products of such a system? Could it be that when we consume the flesh and eggs of these poor animals, something of the sickness, misery and terror of their lives enters us? Could it be that when we take their flesh or eggs into our bodies, we take in as well something of the kinds of lives they have been forced to endure? Instinctively, I can't help but believe this is so.

IN SEARCH OF THE NATURAL BIRD
You may wonder whether you'd be better off eating turkey. Sorry, but the methods applied to the factory production of poultry and eggs are also applied today to other birds, such as turkeys, geese and ducks. [53] These birds are treated with equal disdain for their natural urges and needs, and equal fixation on using them for profit. Turkeys are de-beaked, stuffed in wire cages, and fed the same sort of unnatural diet as chickens, complete with chemicals, drugs and antibiotics. [54]

There are, however, alternatives. One is to consume only "free range," "organic," or "natural" poultry products. Natural food stores often carry items so labeled, but you have to be awfully careful. Words like "organic" and "natural" and "free range" mean different things to different people, and much money has been made by people lying about such terms. The USDA has regulations governing the use of the word "natural," but these regulations are so loose that virtually anything can be so labeled. There are no restrictions at all on the use of antibiotics, or on the housing conditions the animals must endure.

Some health food store owners are more scrupulous than others, but even the best of them may not know all the facts. Many in California carry "Happy Hen Ranch Fresh Eggs," which come in a carton with a picture of a cheerful hen in the midst of luxurious fields. However, I've seen the so-called "happy hens" of the Happy Hen Egg Ranch (near San Jose, California) however, and they do not look very happy to me. They do not live in the spacious fields depicted on the egg carton. They are kept in cages.

In 1986, *East-West* published a conscientious report titled "In Search of the Natural Chicken." Their research found that almost all the poultry products currently sold in the United States as "natural or "organic" come, unfortunately, from chickens whose living conditions are hardly better than the industry norm. Summarizing the investigation, the author noted, none-too-encouragingly:

> *"Some eggs sold as 'fertile, laid by free-range hens' are produced by hens that actually are kept in barns in a space no greater than those kept in cages . . . (With only two exceptions) no sellers of natural poultry products that we contacted suggested that their chickens enjoyed anything resembling a free-range existence."* [55]

The best bet, if you really want to eat poultry products, is to raise them yourself or buy them from someone you know personally. A distant second would be to buy them from a natural food store, but you had better be willing to make a nuisance of yourself with lots of uncomfortable questions. The people who run the store should know the details of how the chickens whose eggs and flesh they sell have been raised and fed. If they don't know, or if their answers are vague or evasive, then, unfortunately, the truth is likely not what you would wish it to be.

The Farm Animals Concern Trust (FACT) has established humane standards for keeping layer hens without cages. Farms comply-

ing with these standards are given use of the FACT trademark—
NEST EGGS®. Though this is not yet widely available, if you buy
eggs bearing this trademark you can be sure you are not partaking of,
or contributing to, the conditions described in this chapter.

An alternative many informed people are taking is to stop eating
poultry products altogether. If you wonder whether you could satisfy
your protein and other nutritional needs if you did not partake of the
products of chicken factories, the answer, as chapters six through ten
will show, is an emphatic yes. The most rigorous scientific research
has determined that these foods are far from the ultimate nutritional
cornerstones the industry would like us to believe. In fact, they contribute mightily to the ravages of heart disease, cancer, strokes, and
many other serious diseases.

I have too much respect for the human journey to take it upon
myself to decide for you what you should or shouldn't eat, and where
you should draw the line. We are each unique. We have different
needs, different emotional associations to different foods, and different
biochemistry. We have our individual life situations to deal with, and
our individual paths to forge. We are each of us responsible for our
own choices, and for the consequences of our choices. However, the
better informed we are, the more intelligently we are able to make food
choices that serve our true needs.

NOW WHAT?

The poultry producers consider themselves innocent of any wrong
doing. They say they do what they do to bring down the price we pay
for our eggs and poultry. To that end, they claim they are simply
people committed to a well-defined sense of purpose, which is to raise
"broilers" for the slaughterhouse and "layer" hens for eggs by the
most cost-effective means possible. That this should happen to involve
the brutalization of billions of innocent animals is, as far as they are
concerned, irrelevant.

The agribusiness companies have their eyes firmly set on the bottom line. But they cannot see there is yet a deeper bottom line. Although they cannot see the more far-reaching consequences of their
actions, these consequences nonetheless exist. None of us is immune

from the repercussions of our actions and choices. As we sow, so shall we reap.

> *"There is a destiny that makes us brothers,*
> *None goes his way alone—*
> *All that we send into the lives of others*
> *Comes back into our own."*

(AUTHOR UNKNOWN)

I don't know what shall be the destinies of those responsible for the animal factories of today. But regardless of the future, it is already sadly true that they live in a heartless world. Treating animals like machines, they are profoundly separated from nature, deeply alienated from kinship with life. They are already in a kind of hell.

If we buy and eat the products of this system of food production, are we not colluding with them in creating this hell?

Is that how we want to vote with our lives?

THE MOST UNJUSTLY MALIGNED OF ALL ANIMALS

"Whenever people say 'we mustn't be sentimental,' you can take it they are about to do something cruel. And if they add, 'we must be realistic,' they mean they are going to make money out of it."

(BRIGID BROPHY)

"There is a single magic, a single power, a single salvation, and a single happiness, and that is called loving."

(HERMAN HESSE)

IN OUR HUMAN blindness concerning the feelings, intelligence, and sensitivity of animals, there is one in particular about whom we've been most wrong. If it were possible to measure our misunderstanding about our fellow creatures on some giant scale, our ignorance of this particular animal might well be the greatest of all. This is an animal who has been abused and ridiculed by people for centuries, but who is actually a friendly, forgiving, intelligent and good natured animal when he isn't mistreated. I am talking, you may be surprised to find out, about the pig.

THE HIDDEN TRUTH ABOUT PIGS
To call a man a "pig," or a woman a "sow," is one of the worst insults in our common speech. This fact testifies not to the nature of pigs, but to our beliefs about them, and only shows how far out of touch we are with these animals. The commonly held image of pigs as greedy, fat, and filthy creatures, gross beasts who eat anything that isn't fastened down, and who selfishly indulge their basest instincts without a trace of sensitivity, could hardly be further from the truth.

Pigs actually have one of the highest measured I. Q.'s of all animals, surpassing even the dog. They are friendly, sociable, fun-loving beings as well. One person very familiar with pigs was naturalist W. H. Hudson. He wrote in his acclaimed *Book of a Naturalist*:

> *"I have a friendly feeling towards pigs generally, and consider them the most intelligent of beasts, not excepting the elephant and the anthropoid ape . . . I also like his attitude towards all other creatures, especially man. He is not suspicious, or shrinkingly submissive, like horses, cattle and sheep; not an impudent devil-may-care like the goat; nor hostile like the goose; nor condescending like the cat; nor a flattering parasite like the dog. He views us from a totally different, a sort of democratic standpoint as fellow-citizens and brothers, and takes it for granted, or grunted, that we understand his language, and without servility or insolence he has a natural, pleasant, camerados-all or hail-fellow-well-met air with us."* [1]

In the common mind, pigs are disgusting creatures, but in fact the only thing disgusting about pigs is our attitude towards them. They are playful, sensitive, friendly animals, who like to roll around and rub on things, and consider the earth their home and not something with which to avoid contact. In a state of nature, pigs love to wallow in the mud, just as stags and buffaloes and many other animals do, especially in the hot days of summer when flies are most troublesome. But pigs don't love mud for its own sake. They use it to cool themselves off, and to gain relief from the flies. They enjoy themselves exuberantly because it is their way to enjoy what they do with robust good nature. People who have seen them in mud have accused them of being filthy animals, not understanding their simple love of the earth. However, when living in anything even remotely resembling their natural conditions, pigs are as naturally clean as any other forest creature. [2] If at all possible, they will never soil their own bedding, eating, or living areas.

But for many years it was the belief in Europe that the filthier the state in which a pig was kept, the better tasting the pork would be. Hence it became commonplace for pigs to be kept in a fashion that made it impossible for them to stay clean. Even then, though, they would often go to great lengths to maintain as clean a living situation as they could manage.

HUDSON'S PIG

Did you know that pigs recognize people, remember individuals clearly, and appreciate human contact when it is not hostile? The naturalist W. H. Hudson wrote a beautiful account of a pig who:

> "... not knowing my sentiments, looked askance at me and moved away when I first began to visit him. But when he made the discovery that I generally had apples and lumps of sugar in my coat pockets he all at once became excessively friendly and followed me about, and would put his head in my way to be scratched, and licked my hands with his rough tongue to show that he liked me. Every time I visited the cows and horses I had to pause beside the pigpen to open the gate into the field; and invariably the pig would get up and coming towards me salute me with a friendly grunt. And I would pretend not to hear or see, for it made me sick to look at his pen in which he stood belly-deep in the fetid mire; and it made me ashamed to think that so intelligent and good-tempered an animal should be kept in such abominable conditions ...
>
> "One morning as I passed the pen he grunted—spoke, I may say—in such a pleasant friendly way that I had to stop and return his greeting; then, taking an apple from my pocket I placed it in his trough. He turned it over with his snout, then looked up and said something like 'Thank you' in a series of gentle grunts. Then he bit off and ate a small piece, then another small bite, and eventually taking what was left in his mouth he finished eating it. After that, he always expected me to stay a minute and speak to him when I went to the field; I knew it from his way of greeting me, and on such occasions I gave him an apple. But he never ate it greedily; he appeared more inclined to talk than to eat, until by degrees I came to understand what he was saying. What he said was that he appreciated my kind intentions in giving him apples. But, he went on, to tell the real truth, it is not a fruit I am particularly fond of. I am familiar with its taste as they sometimes give me apples, usually the small unripe or bad ones that fall from

*the trees. However, I don't actually dislike them. I get skim milk
and am rather fond of it; then a bucket of mash, which is good
enough for hunger; but what I enjoy most is a cabbage, only I don't
get one very often now. I sometimes think that if they would let me
out of this muddy pen to ramble like the sheep and other beasts in
the field, or on the downs, I should be able to pick up a number of
morsels which would taste better than anything they give me. Apart
from the subject of food, I hope you won't mind me telling you that
I'm rather fond of being scratched on the back.*

*"So I scratched him vigorously with my stick and made him
wriggle his body and wink and blink and smile delightedly all over
his face. Then I said to myself: 'Now what the juice can I do more
to please him?' For though under sentence of death, he had done no
wrong, but was a good, honest-hearted fellow mortal, so that I felt
bound to do something to make the miry remnant of his existence a
little less miserable.*

*"I think it was the word 'juice' I had used—for that was how
I pronounced it to make it less like a swear-word—that gave me an
inspiration. In the garden, a few yards back from the pen, there
was a large clump of old eldertrees, now overloaded with ripening
fruit—the biggest clusters I had ever seen. Going to the trees, I
selected and cut the finest bunch I could find, as big round as my
cap, and weighing over a pound. This I deposited in his trough and
invited him to try it. He sniffed at it a little doubtfully, and looked
at me and made a remark or two, then nibbled at the edge of the
cluster, taking a few berries into his mouth, and holding them some
time before he ventured to crush them. At length he did venture,
then looked at me and made more remarks, 'Queer fruit this!
Never tasted anything like it before, but I really can't say yet
whether I like it or not.'*

*"Then he took another bite, then more bites, looking up at me
and saying something between the bites, 'til, little by little, he had
consumed the whole bunch; then, turning round, he went back to
his bed with a little grunt to say that I was now at liberty to go on
to the cows and horses.*

*"However, the following morning he hailed my approach in
such a lively manner, with such a note of expectancy in his voice,*

*that I concluded he had been thinking a great deal about
elderberries, and was anxious to have another go at them.
Accordingly, I cut him another bunch, which he quickly consumed,
making little exclamations the while—'Thank you, thank you, very
good, very good indeed!' It was a new sensation in his life, and
made him very happy, and was almost as good as a day of liberty
in the fields and meadows and on the open green downs.*

*"From that time on I visited him two or three times a day to
give him huge clusters of elderberries. There were plenty for the
starlings as well; the clusters on those trees would have filled a cart.*

*"Then one morning I heard an indignant scream from the
garden, and peeping out saw my friend, the pig, bound hand and
foot, being lifted by a dealer into his cart with the assistance of the
farmer . . ."* [3]

It made Hudson happy to feel he could bring cheer to the last days of
this sociable and sensitive animal, destined though he was for the
butcher. Of course, it is not to be expected that the average person
should be quite as sensitive in translating the grunts and growls as a
trained naturalist. Nevertheless I want to stress the good-naturedness
of pigs because we have done them such a terrible injustice in the way
we think of them, even to using their name as a vile insult.

But why have we given such a bad name to an animal who is full
of intelligence and honest-hearted zest for life; why have we so de-
meaned a creature capable of endearing and lasting friendships with
human beings? It would perhaps be easier to understand if we did this
to the crocodile, for example, who historically has been a real threat to
our lives, and seems to have something about him of the darkness. But
the pig? The loyal, friendly, likeable pig?

Part of the answer, at least, is rather simple. The pig is guilty of
having flesh that human beings find tasty.

*"Man has an infinite capacity to rationalize his rapacity, especially
when it comes to something he wants to eat . . ."*

(CLEVELAND AMORY)

Since few of us have any direct experience with pigs anymore, we can think and speak of them as foul and unwholesome beasts without being disturbed by the facts of the matter. But down through the ages, people who have kept pigs have sensed their undeniable intelligence and friendliness. Only by looking the other way could human beings manage to justify what they have done in order to have bacon and ham, just as black humans were dehumanized in the minds of whites in order to justify their oppression and slavery.

SCHWEITZER'S PIG

When Albert Schweitzer was in Africa running a volunteer hospital, he had a standing offer out to the natives that if they brought him an animal which they would otherwise have killed, he'd pay them for it. In such manner did he save numerous animal lives, create an entourage of assorted critters around him, and show the natives new possibilities of interacting with the local animals. He wrote a remarkable account of meeting a pig.

> *"One day a Negro woman brought me a tame wild boar about two months old. 'It is called Josephine, and it will follow you around like a dog,' she said. We agreed upon five francs as the price. My wife was just then away for a few days. With the help of Joseph and n'Kendju, my hospital assistants, I immediately drove some stakes into the ground and made a pen, with the wire netting rather deep in the earth. Both of my black helpers smiled.*
>
> *" 'A wild boar will not remain in the pen; it digs his way out from under it,' said Joseph. 'Well, I should like to see this little wild boar get under this wire netting sunk deep in the earth,' I answered. 'You will see,' said Joseph.*
>
> *"The next morning the animal had already gotten out. I felt almost relieved about it, for I had promised my wife that I would make no new acquisition to our zoo without her consent, and I had a foreboding that a wild boar would not, perhaps, be to her liking.*
>
> *"When I came up from the hospital for the midday meal, however, there was Josephine waiting for me in front of the house, and looking at me as if she wanted to say: 'I will remain ever so*

*faithful to you, but you must not repeat the trick with the pen.'
And so it was.*

*"When my wife arrived she shrugged her shoulders. She never
enjoyed Josephine's confidence and never sought it. Josephine had a
very delicate sensibility about such things. In time, when she had
come to understand that she was not permitted to go up on the
veranda, things became bearable. On a Saturday some weeks later,
however, Josephine disappeared. In the evening the missionary met
me in front of my house and shared my sorrow, since Josephine
had also shown some attachment to him.*

*" 'I feel sure she has met her end in some Negro's pot,' he said.
'It was inevitable.'*

*"With the blacks a wild boar, even when tamed, does not fall
within the category of a domestic animal but remains a wild
animal that belongs to him who kills it. While he was still
speaking, however, Josephine appeared, behind her a Negro with a
gun.*

*" 'I was standing,' he said, 'in the clearing, where the ruins of
the former American missionary's house are still to be seen, when I
saw this wild boar. I was just taking aim, but it came running up
to me and rubbed against my legs! An extraordinary wild boar!
But imagine what it did then. It trotted away with me after it,
and now here we are. So it's your wild boar? How fortunate that
this did not happen to a hunter who is not so quick-witted as I.'*

*"I understood his hint, complimented him generously, and gave
him a nice present. . ."*[4]

Later, writing of the same boar, Schweitzer spoke of her coming to
church and causing an uproar by behaving like a wild pig, but then
gradually learning to "behave more properly in church." Struck again
and again by the spirit of this animal, Schweitzer wrote:

*"How shall I sufficiently praise your wisdom, Josephine! To avoid
being bothered by gnats at night, you adopted the custom of
wandering into the boy's dormitory, and of lying down there under
the first good mosquito net. How many times because of this have I*

had to compensate, with tobacco leaves, those upon whom you
forced yourself as a sleeping companion. And when the sand fleas
had so grown in your feet that you could no longer walk, you
hobbled down to the hospital, let yourself be turned over on your
back, endured the knife that the tormentors stuck into your feet,
put up with the burning of the tincture of iodine, with which the
wounds were daubed, and grunted your sincere thanks when the
matter was once and for all done with. "[5]

THE FRAGRANCE OF THE FARM

Since I have found that pigs are such endearing and friendly chaps, I
don't look at pork chops the way I once did. And there's something
else I've learned that has forever changed the way I feel about such
things as bacon and ham.

What I have learned is that the pork farmers have by and large
followed the lead of the poultry industry in recent years. Instead of pig
farms, today we have more and more pig factories.

The result is not a happy one for today's pigs.

Some of today's pig factories are huge industrial complexes, with
over 100,000 pigs. You might think that would require an awful lot of
pigpens. But the pigpen, like the chicken yard, is rapidly becoming a
thing of the past. Every day, more and more of these robust creatures
are placed in stalls so cramped that they can hardly move.

If you were to peek inside one of the buildings in which these stalls
are kept, you'd see row upon row upon row upon row of pigs, each
standing alone in his narrow steel stall, each facing in exactly the same
direction, like cars in a parking lot.

But you would hardly notice what you saw, because you'd be so
overwhelmed by the stench. The overpowering ammonia-saturated air
of a modern pig factory is something no one ever forgets.

You see, many modern pig stalls are built on slatted floors over
large pits, into which the urine and feces of the animals fall automatically. Thousands of this type of confinement systems are in operation,
in spite of the fact that many serious diseases are caused by the toxic
gases (ammonia, methane and hydrogen sulfide) that the excreta produce, and which rise from the pits and become trapped inside the
building.[6]

Pigs have a highly developed sense of smell and their noses are, in a natural setting, capable of detecting the scents of many kinds of edible roots, even when those roots are still underground. In today's pig factories, however, they breathe night and day the stench of the excrement of the hundreds of pigs whose stalls are in the same building. No matter how much they might want to get away, no matter how hard they might try, there is no escape.

The pig factory I am describing is unfortunately not an isolated bad example. It's par for the course today. Just a couple of years ago, the owner of Lehman Farms of Strawn, Illinois, was chosen Illinois Pork All-American by the National Pork Producers Council and the Illinois Pork Producers Association. The Lehman farm is considered an industry model, and it is, in fact, one of the more enlightened swine management programs around today. But it seems to leave a little bit to be desired from the point of view of the pigs who call it home. When a "herdsman" at Lehman Farms, Bob Frase, was asked about the effect the ammonia saturated air had on the pigs, he replied:

> *"The ammonia really chews up the animals' lungs. They get listless and don't want to eat. They start losing weight, and the next thing you know you've got a real respiratory problem—pneumonia or something. Then you'll see them huddled down real low against one another trying to get warm, and you'll hear them coughing and gasping. The bad air's a problem. After I've been working in here awhile, I can feel it in my own lungs. But at least I get out of here at night. The pigs don't so we have to keep them on tetracycline . . ."* [7]

"FORGET THE PIG IS AN ANIMAL"

In my visits to modern pig factories, I keep thinking about pigs I have met, social critters much like Albert Schweitzer's Josephine, very capable of warm relationships with people. I remember their friendly grunts and their enjoyment of human contact. This is why I have such a hard time accepting the advice of contemporary pork producers:

> *"Forget the pig is an animal. Treat him just like a machine in a factory. Schedule treatments like you would lubrication. Breeding*

*season like the first step in an assembly line. And marketing like
the delivery of finished goods."*

(*HOG FARM MANAGEMENT*, SEPTEMBER, 1976)[8]

Modern pig farmers, who like to be called "pork production engineers," pride themselves on having a clear purpose. The trade journal
Hog Farm Management put it concisely:

*"What we are really trying to do is modify the animal's
environment for maximum profit."*[9]

Even if an individual pig raiser feels an empathy with the animals in
his charge and has a desire to do things in a more natural way, he is
today practically forced to go along with the agribusiness momentum.
The trend is set. Trade journals like *Hog Farm Management*, *National
Hog Farmer*, *Successful Farming*, and *Farm Journal* are constantly telling farmers to "Raise Pork the Modern Way."

The trade journals tend to be downright hostile to anything but
the most mechanized agribusiness ways of producing pork. Recently,
National Hog Farmer became irate at the USDA, and editorialized,
"Why don't we just turn the Department of Agriculture over to the
do-gooders?"[10] What on earth had the USDA done to provoke such a
terrifying thought? It had proposed spending two hundredths of one
percent of its budget for two small projects that would have encouraged small-scale, local production of food, such as roadside markets
and community gardens in urban areas.

The trade magazines, it must be remembered, derive their income
from advertisers, and these are just the people who profit from the
swing to total confinement systems of pork production—the huge commercial interests who sell equipment and drugs to the farmers. They're
the ones who take out full page ads and pay for space in the journals
which tell the farmers "How To Make $12,000 Sitting Down!"[11]
That's quite a way to catch the attention of an exhausted farmer, who is
only too glad to sit down at all after laboring on his feet all day.

So he reads on. And what does he find? The way to success in
today's pork production world is through buying a "Bacon Bin."[12]

This wonderful new doorway to success, he is told, "is not just a confinement house . . . It is a profit producing pork production system."[13]

Actually, the Bacon Bin is a completely automated system whose designers clearly have overcome any vestiges of the anachronistic idea that pigs are sentient beings. In a typical Bacon Bin setup, 500 pigs are crammed into individual cages, each getting seven square feet of living space. It's difficult for us to conceive how confined this is. Every pig spends his entire life cramped into a space less than one-third the size of a twin bed.

The Bacon Bin system comes complete with slatted floors and automated feeding systems, so that it takes only one person to run the whole show. Another advantage of the system is that, with no room to move about, the pigs can't burn up calories doing "useless" things like walking, and that means faster and cheaper weight gain, and so more profit.

A typical example of Bacon Bin farming was happily described in *The Farm Journal* beneath the title: "Pork Factory Swings Into Production."[14] The article begins proudly:

"Hogs never see daylight in this half-million dollar farrowing-to-finish complex near Worthington, Minnesota."[15]

This is something to brag about?

PIGS' FEET MODERN STYLE

Pigs' feet and legs were designed to scratch for food, to kick or claw if needed for defense, and to stand and move on different kinds of natural terrain. But in today's pig factories, the floors are either metal slats or concrete. Peter Singer and Jim Mason, authors of *Animal Factories*, the classic book on contemporary food-animal raising, have described what happens to pigs' feet under these conditions.

"Pigs are cloven-hoofed animals, and, in most, the outer half of the hoof ('claw') is longer than the inner half. Outdoors, the extra length is absorbed by the natural softness of the soil. On the concrete or metal floors of the factory pen, however, only the tissue in the

*foot can 'give.' As a result, many confined pigs develop painful
lesions in their feet which can open and become infected. Pigs with
these foot sores usually develop . . . abnormal posture in an attempt
to relieve the pain. Eventually, the crippling may worsen when this
abnormal movement and weight distribution overworks joints and
muscles in the legs, back, and other parts of the pig."* [16]

One Nebraska study showed that nearly 100% of all pigs raised on
concrete or metal slats had damaged feet and legs.[17] Providing bedding
can reduce the problem,[18] but bedding is rarely provided in the modern
homes of the pigs destined to become America's pork chops, because
straw costs money, and the pain and suffering the pigs endure from
damaged feet and legs is not figured into the financial equations that
determine policy. Of course, the pork producers are aware that the
animals are crippled by the flooring, but they are not disturbed. As the
editors of *Farmer and Stockbreeder* explain:

> *"The slatted floor seems to have more merit than disadvantage.
> The animal will usually be slaughtered before serious deformity sets
> in."* [19]

In other words, the pigs are usually slaughtered before their deformities become so extreme as to effect the price their flesh will fetch. One
producer summarized industry thinking rather colorfully.

> *"We don't get paid for producing animals with good posture around
> here. We get paid by the pound!"* [20]

As I look at the situation, I doubt whether the pigs who spend their
painful lives on these devastating floors, hobbling about on distorted
skeletons, are able fully to appreciate this kind of logic.

IMPROVING ON MOTHER NATURE
It may not be wise to tamper with nature. It may even be disastrous.
But you can be sure that if it's profitable, someone is certain to give it a
try. The leading edge in pork production these days is in getting more

pigs per sow per year. The idea is to turn sows into living reproductive machines.

"The breeding sow should be thought of, treated as, a valuable piece of machinery, whose function is to pump out baby pigs like a sausage machine."

(*NATIONAL HOG FARMER*, MARCH, 1978)[21]

In a barnyard setting, a sow will produce about six piglets a year. But modern interventions have cranked her up to over 20 a year now, and researchers predict the number to reach 45 within a short time.[22] Producers rave about the prospect of being able to force sows to give birth to over seven times the number of children nature designed them for.

They've got it down to a science. First of all, piglets are taken away from their mothers much earlier than would ever occur in any natural situation. Without her babies to suck the milk from her breast, the sow will soon stop lactating, and then, with the help of hormone injections, she can be made fertile much sooner. Thus, more piglets can be extracted from her per year.

Unfortunately, the poor sow is not up-to-date enough in her thinking to appreciate the wonders of a system in which she will spend her whole life producing litter after litter, only to have her babies taken away from her as soon as possible after each birth. The sow calls and cries for them, though her distressed sounds always go unheeded. Not having gotten the hang of modern factory life, she only knows that her whole being is filled with an inexorable instinct to find her lost babies and care for them.

Most pork producers have found that they have to let the piglets suckle from their mother for a couple of weeks before taking them away, or else they die, which, of course, defeats the whole purpose. But at least one large manufacturer of farm equipment sees the waste in such an operation, and is now strongly promoting a device it calls "Pig Mama."[23] This is a mechanical teat that replaces the normal one altogether, and allows the factory manager to take the piglet away from his mother immediately, and get her back to the business of being pregnant, just a couple of hours after birth. Noting this development, *Farm Journal* said it was looking forward to "an end to the nursing phase of pig production."[24] The result, they predicted gleefully, would be a:

> ". . . *tremendous jump in the number of pigs a sow could produce in a year.*"[25]

For years now, pork breeders have also been hard at work developing fatter and fatter pigs. Unfortunately, the resulting products of contemporary porkbreeding are so top-heavy that their bones and joints are literally crumbling beneath them.[26] However, factory experts see nothing amiss in this because there is additional profit to be made from the extra weight.

There are, however, a few problems with the "new model pig" rolling across the assembly line in today's pork factories which do concern the factory experts. Singer and Mason point out a few of these problems in *Animal Factories.*

> *"The pig breeders' emphasis on large litters and heavier bodies, coupled with a lack of attention to reproductive traits, has produced . . . high birth mortality in these pigs. These new, improved females produce such large litters that they can't take care of each piglet. To cure this problem, producers began to select sows with a greater number of nipples—only to discover that the extra nipples don't work because there's not enough mammary tissue to go around.*"[27]

Not to be dismayed, however, the genetic manipulators are continuing their efforts to "improve" the pig, and convert this good-natured and robust creature into a more efficient piece of factory equipment.

> *"Breeding experts are trying to create pigs that have flat rumps, level backs, even toes, and other features that hold up better under factory conditions.*"[28]

HORMONE CITY
What they can't accomplish with genetics, today's pork producers shoot for with hormones. Hormones, as you may know, are incredibly

potent substances which are naturally secreted, in minute amounts, by the glands of all animals, pigs and humans included. It takes minuscule amounts of these substances to control our entire endocrine and reproductive systems. If our taste buds were as sensitive to flavor as our target cells are to hormones, we could detect a single grain of sugar in a swimming pool of water.[29]

Given the immensely powerful effects hormones have on animals reproductive systems, even in concentrations so low they are discernible only by the most sophisticated laboratory technology, many scientists are extremely concerned about their use in animal farming, acknowledging that we know very little about many of the potentially dangerous effects of these substances. The factory experts, however, look through very different eyes. When they first realized the new drugs gave them the power to control a sow's estrus, and thus to induce or delay her fertility, they were overjoyed.

"Estrus control will open the doors to factory hog production. Control of female cycles is the missing link to the assembly line approach."

(*FARM JOURNAL*)[30]

One pork producer was so taken with this new development that he called it the . . .

". . . greatest advance in hog production since the development of antibiotics."[31]

Another new innovation which has the industry astir is called embryo transfer.[32] Here a specially chosen sow is dosed with hormones to cause her to produce huge numbers of eggs, rather than the usual one or two. These eggs are fertilized by artificial insemination, then surgically removed from the sow and implanted in other females. It is not uncommon for a breeder sow to go repeatedly through this unnatural violation until the stress kills her.

At the University of Missouri, work is being done in test tubes to combine sperm and eggs which have been taken from specially selected breeding animals.[33] The newly fertilized eggs are then implanted surgically in ordinary females.

Once a sow in today's pork factories is pregnant, she is injected with progestins or steroids to increase the number of piglets in her litter. She will also be given products like the new feed additive from Shell Oil Company. Called XLP-30, it is designed to "boost pigs per litter,"[34] though it has a name that makes it sound like it should be added to motor oil instead of animal food. Incredibly, a Shell official acknowledges—"we don't know why it works."[35] Undeterred by such ignorance, however, the industry is not at all reluctant to tamper with the reproductive systems of the animals whose flesh is designed for human consumption. Anything that can speed up the assembly line and improve profits is considered fair practice.

A LIFE OF SUFFERING
It is difficult for us to fathom the suffering of today's pigs. They are crammed for a lifetime into cages in which they can hardly move, and forced against their natures to stand in their own waste. Their sensitive noses are continuously assaulted by the stench from the excrement of thousands of other pigs. Their skeletons are deformed and their legs buckle under the unnatural weight for which they have been bred. Their feet are full of painful lesions from the concrete and slatted metal floors on which they must stand.

I have looked into their eyes and I can tell you it's a terrifying sight. These sensitive, tortured creatures, have been literally driven mad.

In this respect, they are similar to the chickens who live in today's "chicken heavens." Chickens, you may remember, when forced into unbearably crowded conditions, go crazy and develop "vices" such as feather-pecking and cannibalism. Forced into equally bizarre conditions, pigs are likewise driven completely out of their minds. One reporter noted:

> *"Some animals may become so fearful that they dare not move, even to eat or drink. They become runts and die. Others remain in constant, panicked motion, neurotic perversions of their instinct to escape. Cannibalism is common in swine . . . operations."* [36]

One of the most common problems in modern pork factories is known in the trade as "tail-biting." The trade journals are full of discussions about "tail-biting," and what to do about it. When I first heard the phrase "tail-biting" I rather naively pictured some kind of playful nipping at little, curly, pink tails. But I have since learned how very far from the mark I was. "Tail-biting" is the industry's term for the deranged and desperate actions of powerful animals driven berserk by the frustration of every single one of their natural urges.

> *"Acute tail-biting . . . frequently results in crippling, mutilation, and death . . . Many times the tail is bitten first, and then the attacking pig or pigs continue to eat further into the back. If the situation is not attended to, the pig will die and be eaten."* [37]

Tail-biting, naturally, disturbs the managers of the pork factories, who can't sell a pig that's been eaten by another pig. Not being the types to sit back and let a disaster like that occur, they've come up with a number of bizarre solutions.

One strategy is to keep the pigs in total darkness. A March, 1976 edition of *Farm Journal* carried an article titled "Cut Light and Clamp Down On Tail Biting." This report reassured pork producers:

> *"They can still eat—total darkness has no effect on their appetites."* [38]

The preferred method of preventing tail-biting in today's pork factories, however, is a trick the pork producers picked up from the poultrymen. They can't, of course, de-beak pigs, because pigs don't have beaks. But they have found another way of preventing tail-biting which, like chicken de-beaking, does absolutely nothing to correct the grotesque conditions that give rise to the behavior in the first place.

They cut off the pigs' tails.

This practice, known in the trade as "tail-docking," is now standard operating procedure in United States pork production. [39] Its application is nearly universal today, despite the fact that it causes severe pain to the animals, and drives them even crazier. I asked one pork farmer about tail-docking, and he replied, somewhat angrily:

"They hate it! The pigs just hate it! And I suppose we could probably do without tail-docking if we gave them more room, because they don't get so crazy and mean when they have more space. With enough room, they're actually quite nice animals. But we can't afford it. These buildings cost a lot." [40]

This farmer's remarks don't reflect his thoughts alone. They are typical of the rationale behind virtually all of the steps being taken today towards even more mechanized pork production. Having invested great sums of money in confinement buildings and automated feeding systems, today's producers feel they must use every trick in the book to get the maximum number of piglets per sow and cram as many pigs as possible into the buildings. [41]

In fact, the trade journal *Hog Farm Management* has an even better idea than the parking lot-like stalls. How about stacking the pigs in cages, one on top of each other, like shipping crates? Just think how many more animals you could get in a building this way. Explaining the brilliance of having not only wall-to-wall pigs, but floor-to-ceiling pigs as well, the journal reasoned:

"There's too much wasted space in a typical controlled-environment single-deck nursery. The cost of the building is just too big a cost factor. Stacking the decks spreads the building cost out over more pigs." [42]

A number of today's largest pig factories have been so impressed with this idea that they've wasted no time in employing it. You might not think that it would make that much difference to a pig who is already crammed into a cage so small he can hardly move, whether there are other pigs above him in the same plight. But it does. The excrement from the pigs in the upper tiers falls steadily on the pigs in the lower tiers.

ANGER AND TEARS FROM A PORK PRODUCER
It's actually gotten to the point where many of today's pig farmers are being forced to do things even they find abhorrent. I'm not talking

now about people who are particularly empathic towards animals. I'm referring to people who long ago came to accept bashing an animal's brains out, or slitting its throat, as all in a day's work. These are hardened veterans of the everyday brutalities of animal farming, but even they are increasingly disgusted by what is happening today.

In a 1976 issue of *Farmer and Stockbreeder*, a letter appeared which expressed the concern of such an old-timer. He was writing in response to a report on a new cage system for pigs.

> *"May I dissociate myself completely from any implication that this is a tolerable form of husbandry? I hope many of my colleagues will join me in saying that we are already tolerating systems of husbandry which, to say the least of it, are downright cruel . . . Cost effectiveness and conversion ratios are all very well in a robot state; but if this is the future, then the sooner I give up both farming and farm veterinary work the better."* [43]

The same year, a retired farm veterinarian sent a thoughtful letter to the factory farming journal *Confinement*.

> *"More and more I find myself developing an aversion to the snow-balling trend toward total confinement of livestock . . . If we regard this unnatural environment as acceptable, what does it portend for mankind itself? . . . How can a truly human being impose conditions on lower animals that he would not be willing to impose on himself? Freedom of movement and expression should not be the exclusive domain of man . . . What (then) of human behavior (in the future)? Will it sink to the nadir of contempt for all that is naturally bright and beautiful? Will all of us become tailbiters without recognizing what we have become?"* [44]

These two letters were written in 1976, just as total confinement systems for pork production were gathering steam. Since then, despite the pleas of these and other warning voices, the trend has continued: more total confinement, more frustration of all the animals' natural urges, more farming by automation and technology, more drugs, and more assembly-line pork.

And what happens to those farmers who just can't stand to do this to animals whom they know are intelligent and capable of lasting friendships with people? Most have quit the whole affair in disgust and failure. Others have continued on, often with an aching sense of frustration and defeat as they capitulate time and time again out of financial necessity to the harsh economic reality of modern "farming." One such pig farmer told me, angrily:

"Sometimes I wish you animal lovers would just drop dead! Just go and fall off a cliff or something. It's hard enough to make a living these days without having to be concerned about all this stuff!"

Later that night, after dinner and a long talk in which he opened up to his true feelings, this same farmer told me, with tears in his eyes:

"I'm sorry I got so mad at you before. It's not your fault. You are just showing me what I already know, but try not to think about. It just tears me up, some of the things we are doing to these animals. These pigs never hurt anybody, but we treat them like, like, like I don't know what. Nothing in the world deserves this kind of treatment. It's a shame. It's a crying shame. I just don't know what else to do."

THE AMERICAN PORK QUEEN SPEAKS

The National Pork Council and related organizations spend millions of dollars a year to convince the public that today's pigs are happy as can be with the way they are raised. In May, 1987, the Council officially and unabashedly proclaimed that pork producers "have historically treated their farm animals with the utmost care and respect." Each year, the Pork Council sends an official "American Pork Queen" out across the country to enlighten schools and community groups about the joys of modern pork production. Speaking about her work, one year's American Pork Queen, Pam Carney, explained:

"Well, I kind of told about myself from the perspective of being a pig . . . You see, we are getting a lot of questions from people now who are for animal rights and who are worried about pigs being

put into small pens and farrowing crates. So, I talked about how much we pigs like the new confinement barns as opposed to living outside in the natural environment, because a herdsman can keep a close eye on us, watch for disease, give us warmth, good feed, and clean water . . . "[45]

The American Pork Queen reassures us today's pigs receive "good feed and clean water." But the truth, as you might guess, is a little different. In nature, pigs live with gusto and passion, foraging in the earth for their food. Even in a barnyard setting they root around as much as they can, and their diet consists of table scraps along with the foods they can root from the earth. But today, they are fed a completely unnatural diet designed with one thing alone in mind—to make them as fat as possible, as cheaply as possible. Their feed is routinely laced with antibiotics, sulfa drugs, and countless other products of the laboratory. It is a menu that often features recycled waste.

One modern pig farmer proudly announced in *Hog Farm Management* that in his system pregnant sows don't need to be fed for 90 days. Presenting his ingenuity as a model for the forward thinking pig man, he boasted that he simply allows them only what they can find in the manure waste pits beneath the slatted floor cages where young pigs are being fattened for slaughter. His excitement about how much money he saves was not dampened by the fact that during pregnancy the nutritional needs of pigs, like any mammal, are especially critical.

The industry norm isn't much better. Today's pigs are routinely fed recycled waste, even though this waste consistently contains drug residues and high levels of toxic, heavy metals, such as arsenic, lead and copper.[46] Often the helpless creatures are simply given raw poultry or pig manure.[47]

I don't know about you, but the idea of feeding pigs their own excrement doesn't strike me as an ideal diet.

But if what today's pigs are fed leaves a little to be desired, it's almost a picnic compared to the water they receive to drink. Sometimes the only water they get comes from an:

". . . oxidation ditch, which channels the liquid wastes from factory manure pits back to the animals; they have to drink it because it's the only 'water' offered to them." [48]

Interestingly enough, the industry's public stance is that the health and well-being of today's pigs is better than ever.

But over 80% of today's pigs have pneumonia at the time of slaughter. One Minnesota plant found pneumonia in the lungs of 95% of the pigs inspected. In 1970, 53% of all U.S. pigs had stomach ulcers. The Livestock Conservation Institute reports that pig producers lose more than $187 million each year from dysentery, cholera, abscesses, trichinosis, and other swine diseases.[49] A disease known as pseudo-rabies has been wiping out whole herds of factory pigs in the midwest since 1973.[50] The National Pork Council wants the government to pay for a five-year program to eradicate pseudo-rabies. *Hog Farm Management* thinks this would cost taxpayers $90 million.[51]

Of course, that's not a lot of money compared to the bill for another disease, African Swine Fever, which is beginning to infect pigs raised the modern way in this country. *National Hog Farmer* expects the cost of coping with this disease to be in the neighborhood of $290 million.[52]

The pork industry says these diseases amount to only minor technical problems in the assembly-line production of pork. With the help of taxpayers money, and the application of more drugs, they say, the problems can be solved in no time. As to the possibility that today's pigs are not really all that healthy, the industry points to the impressive weights the animals attain as proof they are as robust as can be. This is a remarkable argument, in that it attempts to equate systematically-induced obesity with good health. That's certainly not true for humans, why should it be true for pigs?

AND THEN
The pigs I've known have been friendly and sensitive critters, like Albert Schweitzer's Josephine. They can be good friends, playful, loyal and affectionate. Watching what happens to these good-hearted creatures in today's pig factories has not been at all easy for me. At each stage of the assembly line they are treated with complete disdain for the fact that they are our fellow creatures. But they are sentient beings, and they remain so to the end.

"Before they reach their end, the pigs get a shower, a real one. Water sprays from every angle to wash the farm off them. Then they begin to feel crowded. The pen narrows like a funnel; the drivers behind urge the pigs forward, until one at a time they climb unto a moving ramp . . . Now they scream, never having been on such a ramp, smelling the smells they smell. I do not want to overdramatize because you have read all this before. But it was a frightening experience, seeing their fear, seeing so many of them go by. It had to remind me of things no one wants to be reminded of anymore, all mobs, all death marches, all mass murders and extinctions . . . "[63]

THE NEW QUESTION

Seeing what happens to today's pigs is especially difficult for me because I know what friendly animals they can be by nature. We have come to know pigs as fat only because we have bred and fed them that way. We have come to know pigs as mean only because we have tortured them and deprived them of any conceivable expression of their energies. We have made them what they are.

Could it be then, that when we eat the flesh of animals who have been treated with such complete contempt, that we assimilate something of their experience and carry it forward into our own lives? Could it be that eating the products of such an insane system may contribute significantly to the feeling pervading mankind today that this earth sometimes resembles the lunatic asylum of the universe?

People of the stature of Plato, Tolstoy and Gandhi have also refused to eat meat. But today the question of meat eating has taken on a far more urgent significance than ever before. There is something uniquely painful happening in the way contemporary animals are being raised for meat. Animals have been treated cruelly before, and in some cases sadistically—but the process has never before been institutionalized on such an overwhelming scale. And never before has the cold expertise of modern technology and pharmacology been employed to this end.

Throughout history, there have been people who sensed that eating the flesh of animals killed unnecessarily was not the best thing we

could do towards the goal of bringing peace to ourselves and to the
world. The more I've learned of modern meat production, the more
I've felt that their message is even more vital today.

*"While we ourselves are the living graves of murdered beasts, how
can we expect any ideal conditions on this earth?"*

(GEORGE BERNARD SHAW)

*"I have no doubt that it is part of the destiny of the human race in
its gradual development to leave off the eating of animals, as surely
as the savage tribes have left off eating each other when they came
into contact with the more civilized."*

(THOREAU)

*"The time will come when men such as I will look on the murder
of animals as they now look on the murder of men."*

(LEONARDO DA VINCI)

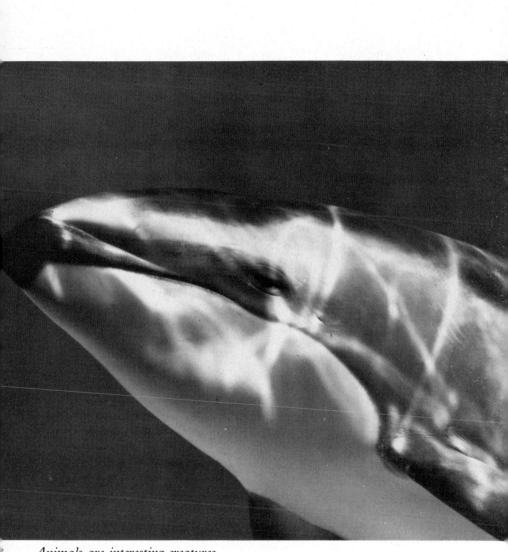

Animals are interesting creatures . . .

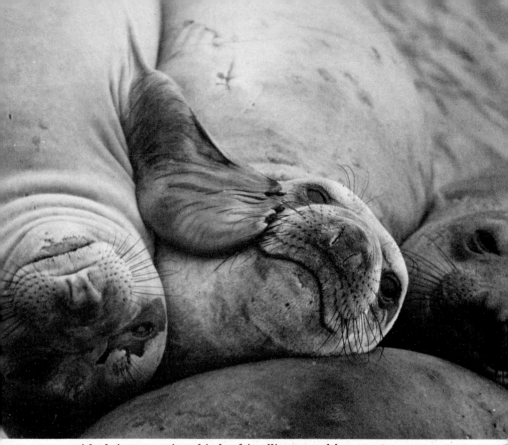

with their own unique kinds of intelligence and beauty . . .

When treated well, most kinds of animals are friendly to people . . .

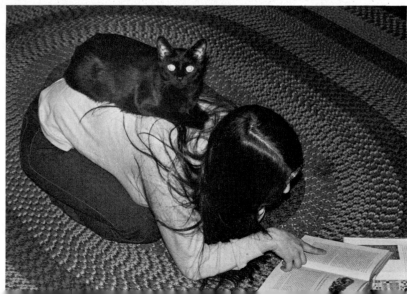

Photograph: Frank S. Balthis

Photograph: Sumner Wm. Fowler

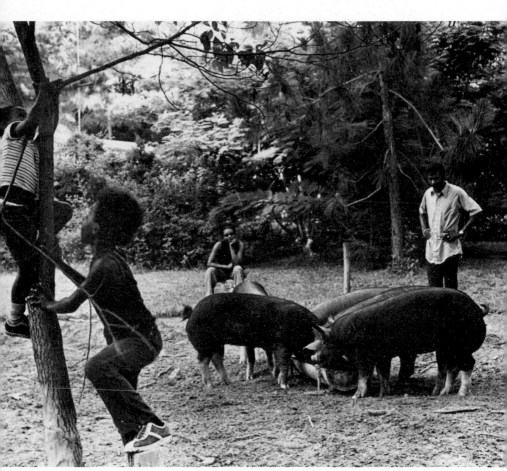

Pigs are as capable of friendship with us as dogs and cats . . .

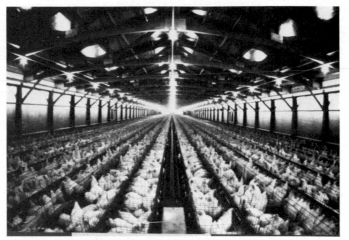

But the animals raised for meat, eggs, and dairy products in the United States today . . .

are treated terribly . . .

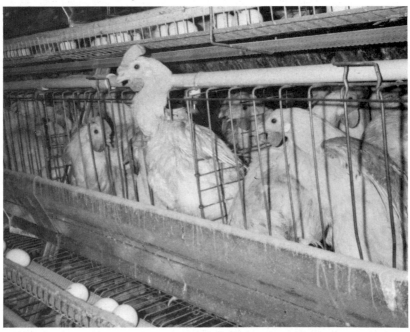

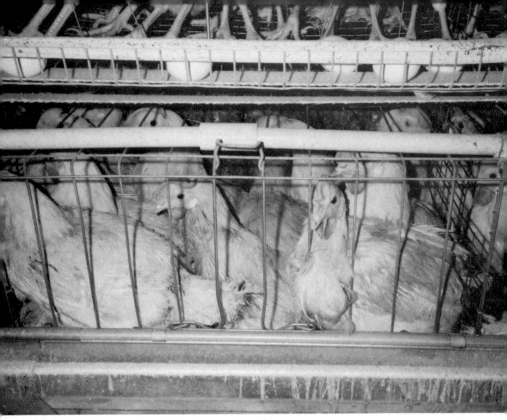

Chickens are crammed into cages so tightly
they can barely move and are driven insane . . .

From below, the view is nothing to put on a picture postcard.

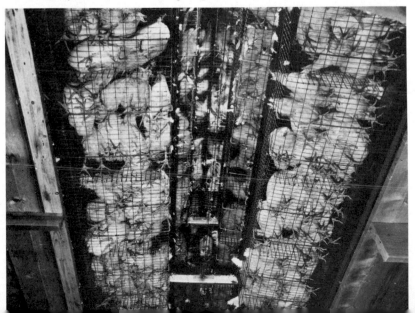

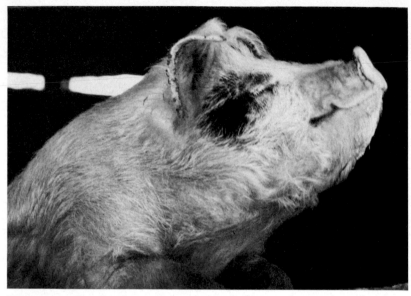

When treated well, pigs are remarkably happy . . .

and friendly creatures . . .

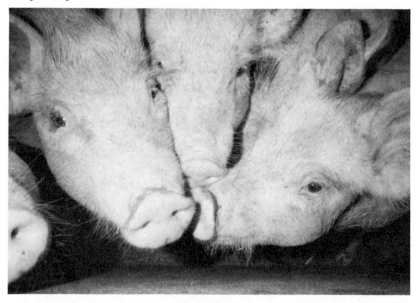

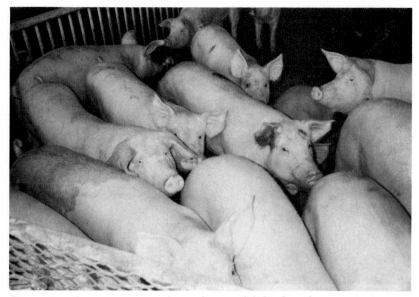

But today they are crammed together so tightly that they go crazy . . .

and often bite each other's tails and rears, even killing each other . . .

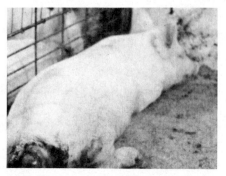

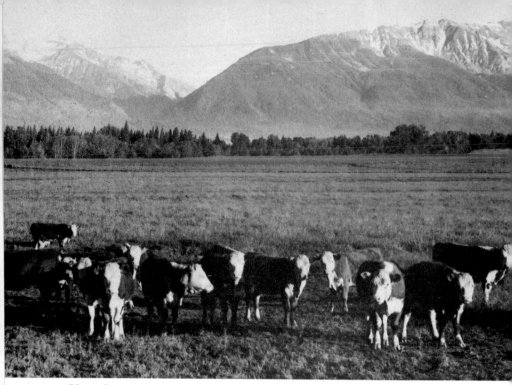

Yesterday's cows spent their whole lives grazing happily in pastures . . .

But today this is no longer the case . . .

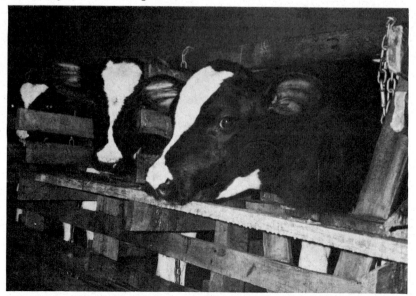

USDA Photograph; Earl R. Baker

Photograph; R. Miller Humane Farming Association

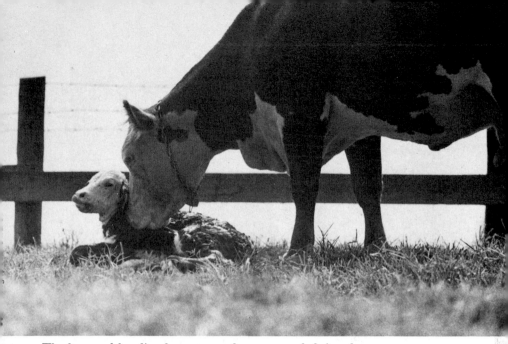

The love and bonding between mother cows and their calves . . .

is strong and deep . . .

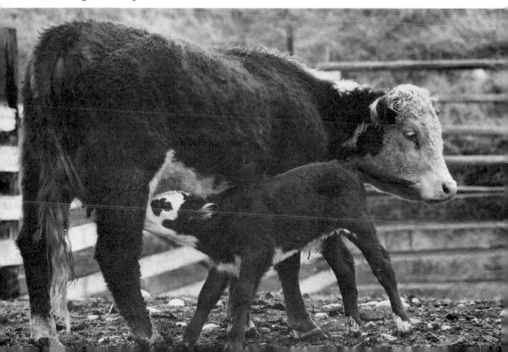

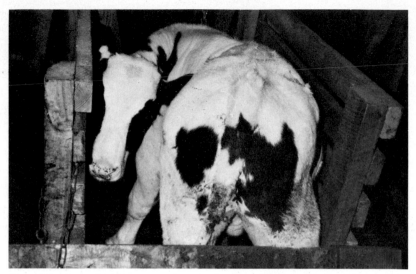

But today's veal calves are taken away from their mothers as soon as they are born . . .

and forced to live their entire lives in unspeakably miserable conditions . . .

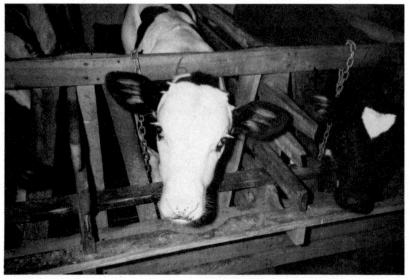

Photographs: B. Miller, Humane Farming Association

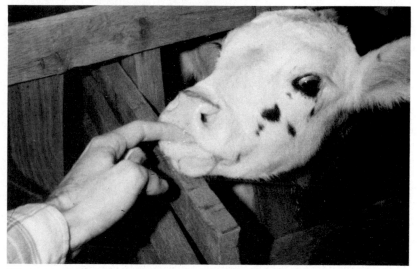

These are little babies, separated from their mothers, and they desperately seek anything to suck on . . .

But they are never allowed to suck, and instead fed a diet deliberately designed to make them anemic. Anyone who treated a dog or cat the way millions of baby veal calves are treated today would be arrested . . .

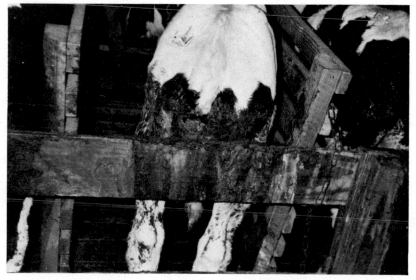

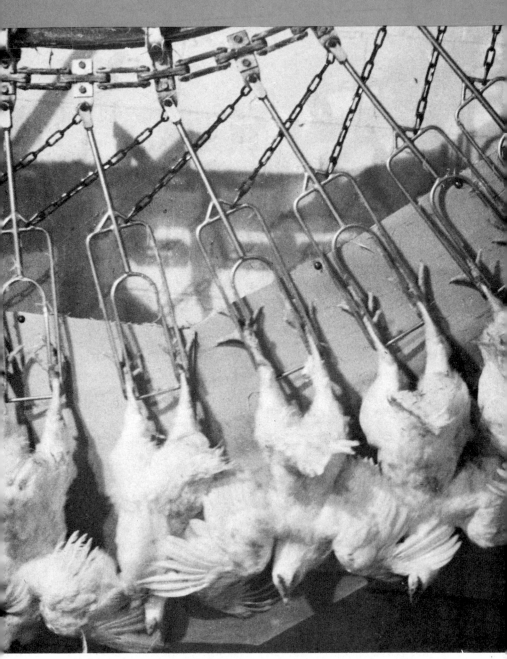

We prefer to numb ourselves psychically to the fact of the slaughterhouse. We don't like to remember that a hamburger is a ground up cow . . .

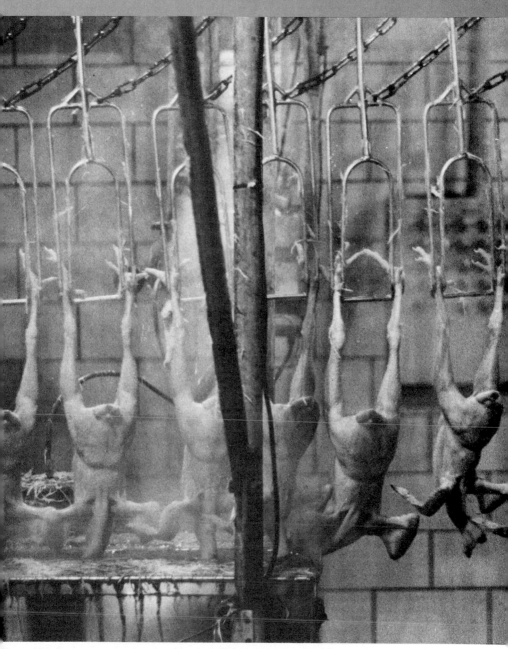

In fact, some people evidently think chickens are vegetables.
When someone says they are a vegetarian, these people say:
"Yes, but you do eat chicken don't you?"

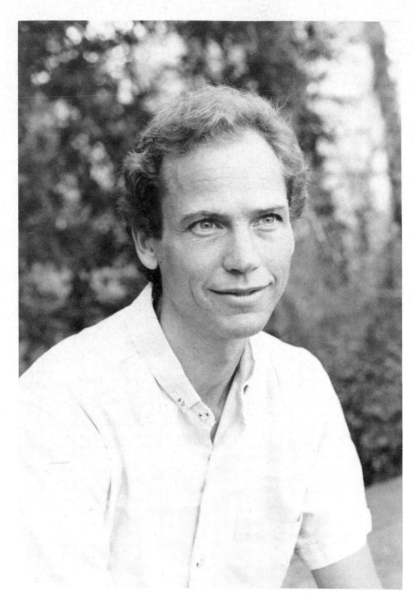

The author of Diet for a New America, *John Robbins shows us how our health, happiness, and the future of life on earth depend on our shifting to a compassionate way of eating.*

HOLY COW

*"I tremble for my species when I reflect that
God is just."*

(THOMAS JEFFERSON)

*"Each man is haunted until his humanity
awakens."*

(BLAKE)

A S I'VE learned what is being done to today's farm animals I've
become increasingly distressed. If our society is to reflect any
kind of compassion and respect for life, how can we allow
such extreme abuses of sentient beings to continue?

The problem is that the behemoths of modern agribusiness seek
profit without reference to any ethical sensitivity to the animals in their
keeping. And at present we have virtually no laws restraining cruelty
to animals being raised for food.

I look forward to the day when this has been corrected, when our
society is at peace with its conscience because it respects and lives in
harmony with all forms of life. I look forward eagerly to the enactment
of laws against such cruelty to animals, laws that will guide humankind
to actions consistent with an ethic of appreciation for Creation, and
respect for the lives of our fellow creatures.

Though I have felt anger at the outrages inflicted on innocent
animals, I know that many of today's farmers are basically decent human beings who have become caught in a vicious circle of economic
necessity, seeing no choice but follow the lead of the multinational
agrichemical conglomerates.

The laws that are needed to restrain those who would in their insensitivity abuse animals will not arise out of ill will towards those who have become instruments of such cruelty. True justice never punishes for the sake of punishment, but instead seeks to provide the experiences that will educate and reform. Since insensitivity to nature is the real problem, our intent should not be to blame, but to guide these unfortunate people to an awareness of the lives and needs of other living creatures, and thus to their own potential for living in an ethical relationship to the rest of life.

Those who are so alienated from other beings that they would mistreat them are in need of a deeper respect for life, for themselves, and for a more meaningful sense of their own value and integrity. We need laws against cruelty to animals, not just for the animals' sake.

Interestingly, legend has it that there was once a time when such a form of justice actually prevailed. This was a time, it is said, when an ancient people sought to live in accord with the laws of Creation. As a result, when disputes and conflicts arose, the remedy was often remarkable.

Here is such a case, chronicled from ancient Egypt. The times are different, but the message is the same. A fifteen-year-old boy has gotten himself in trouble time after time for his cruelty to animals. In spite of repeated punishments from his father, however, his actions have persisted. Neighbors have finally appealed to the judge for help, and he has decreed that the boy be watched without his knowledge. This is done, and the boy is seen burying a cat alive. When confronted with his action, the boy shows no sense of shame or remorse, and says defiantly, "You can beat me, but I won't mind. I'm used to being beaten, but you can never make me scream!" He pulls off his shirt, and displays a back that is deeply scarred from the previous beatings his father has administered. To the counselor who comes in to see him he brags about the number of animals he has tortured, and the amount of pain which has been inflicted upon him in return. It is not an easy case for the judge to handle. But fortunately, there is a seer who can look into the boy's psyche, and see what has occurred that has made him this way. The seer understands the pattern the boy is locked into. He understands that in the boy's clouded mind, his cruelty to animals is actually part of an effort to expiate the guilt he feels for his mother having died during his birth, something his father never lets him forget. It is plain to the seer that it would be pointless to punish the boy, for to do so would simply reinforce the guilt that motivated the whole behavior in the first place.

The seer decides to take drastic steps.

The next day, in the boy's food there is mixed a violent cathartic. As soon as the boy's bowels start cramping he is told that he has a rare and dangerous disease, and is warned that unless he is both brave and obedient he will likely die. Over the next few days he is given other concoctions, which keep him intermittently in pain, and also make him sufficiently weak to prevent him from having any desire to exert his independence and reconstruct his accustomed self-image. Exactly as though he is suffering from a very serious disease, he is cared for by one who is in training to become a true healer, a girl of twenty who is both beautiful and compassionate. She holds his hand to help him bear the pain, and smooths his forehead until he falls asleep. She washes and feeds him as though he is a baby, and when he grows a little stronger, she tells him stories of the ways of peace and love.

As he convalesces, he conceives a deep devotion and gratitude to his nurse, and asks that he might be allowed to serve her in however humble a capacity. She tells him that one of her duties is to look after the geese, that the geese are very special to her, and that it would be a great help if he would do this for her. Her words cause him to remember his many cruelties, and he begins to cry bitterly, and says that he dare not do what she asks, for sometimes almost against his will he has been cruel to animals, and so he is very afraid that he might attack her geese, an act which, to him now, would be like causing her personal injury.

She says to him: "You were so ill that you might have died. I asked the Gods that you might be born again; they listened, and you recovered. The cruelty which you once afflicted, and the pain you suffered, are as though they had never been. They are dead, but you are alive. Because of the link between us, you will never forget again the link between you and your younger brothers and sisters."

The boy is filled with hope, but even so does not entirely believe her. She brings him a kitten, but he protests, saying he can't be trusted with the kitten. She smiles, and teaches him how to scratch the kitten's throat and ears, and points out how loudly it purrs when he does so. "It likes you," she says. "It knows you can be trusted, and I know you can be trusted, too, so I will leave you alone with the kitten now."

The boy doesn't know what to think, and protests, but she just smiles and kisses his forehead.

When she returns, several hours later, she finds the boy asleep, with the kitten curled up beside him, purring.

The boy grows to become one of the kindest veterinarians in all the land, and his manner with animals is so gentle and clear that even the most terrified and injured of them instinctively know they can trust him.[1]

It looks to me as if many of the people who mistreat the animals raised for today's meats and eggs are not that different from this boy, likewise crying out for wise and compassionate help. The lack of caring they display for the animals in their keeping stems from an alienation from themselves and from life, not from innate cruelty. Merely blaming and hating them does nothing to heal the separation and isolation out of which their cruelties spring. Our goal should be to help them learn to act according to an authentic respect for other creatures, for in so doing they can come to feel a kinship with life, and their own value as part of Creation. We urgently need laws that would guide them in this direction.

Of course, in some instances it may take a serious remedy to be effective. Sometimes only a severe corrective is able to produce the needed empathy in someone who otherwise remains indifferent to the suffering of his fellow creatures. Here is another such case from ancient times.

A man is accused of mistreating his oxen. The judge inspects the animals and sees that they are indeed in bad condition, and have deep sores upon their shoulders from an ill-fitting yoke. He tells the owner that this is not good, thinking that perhaps the man is ignorant, or stupid, and has not seen the hurt done to animals. But the man protests defensively that his oxen are thin because they are too lazy to eat, that the work they do in the fields is light enough for a child, and that he envies the oxen their contentment. And the judge says: "There shall be no longer any need for you to have to envy them. For now you will have the opportunity to share their contentment, by doing yourself this work you say is 'child's play.' Tomorrow you shall be yoked to the plow, and you will draw it back and forth under the hot sun until the field is furrowed."

The judge gives the man's oxen to a neighbor whose animals are well cared for, and says that the man may regain his oxen when he has finished furrowing the field. Furthermore, his oxen will be inspected thereafter, and if it is found that he has mistreated them, he will receive unto himself whatever treatment he has given unto them. But if it is found that he now treats them well, then it will be known that he can be trusted with oxen, and so his herd will be expanded.[2]

If a person refuses time and again to imagine how he would feel in another creature's shoes, sometimes the only remedy that will bring about the needed empathy is to physically place him there.

In some cases the conditions suffered by today's food animals arise simply because greed has clouded the eyes of those responsible, and they can no longer see the pain of their fellow creatures. In such cases, the best justice may be that which serves not only to right the wrong that has been done, but also to clear the vision that has become so clouded.

Here is one more case of ancient wisdom, uniquely pertinent to the issue of greed. In one village there are two men who dispute ownership of a wild ass. Both claim ownership by right of having seen the animal first. One of the men is more prosperous than the other, yet he keeps bemoaning his poverty, the number of his children and the poorness of his fields and he protests that the ass should be given to him because his is by far the greater need. A wise judge says to him: "You tell me that your need is the greater because you are poor and this other man is far wealthier than you; and when he says he is the poorer you say he is lying. Therefore I shall give a judgment that will adjust the wrong that he does to you. You, who are the poorer man, shall have the wild ass. And to show you how much you are favored, you and this other man shall exchange all your possessions."

Now the man cries out in self-pity, and says he has been robbed. At this, the judge pretends to be surprised. "Robbed? When I have given to you the greater possessions of your neighbor? Surely you don't believe his claim that his possessions are meager, when you yourself have just assured me that he lies and his holdings are great. As an honest man, you must admit the exchange has indeed favored you."³

A COW TESTIFIES IN COURT
In our own times, courtroom justice is not always so poetic or profound. But our judges sometimes manage to come up with creative ways of getting to the truth of a dispute.

On July 6, 1953, a California man named Mike Perkins was formally accused of stealing a calf from his neighbor's ranch, and then branding it with his own ranch's insignia, to conceal the theft. Mike stood before the judge and vehemently denied the charges, saying his neighbor had made the whole thing up out of jealousy.

The judge was going to find Perkins innocent, because the only evidence against him was the other farmer's word. But then he had an idea: he sent the sheriff out to Perkin's ranch, and had him bring to a yard adjacent to the courthouse all of Perkin's calves who were about the age the allegedly stolen calf was reputed to be. Then he sent the sheriff out to the accusing neighbor's ranch, and had him bring to the yard the cow who was alleged to be the mother of the stolen calf.

When the mother cow arrived, she began calling loudly, and seemed to be trying to move towards the roped-in calves. The judge decreed that she be allowed freedom of movement. When she was let go, the cow gave her testimony to the court in no uncertain terms. She went directly over to the calves, nudged her way to one in particular, and began to lick it over and over, right on the hip, where Perkin's brand "P" was located.

I probably don't have to tell you Mike Perkins was found guilty.

WHAT THEY'RE REALLY LIKE
When I first heard what happened in this California court, I was surprised. There was an image in my mind what cows could and couldn't do, and I wouldn't have thought this kind of thing possible. I was still , more than I knew, a prisoner of the common notion that animals are automata, with perhaps a dash of intelligence. But everything I have learned since then has shown me how wrong I was.

The truth is that cows have a special kind of intelligence and sensitivity. But because they are such patient and gentle souls who rarely hurry or make a fuss about things, we tend to think they are dumb, and don't recognize their unique presence. Rooted deeply in the rhythms of the earth, they move through life with a peacefulness that is not easy to disturb. They are not troubled by much of what bothers us, and when they are alarmed—usually by things we cannot see—they are still slow to panic, and rarely overreact.

Aldous Huxley once said that in this century we have added onto the seven original deadly sins an eighth that is just as deadly—the sin of hurry. In terms of this sin, at least, cattle are saints.

Few of us, today, have much opportunity to experience for ourselves what kind of creatures cattle are, and so we are easy prey to the common prejudices about them, which are born and thrive in ignorance. But a naturalist who knew cows well, W. H. Hudson, spoke movingly of:

". . . the gentle, large-brained, social cow, that caresses our hands and faces with her rough blue tongue, and is more like man's sister than any other non-human being—the majestic, beautiful creature with the Juno eyes . . ." [4]

People of less sophisticated times, living in closer contact with the earth, had great respect for these patient and gentle souls. 2,000 years ago, the poet Ovid wrote:

"Oh ox, how great are thy desserts! A being without guile, harmless, simple, willing for work . . ." [5]

HOW NOW BROWN COW?

For centuries, these animals have pulled our plows, sweetened our soils, and given their milk to our children. Today, however, these peaceful and patient creatures have been rewarded for their centuries of service by being treated in much the same way as today's chickens and pigs. You might think there are laws requiring them to be treated humanely. But harkening back to darker times, the Animal Welfare

Act specifically excludes creatures intended for use as food from its regulations governing the "humane" treatment of animals.[6] And though this law places some restrictions on how cruelly animals can be treated, cows, pigs, and chickens, however, are evidently not considered animals within the meaning of the Act. The current philosophy is that you can be as cruel as you like, as long as the animal is later going to be eaten.

The result isn't very pretty.

You may wonder, as I have, how the people who actually handle the animals rationalize what they do. I asked a livestock auction worker named George Kennedy if he were ever uncomfortable with the way the animals were handled. He replied:

> *"Look, if you want beef, this is the only way you can have it. There's no room in this business for a 'be nice to animals' attitude. There's work to be done, and that's all there is to it."*

Later, I talked with the owner of the auction, a man named Henry F. Pace. I asked him how he felt about the charges from animal rights groups that the auctions were cruel to the cattle. He sized me up for a moment, then answered:

> *"It doesn't bother me. We're no different from any other business. These animal rights people like to accuse us of mistreating our stock, but we believe we can be most efficient by not being emotional. We are a business, not a humane society, and our job is to sell merchandise at a profit. It's no different from selling paper-clips, or refrigerators."*

In the eyes of the law, Henry Pace is right. There are almost no legal limits on what can be done to the animals destined for our dinner tables.

A federal law, passed in 1906, does put certain basic restraints on the way cattle can be shipped by railroad. This law was passed to curb the cruelty that most of us would like to think belonged to a less-enlightened time. But this law puts no restraints on the way animals can be shipped by truck, because trucks did not yet exist at the time this act was passed, and apparently the cattle industry has managed through the years to block the passage of any legislation which might extend the cow's protection to include more modern transportation.

With a sharp eye for this kind of loophole, the meat industry today almost always ships cattle by truck. The journey, as you could probably guess by now, is a horror from start to finish.

If you were to step inside one of these trucks you'd be immediately struck by the smell. It wouldn't take you very long to know that the ventilation is terrible. And you'd soon find out that the temperatures are scorching hot in the summer, and bitterly cold in the winter. You'd see that these animals—ruminants whose stomachs only function properly with a more or less continuous supply of food—may spend as much as three days and nights without being fed or watered. One authority wrote:

> *"It is difficult for us to imagine what this combination of fear, travel sickness, thirst, near-starvation, exhaustion, and (in winter) . . . severe chill feels like to the cattle. In the case of young calves, which may have gone through the stress of weaning and castration only a few days earlier, the effect is still worse."*[7]

Today's cattlemen regard it as a normal part of the business that some of the animals will die in transit. It's a calculated loss. They find it more profitable to absorb the loss due to deaths and injuries than to handle the animals differently. They fully expect to find some of the animals dead on arrival, and they calculate the loss simply as one of the costs of transporting the animals, along with the price of gasoline.

Most of the deaths are caused by a form of pneumonia known quite appropriately as "shipping fever."[8] More than one animal dies of this disease for every hundred cattle that reach market. The Livestock Conservation Institute has called it the most costly animal disease in the United States today.[9] Accordingly, livestock producers today routinely use a dangerous antibiotic called chloramphenicol to treat shipping fever. It helps keep shipping fever deaths down and profits up.

The Food and Drug Administration, however, is not very happy about the use of chloramphenicol in the beef industry, and frankly, I don't blame them. The Book of Lists #2 has a remarkable listing titled "Nine Travesties of Modern Medical Science," which ranks chloramphenicol right along with the thalidomide tragedies and other horrors.[10] The reason is that in a small but significant percentage of people even minute quantities of chloramphenicol cause a fatal blood disorder called aplastic anemia. Chloramphenicol has legitimate medical uses in extreme cases where human lives are at stake and no other antibiotic will work. But it is an extremely dangerous drug. Even infinitesimal amounts will kill susceptible human beings by preventing their blood marrow from producing red blood cells. And there is no way to know who is susceptible! Dr. Joseph A. Settepani, a veterinarian who works for the FDA in the area of human food safety, says amounts as low as 32 milligrams of chloramphenicol have killed human beings. This is an amount you would ingest from consuming a quarter-pound of meat with a residue count of 8 parts-per-million. Commercial beef from animals treated with chloramphenicol for shipping fever has been found to have residue counts 100 times that high.[11]

If you were to watch today's cattle being shipped, you'd see that shipping fever is only one cause of death for cattle in transit. There are other causes too and none of them leads to a particularly easy death for these gentle animals. You'd see cattle freeze to death in the winter. You'd see them collapse and die from heat prostration and severe dehydration in summer. You'd see them suffocate when other animals pile on top of them as the overcrowded trucks go around curves.

If you were on hand when the animals arrive at their destination you'd see that those who survive the journey are not in the best of shape either. Not only may they have contracted shipping fever, but they have suffered a great deal of bruising and may be crippled from the pounding they have taken. Incidentally, the trade definition of a "cripple" is:

". . . an animal that must be carried or dragged from the vehicle." [12]

In other words, an animal that can manage to limp along even though its legs are mangled and broken is not a "cripple." By the same token, an animal is not considered officially "bruised" unless its injuries are so bad its flesh must be condemned as unsuitable for human consumption. Apparently bruising counts only when it affects the pocketbook.

HOME SWEET HOME?

For the animals who survive the journey, arrival does not immediately signify it's time to relax and enjoy life again. Exhausted, depleted, and ill, bewildered by the harsh handling they have received, these peace-loving creatures may be welcomed to their new home by being dipped in a trough full of insecticides. Then they may be castrated, de-horned, branded, and injected with various chemicals.

All in all, it's a little less than the ideal homecoming.

Castration is the removal of the testicles of a bull in order to produce a steer, and is an extremely painful process for the animals to undergo. I had thought it was done to produce more docile, easier-to-handle animals, and this is, in fact, one of the reasons for the operation. But the main reason is that steers have a higher percentage of body fat than bulls and the industry grades meats according to fat content, with the most expensive grades being those with the most fat marbled through the flesh, where it cannot be trimmed off. To a meat producer, that's sufficient reason to inflict any degree of pain. Castrated animals have more fat, and so fetch a higher price.

Removing the testicles of a bull substantially reduces its natural hormone production. But this presents no problem to today's cattlemen. The steers are simply implanted with synthetic hormones to offset the natural hormone deficiencies caused by castration.[13] The fact that these synthetic hormones may produce carcinogenic residues in the meat from these animals is rarely seen by the industry as anything other than a public-relations issue.

"Castration is a beastly business, even to the hardened pig man," wrote the British trade journal *Pig Farming*.[14] I can't help but wonder, if it's so difficult for the "hardened pig men," how bad it must be on the pig or bull itself. And if it's so "beastly" in Britain, where anesthetics by law must be used, how much worse is it in the United States, where there is no such legislation, and pain-killers are rarely used.

The farmers who actually do the work know what is involved. A California cattleman, Herb Silverman, told me:

"I hate castrating them. It's really horrible. After you put the ring on its scrotum the calf will lie down and kick and wring its tail for half an hour or more, before the scrotum finally goes numb. It's obviously in agony. Then it takes about a month before its balls fall off. You can do it faster with a special kind of pliers, but I can't bear to use those because I can't take how they carry on."

By nature the most mellow and easy going of animals, cattle do not usually become riled unless a great deal of pain has been systematically applied to get them upset. If you have been to a modern rodeo, with events like bull riding and steer wrestling, you've seen what appear to be vicious, mean and ornery animals. You've heard them described by the rodeo announcers as "rampaging brute fury," or some other term designed to make you tremble in your seat. And though you may have felt the carnival atmosphere of the proceedings, and sensed that their meanness was in some way hyped-up, you probably didn't know to what extreme measures rodeo personnel have to resort to make these animals—placid by nature—into a living picture of fury and agitation.

To this end, they fit an animal with a "flanking strap," which causes him immense pain, and from which he does everything in his power to gain release. He doesn't buck because he is a wild and furious beast, but because an excruciatingly painful strap has been cinched, tightly, in the areas of his genitals and intestines. Sometimes a nail, tack, piece of barbed wire or other sharp metal object has been placed under the strap, to further infuriate him. And just before the animal is let out of the chute, an electric prod known in the trade as the "hot shot," is applied to his rectum, all to provoke this gentle animal into dashing madly into the arena, to put on an "exciting" exhibition that is really nothing but the poor fellow's pain and panic.

Cattlemen acknowledge that except in extremely crowded conditions there is no need to de-horn cattle, because these peaceful animals will not hurt each other unless they are crammed so tightly together that they cannot help it. And cattlemen also know the process is extremely painful to the animals, often resulting in hemorrhage, maggot infestations and infections.[15] But today's cattle are routinely de-horned because today's cattle feedlots, where the great majority of today's cattle spend the last half of their lives, are unbelievably overcrowded.

And they are not likely to become less crowded in the foreseeable future. The trend is toward ever increasing crowding, known in the jargon of the trade as "stock density."[16] Studies at the University of Minnesota suggest maximum profits can be obtained by allowing each of these large animals fourteen square feet of living space.[17] To realize what this means, consider that a typical 12' × 15' bedroom is 180 square feet. Imagine thirteen half ton steers in your bedroom and you've got the picture.

THE PHARMACEUTICAL FARM

Most of us, with images in our minds of the cows of yesteryear, could hardly believe the extent to which the meat industry today relies on chemicals, hormones, antibiotics and a plethora of other drugs.[18] It is a business, and a very competitive one. Even the small cattlemen are eager to use anything the drug companies can convince them will make their work easier, make their animals gain weight faster, or enable them to mask the signs of disease and gross stress in their animals so they can be sold to the slaughterhouse—anything to give them an edge in the marketplace.

I asked cattleman Herb Silverman how he felt about the high levels of drugs fed to today's cattle. He replied:

> *"It's not good. Instead of improving husbandry practices, which would make the animals healthier, we just shoot 'em up with drugs. It's cheaper that way, and because this is a competitive business I've got to do it, too. But in the meantime the general public is catching on, and getting afraid of residues in the meat. And I'll tell you something. I don't blame them."*

The avalanche of drug usage has occurred in the last 20 to 30 years, coincidental with the shift in production methods from range grazing to feedlots. Before 1950, almost all the nation's cattle spent their lives grazing and foraging for their food in something like the wide open spaces most of us picture as "cattle country." But no more. By the early 1970's, three-quarters of U. S. cattle were trucked off to spend half their lives in feedlots.[19]

Some of the larger feedlots have as many as 100,000 "units." Here the animals are fed a diet designed for one purpose only—to fatten them up as cheaply as possible. This may include such delicacies as sawdust laced with ammonia and feathers, shredded newspaper (complete with all the colors of toxic ink from the Sunday comics and advertising circulars), "plastic hay," processed sewage, inedible tallow and grease, poultry litter, cement dust, and cardboard scraps, not to mention the insecticides, antibiotics and hormones. Artificial flavors and aromas are added to trick the poor animals into eating the stuff.[20]

Meanwhile, scientists at the University of Arizona are studying the biological processes that curb a cow's appetite. Their reason?

"Obviously, if the thing that turns a beef animal away from the feed bunk were found, and could be overcome, it would mean a lot."[21]

It sure would, because the whole idea is to make them as fat as possible as cheaply as possible. The massive agribusiness conglomerates which own the feedlots are very excited about the prospect of having chemicals that would give these placid animals insatiable appetites.

The industry recognizes that major health problems ensue from the way today's cattle are fed. But it doesn't matter to them if the animal is ill, even if the illness is so severe it is dying, so long as it can be kept alive with drugs long enough to be slaughtered and sold to the consumer.

MILK FROM CONTENTED COWS?

If life in today's feedlots isn't the greatest thing that could ever happen to a cow, neither is life in a modern milk factory.

The trouble seems to stem from the modern cow's insistence in asserting her fundamental nature. She still wants to do what cows have always done: devotedly care for her young, quietly forage and ruminate, and patiently live with the rhythms of the earth.

Such outdated ideas, of course, put her at cross purposes with an industry that looks upon her as a four-legged milk pump, a machine whose purpose is to provide milk for profit. She is bred, fed, medicated, inseminated, and manipulated to a single purpose—maximum milk production at minimum cost.

The industry points today with considerable pride to the fact that the average commercial cow now gives three or more times as much milk in a year as her bucolic ancestors. They don't mention that her udder is so large that her calves would have a hard time suckling from it, and might easily damage it if they were allowed to try. Nor do they mention that under natural conditions Old Bessie would live 20 to 25 years. In the unbelievably stressful world of today's dairy factories, however, she is so severely exploited that she will be lucky if she sees her fourth birthday.

Old Bessie may spend her whole life in a concrete stall, or, worse yet for her legs and feet, on a slatted metal floor. She is pregnant all the time, and her nervous system has been made so ragged by breeding practices devoted exclusively to milk production and a lifestyle that affords her no exercise, that this most mellow and patient of animals has become something else. She is today so tense, nervous and hyperactive that she often has to be given tranquilizers.

If Old Bessie lives in a factory that brings portable milking machines to the cows, she may remain for months in her cramped, narrow stall, chained at the neck. On the other hand, she may call home the type of dairy factory that wishes her to come to the milking apparatus. One method for transporting Old Bessie to the equipment has been designed by Alfa-Laval, a Swedish agricultural company.

"Each cow is placed in a contraption called 'Unicar' which is a kind of cage on wheels that moves along a railway line. The cages, with cows in them, spend most of their time filed in rows in a storage barn. Two or three times a day, the farmer pushes a button in the milking parlor. Rows of cows then move automatically up to the milking parlor like a long train. As they go, their car wheels trip switches which feed, water, and clean the cars. After milking, the cows, still in the cages, roll back to the storage area. The cows live in the cages for ten months of the year, during which time they are unable to walk or turn around." [22]

Today's dairy cows are commonly implanted with hormones to promote milk production, but after a while, under these conditions, their output inevitably drops. Then it is time for Old Bessie, exhausted and depleted, to climb into the truck for one last journey.

HER BABIES

Old Bessie never knows what becomes of the babies who are taken from her at birth. And it is probably a good thing she doesn't. For the most part, her daughters are raised to follow in her hoof-steps. But her sons, the little boy calves, cannot be converted into four-legged milk pumps. So another fate lies in store for them.

These little fellows are sent to auctions when they are all of a day old. There, bewildered and terrified, barely able to stand, their umbilical cords still attached, they are purchased to be "made" into veal, a process which takes about four months.

It is a process which to my eyes may be the most obscene of all the cruelties I've seen in modern animal factories.

Anyone who has struggled with young calves, perhaps striving to teach them to drink milk from a bucket, knows how strong, wayward and vital these creatures can be. They suck at a finger pushed into their mouth, gulp the milk, toss their head, tug at whatever they can. Young calves are playful and exuberant, with a powerful desire to frolic. Newborn, they are utterly vulnerable, and their eyes are beautiful with a special kind of innocence and awe.

But in today's dairy factories these little fellows are placed onto a veal production assembly-line within hours of their births. Most meat-eaters think the pale, tender flesh they eat comes from a particular type of calf, bred for veal. But this is not so. It comes from the male calves born to dairy cows.

THE LATEST THING IN VEAL

In a hotel room I stayed in recently there was a menu for the hotel restaurant. In the tradition of "fine dining" to which this hotel aspired there were three "specialties of the house" featured. These were all veal dishes—veal scallopini, veal Oscar, and veal piccata. Veal dishes are expensive, and sound very high class. With an Italian name, they bring to mind the haute cuisine of continental Europe. Few people know that in the last few decades there has been a revolution in the world of veal. Chef James Beard wrote in *American Cookery*:

> *"Good veal has always been difficult to find. But recently a Dutch process has come to our shores and is giving us a limited quantity of much finer veal than was generally available before . . . The calves . . . have delicate whitish-pink flesh and clear fat and are deliciously tender."*
>
> (*JAMES BEARD, AMERICAN COOKERY*)[23]

There is a secret to how this new Dutch process manages to provide veal that is so "delicate whitish-pink" and so "deliciously tender." Learning about this secret has changed me, forever.

The veal that has traditionally been prized by gourmets is whitish, and its tender texture comes from muscles which have never been used. This veal has come from the flesh of a baby calf that has consumed only its mother's milk. Since calves normally start nibbling grass and other solid food within a few day's of their birth, it doesn't take very long before their flesh, whitish when they are born, begins to turn pink. Veal was prized in Europe because of the very fact that it was a rare and expensive commodity.

But then came the revolutionary thinking which originated in Holland after World War II, and was brought to America by Provimi, Inc., of Watertown, Wisconsin. Provimi proudly takes credit for developing this "new and complete concept of veal raising," which totally dominates the industry today. But as we shall soon see, it's not something I'd be all that proud about.

Traditionally, the veal calf had to be slaughtered shortly after his birth, before his flesh acquired color, which meant before he exercised and developed muscles, and before he ate anything besides his mother's milk. Traditionally, veal calves were slaughtered at about 150 pounds, which isn't much more than their birth weight. But the Provimi method enables much more profit to be obtained from each calf, because they have found a way of keeping the calves' flesh white and tender up to a weight of 350 pounds.

The way they manage to fatten these little baby calves while keeping their flesh white and their muscles undeveloped is the heart of the Provimi method.

First of all, the calf is taken away from his mother immediately after birth. Veal producers are aware this deprives the infant calf of the colostrum in its mother's milk, and so renders the little ones very susceptible to disease. But they separate mother and child at birth anyway, because the large udder of today's dairy cow can be damaged by suckling, and the cow will produce more milk if attached to a machine. Additionally, according to Dr. Jack Albright, Professor of Animal Science at Purdue University, and consultant to the veal industry, it is important the calves do not bond with their mother, as they would if she nursed them. If the calves are taken away from their mothers after this bond develops, the cow will cause a great deal of trouble and even try to break down fences to be with her calves.

The newborn calves are taken to veal sheds, and placed in what are euphemistically called "stalls." These stalls will be their homes until they are slaughtered at the age of four months, unless, of course, they die first. A high percentage are not able to survive even four months so horrid are the conditions.

The stalls have been designed to keep the calves' flesh "tender enough to be used for baby food." If the calves were let outside, or even kept in a pen, their frisky nature would lead them to romp around and they would soon develop muscles. This, of course, must not happen. So the infant calves are shut tightly in their stalls, and allowed no exercise whatsoever, right from the start.

Every year, one million newborn calves are shut up in such stalls in the United States, to be raised for veal. These youngsters not only never have a chance to romp or play; they never even walk! Remember these are babies, only a day or so old, cut off from their mothers and imprisoned in this way.

The newborns are isolated in stalls all of 22 inches wide and 54 inches long—far less than the space that can be found in the trunk of the smallest cars.

The stalls are so tiny the animals can hardly move. They are so narrow that in order to lie down the calves must hunch into a position no cow ever normally assumes. They cannot stretch out into their natural sleeping posture. They cannot turn around. Chained around the neck, the baby calves cannot even twist their heads to lick and groom themselves with their tongues, though this is one of their most basic and innate desires. They can move only a few inches back and forth, and side to side. Their stall is as cramped as a shipping crate. As the days pass, and the calves grow, they become even more cramped, so that any movement at all becomes nearly impossible.

THE REAL MEANING OF "SPECIAL-FED"

Keeping infant calves confined to stalls so small they cannot take a single step is Provimi's ingenious method of preventing any muscular development in the calves, and so keeping their flesh "tender enough for baby food." In order to keep the flesh the "whitish-pink" color traditionally associated with prize veal, Provimi has come up with another macabre idea, and created the diet which accounts for the names "special-fed veal," and "milk-fed veal." Provimi is proud of developing this "special" diet, which can bring the calves to a weight of 350 pounds, yet retain the whiteness of flesh of the newborn infant.

When I first heard the phrase "special-fed veal," I got an image of something fancy. Knowing that veal is an expensive "delicacy" supposedly associated with "fine continental cuisine," I surmised that "special fed" veal calves must receive a diet that is better in some way, and probably more expensive, than normal calves. I supposed that "special fed" calves were probably extremely healthy. I had the idea they were in some way the cream of the crop.

I was wrong. The "special" diet fed these calves achieves its objective, which is to keep the calves' flesh white, by systematically inducing anemia in the young animals. It is a diet that is deliberately and profoundly iron-deficient.

Calves are born with stores of iron in their bodies, primarily in the form of extra hemoglobin in the blood, with lesser amounts stored in the liver, spleen and bone marrow. During the four months the veal calf is confined and "special fed," these reserves decline steadily. The veal producers are pleased to have achieved their objective: the calves' flesh remains white while they put on weight.

Producers would like to take the calves to even heavier weights, but by the time four months have passed and they have reached about 350 pounds, the calves have become so seriously anemic that those still alive would soon die in their stalls.

Deliberately deprived of iron, the little calves develop an insatiable craving for the mineral. They lick any iron fittings in their stalls in a desperate effort to obtain some iron, but today's vealers are not ones to be outsmarted by such maneuvers. Provimi tells its producers:

"The main reason for using hardwood instead of metal boxstalls is that metal may affect the light veal color . . . Keep all iron out of reach of your calves." [24]

Vealers are also cautioned to make sure the calves have no access to rusty nails, or any other kind of metal which they might lick. No straw or other bedding material is provided, because in the calf's craving for iron, he would eat it. Producers are told to test the iron level in the water used to mix the animals' feed, and not to hesitate to use an iron filter. All possible sources of iron must be kept from the young calves. This is one of the reasons why the stalls are so narrow, and the calves are chained around the neck.

The results of this treatment are not pleasant. For example, calves, like pigs, will normally not go near their own manure or urine. But because their urine does contain tiny amounts of iron, the calves, in their desperate natural craving for this nutrient, would, if they could, lick the floor where their urine fell. Veal producers, however, are not about to let the baby calves get away with something like that. Accordingly, they have arranged it so the calves cannot turn around and get even the little bit of iron they might obtain in this pitiful way.

With their mothers, baby calves would suckle an average of sixteen times a day. Sucking is perhaps their strongest and most essential instinct and need. Deprived not only of their mothers, but of any conceivable source of stimulation and interest, the little baby calves crave something to suck on. Their urge is strong to begin with, and becomes absolutely ravenous when they are deprived of any opportunity to do so. The result is that they frantically try to suck some part of their stall. But once again the superior intelligence of the veal producers has the upper hand. They have carefully planned the stalls so there is nothing at all for the calves to suck on.

If you move close to a veal calf's head, he will try frantically to suck on your hand, or your elbow, or your shirt, or your purse, or your umbrella, or anything at all he can reach. It is hard to avoid feeling that these calves in bondage are not veal machines, but ill little babies, desperately craving for what might heal their disease.

ACES UP THEIR SLEEVES
It is difficult to imagine how conditions could be made any worse for the wretched animals. Yet today's veal producers have a few other aces up their sleeves which increase the profits they can make from their "units." One of these is to give the calves no water. This way the calves must try to quench their thirst by consuming the only source of liquid they have, the government surplus skim milk and fat mixture they are fed. This clever tactic forces them to consume far more of the stuff than they otherwise would, and so put on weight out of their desire to avoid dying of thirst.

Many of today's veal calves are also exposed to a final insult: they are forced to live in complete darkness except for their two daily feedings. The producers are delighted with this maneuver, seeing it as an effective way to put more fat on the animals. They are not at all disturbed that, under these conditions, many of the calves go blind.

There is some indication, however, that the calves themselves are not all that pleased with the situation, as they quite frequently express their displeasure by dying shortly after losing their sight.

A PICTURE OF HEALTH?
Though the "special" diet the little calves are fed is supposed to keep them alive, the steadily worsening anemia makes the animals extremely susceptible to pneumonic and enteric diseases. Even dosed with a massive and constant supply of antibiotics and other drugs, many of the animals don't survive the four months. Authorities on contemporary veal production say the calves:

> ". . . get sick despite the precautions and must be treated frequently with drugs by mouth and injection. Two of the four most common drugs used are nitrofurazone and chloramphenicol . . ." [25]

Nitrofurazone is a recognized carcinogen. And chloramphenicol, as you may remember from the discussion of shipping fever, causes a fatal blood disorder in a significant percentage of humans, even in infinitesimal concentrations.

Such dangerous drugs must be used to keep the little calves alive because the animals are so extremely unwell, and safer medications are not strong enough.

The Farm Animals Concern Trust (FACT) is an organization trying to improve the lot of today's veal calves. In one of their mailers, they made the following charges against the industry.

> *"Veal calves are:*
>
> * *denied sufficient mother's milk*
> * *trucked to auctions when only a day or two old*
> * *commingled with sick and dying animals*
> * *sold to veal factories where they are chained for life in individual crates only 22 inches wide*
> * *fed government surplus skim milk*
> * *denied solid food to chew on*
> * *made anemic*
> * *kept in the dark to reduce their restlessness*
> * *plagued by respiratory and intestinal disease*
> * *unable to lie down normally*
> * *deprived of any bedding*
> * *unable to walk at all, let alone romp and play."*

A veal producer got hold of the mailer, but didn't know how to counter the statements it made. So he sent the mailer to the editor of the industry's journal requesting an effective rebuttal from the industry experts. The editor of *The Vealer USA*, a man named Charles A. Hirschy, looked over the charges made by the FACT mailer, and then answered as follows.

> *"Thank you for the information about FACT. We've read the information and regret that we are unable to counter their statements."* [26]

The Farm Animals Concern Trust (FACT) has developed a new husbandry method for raising non-anemic veal calves outdoors on pasture.

As yet this far more humane method of raising veal calves is followed by only a few farms. But if you see veal marked RAMBLING ROSE BRAND™, you can trust it was not raised by the Provimi method.

A WOLF IN SHEEP'S CLOTHING

The Humane Society of the United States does not normally concern itself with animals being raised for food. But it has sponsored a "No Veal This Meal" campaign in an effort to educate the public to the darker side of this white "gourmet" meat. It also printed "No Veal" cards, and is asking people to leave them in restaurants. The cards read: "Dear Restauranteur, I enjoyed my meal here, but I did not choose a veal entree because I believe milk-fed veal is inhumanely raised. I would prefer it if you did not offer this veal on your menu."

The Humane Society is not alone in expressing its opposition to contemporary veal-raising practices. The American Society for the Prevention of Cruelty to Animals chose the veal calf as its "1987 Animal of the Year," to bring attention to the cruelties inflicted upon animals raised for food. At the same time, the Humane Farming Association, which is spearheading a campaign against the abuses of factory farming, is coordinating nationwide veal boycott demonstrations in front of restaurants and other establishments which continue to sell anemic veal. These actions have generated nationwide media coverage, and informed the public about the real story behind today's veal. As a result, a number of restaurants have stopped selling the product. Furthermore, the Humane Farming Association has introduced legislation to outlaw the practice of raising veal calves in crates. This is the first legislation which would protect farm animals from intense confinement and immobilization.

Provimi, Inc., whose name is practically synonomous with the veal industry in the United States today, has not been unaffected by the pleas that veal calves be treated humanely. Their response has been to call upon the "farm" community to boycott the Humane Society. And they have pledged $200,000 to fight the "No Veal" campaign.

Meanwhile, the American Veal Association, alarmed at the rising tide of public opposition to veal production practices, has taken a step to quell the objections, though it does not seem likely to improve the fate of today's veal calves. They have hired a public relations firm to improve their public image—Jackson, Jackson, and Wagner.[27]

For a number of years, the industry has had an organization called the "Coalition for Animal Agriculture," whose specific duty it has been to defend factory farming, and present it to the public in a positive light. Losing a bit of ground as of late, due to the Humane Society campaign and the work of many other dedicated individuals and groups concerned for the welfare of animals, the "Coalition for Animal Agriculture" has come up with a brilliant move. It has changed its name to the "Farm Animal Welfare Council," and now presents itself to the public as an organization devoted solely to the welfare of the animals.[28]

The treasurer of the "Farm Animal Welfare Council" is a vicepresident of Provimi, Inc.[29]

In another ploy, John Mahlman, sales manager for Provimi, defended the veal industry by saying: "What we are talking about here is world hunger."[30] Unfortunately, he did not exactly explain the relationship between anemic veal, at $9 - $14 a pound, and world hunger.

Despite such maneuvers to whitewash the veal industry, major TV news shows are beginning to get wind of what's going on and investigate. KARE-TV in Minneapolis and KRON-TV in San Francisco both recently did programs presenting the results of their inquiries. The programs did not please the veal industry apologists, bearing titles such as "Misery On The Menu," and "Unpalatable Treatment." The reports naturally included interviews with the vealers themselves, and these, to my mind at least, proved the old adage in favor of free speech: "The best thing to do in the case of a fool is to encourage him to advertise that fact by speaking."

One vealer, a man named Marv Pratt, told the television audience of his veal calves: "Hey, they live like kings!"

NEVER BEFORE

Today's veal producers are not alone in their crimes. They are only a particularly blatant and grotesque example of an industry gone amuck. All of today's food animals—the proud and passionate chickens, the friendly and steadfast pigs, the gentle-hearted cows—are treated today in a manner that would, I believe, sicken any open-hearted person who had eyes to see what was actually happening.

Throughout history there have been people who have chosen to be vegetarians because they did not feel it was right to kill animals for food when this was not necessary, when there was other nourishing food available. But today, because of the way animals are raised for market, the question of whether or not to eat meat has a whole new meaning, and a whole new urgency. Never before have animals been treated like this. Never before has such deep, unrelenting and systematic cruelty been mass produced. Never before has the decision of each individual been so important.

ANY WAY YOU SLICE IT, IT'S STILL BOLOGNA

"A missionary was walking in Africa when he heard the ominous padding of a lion behind him. 'Oh Lord,' prayed the missionary, 'Grant in Thy goodness that the lion walking behind me is a good Christian lion.'

And then, in the silence that followed, the missionary heard the lion praying too: 'Oh Lord,' he prayed, 'We thank Thee for the food which we are about to receive.'"

(CLEVELAND AMORY)

"Custom will reconcile people to any atrocity."

(GEORGE BERNARD SHAW)

IT HAS OFTEN been pointed out that there were many good-thinking and decent Germans who listened to Adolph Hitler as he rose to power, knew him for what he was, and yet did nothing. They sensed that his campaign rhetoric masked an insatiable drive for power that would stop at nothing to achieve its ends. But they stood silently by and watched the Nazis take over, because they were afraid to open their mouths.

One man who did open his mouth was Edgar Kupfer, and he paid dearly for trying to awaken a sense of conscience in his countrymen. Kupfer was imprisoned in the concentration camp at Dachau during World War II. His crime? He was a pacifist.

In this hell of hells, Edgar Kupfer managed to steal scraps of paper and bits of pencils. Stealthily, he kept a diary. Between the few precious moments when he was able to write in his diary, Kupfer kept his secret work buried underground. He knew what would happen if the Nazis found it.

On April 29, 1945, Dachau was liberated. Edgar Kupfer was free. And so were his buried diaries. The Dachau Diaries of Edgar Kupfer are now preserved in a Special Collection of the Library of the University of Chicago. In one of his essays, called "Animals, My Brethren," Kupfer wrote:

> *"The following pages were written in the Concentration Camp in Dachau, in the midst of all kinds of cruelties. They were furtively scrawled in a hospital barrack where I stayed during my illness, in a time when Death grasped day by day after us, when we lost twelve thousand within four and a half months . . .*
>
> *"You asked me why I do not eat meat and you are wondering at the reasons of my behavior . . . I refuse to eat animals because I cannot nourish myself by the sufferings and by the death of other creatures. I refuse to do so, because I suffered so painfully myself that I can feel the pains of others by recalling my own sufferings . . .*
>
> *"I am not preaching . . . I am writing this letter to you, to an already awakened individual who rationally controls his impulses, who feels responsible, internally and externally, for his acts, who knows that our supreme court is sitting in our conscience . . .*
>
> *"I have not the intention to point out with my finger . . . I think it is much more my duty to stir up my own conscience . . .*
>
> *"That is the point: I want to grow up into a better world where a higher law grants more happiness, in a new world where God's commandment reigns:* **You shall love each other."**[1]

Edgar Kupfer had seen enough of the opposite to want to live in a world where love would reign. May his prayers be granted.

After the war, Edgar Kupfer moved to Chicago. There is a sad irony here, because for years Chicago was the central slaughterhouse of the United States, and is still the location for the killing of millions of animals every year. But what was once the hub of Chicago's animal slaughter industry, the notorious Union Stockyards, is now closed. All that is left of it is the entrance gate, designated a historic landmark by Mayor Daley. Poignantly, this gate is said to "very closely resemble" the gate marking the entrance to the concentration camp in Dachau.[2]

During the war, millions of Germans knew vaguely that Jews, Gypsies and pacifists like Edgar Kupfer were being sent to places like

Auschwitz and Dachau. But they didn't know the immensity of the horror that was done in these places. And most of them, it must be admitted, preferred not to know. In fact, when a few brave souls like Edgar Kupfer tried to tell them, these valiant voices were often silenced for their efforts, for trying to awaken some vestige of dormant humanity in the German psyche.

A web of repression permeated the time, a collective determination to avoid the immense pain that would have come from really seeing what was happening.

In conquered countries as well, the psychic numbing took place. While there were always some people who resisted, who did what they could to save the lives of those hunted by the Nazis, often risking their own lives in so doing, most others tried to ignore the horrors, tried to keep a stiff upper lip and pretend nothing amiss was happening. Though it was hard to avoid knowing at least part of the horrid truth, they found ways of blocking the impact. They busied themselves with other matters, conjured up rationalizations, narrowed their awareness, and looked the other way.

Today, the process of denial is once again rampant. We all know at some level today that our world is in great peril. We all sense the ever-present threat of nuclear war, the increasingly rapid destruction of our life support system, and the growing misery of half the planet's people. We are continuously bombarded by signals of profound planetary anguish, some of which, whether we know it or not, come from the factory farms and slaughterhouses. Often it seems too painful to even think about, so we block it out. We tend to deny the pain we feel because it hurts so deeply, and because it can be so frightening.

Yet the more we succeed in numbing ourselves to our deepest human responses, the more powerless, futile and isolated we feel. The more we avoid our pain for the world, the more disconnected we become and we repress our own painful feelings by filtering out the information that provokes them. Yet this is the very information, painful though it may be, that cries out for our response.

Only by facing the enormity of what is happening can we discover in ourselves the response that will free us from creating such needless horrors, and at the same time, free the animals from such needless pain.

"Each act of denial, conscious or unconscious, is an abdication of our power to respond."

(JOANNA ROGERS MACY)

The healing that is called for asks us to move beyond denial, to acknowledge and express our feelings about these catastrophes without apology or timidity. In the heart of our grief we can find our connection with each other, and the power to act.

As I've learned what is done to animals today, again and again I have had to face my own tendencies to withdraw and go numb. There have been times I felt so overcome with grief and rage that I doubted whether there was any point in continuing to unearth the seemingly endless parade of cruelties. There have been times I seemed to want, with every cell of my body, to forget I had ever heard of a factory farm. But in my willingness to face the immensity of what is actually happening, something just as immense has welled up from the depths of my humanity. A power has arisen in response to the horrors; a power that has transformed isolation, indifference and passivity into a commitment to exposing this madness for what it is.

PHONY BOLOGNA

There are powerful interests today who are profiting from the web of repression about modern farming. It is to their advantage that we not know too much, or be too interested in what goes on in factory farms and slaughterhouses. They don't want us to know what actually happens to the animals whose flesh they sell.

These people are particularly interested in "protecting" young children from the truth. Children aren't as quick to rationalize and numb themselves as adults are. The least repressed among us, they are also the most impressionable. So those who profit from our collective denial go out of their way to make sure our children receive heavily sugar-coated pictures of animal farming. The seeds of denial are thus planted early and deep.

The National Livestock and Meat Board makes it a point to "reach the children of the land at an early age," and "prepare them for a lifetime of meat-eating." As they put it in their 1974-1975 Report:

"The 37 million elementary and 15 million high school students in the United States constitute a special Meat Board audience." [3]

By calling our country's children a "special Meat Board audience" they are not expressing a particularly noble interest in the education of our youngsters. Consider the pictures on page 127, taken from what are called "educational coloring books" for children. These coloring books reassure us they are "factual stories," approved, in one case by the American Egg Board, and in the other by the National Dairy Council and Milk Industry Foundation.

Such nice pictures, aren't they? So sweet and wholesome and appealing. I just wish they were true.

Pictures like these of the lives of chickens and cows are perhaps similar to the ones you carried in your mind before finding out otherwise. Such was certainly the case for me.

Similarly, the American Meat Institute also distributes "educational materials" to thousands of schools. One such title is "The Story of Beef." (See page 128.) You might notice something missing from this fairy tale, however: there is no trace of the animal suffering in any way at any time. At first the calf is shown romping innocently alongside his happy mother; next we see him looking like the very picture of sunshine and cheer in a feedlot; then we see him being happily shipped to the stockyards; and finally we see him evidently delighted as can be as different companies bid for the right to kill him.

The lucky creature, it would seem, is tickled pink at every step of the path to the meat counter.

Other "educational materials" paint equally contrived versions of the animal's experience. In "The Story of Pork," children are shown a pig smiling delightedly all the way until he is "made into eating meat."

The manager of the California Beef Council says that about 800 junior and senior high schools in California, about half of the public schools in the state, receive the Beef Council's "consumer information" program. In a given year, he says, about half a million pieces of literature are distributed in California high schools alone. Over 1,000 teachers are sent "beef teaching manuals, lesson plans, charts, and other such material."

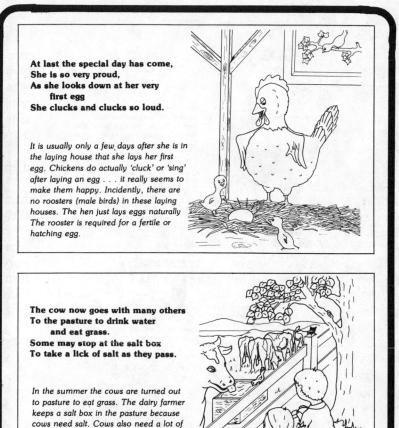

**At last the special day has come,
She is so very proud,
As she looks down at her very
    first egg
She clucks and clucks so loud.**

It is usually only a few days after she is in the laying house that she lays her first egg. Chickens do actually 'cluck' or 'sing' after laying an egg . . . it really seems to make them happy. Incidently, there are no roosters (male birds) in these laying houses. The hen just lays eggs naturally The rooster is required for a fertile or hatching egg.

**The cow now goes with many others
To the pasture to drink water
        and eat grass.
Some may stop at the salt box
To take a lick of salt as they pass.**

In the summer the cows are turned out to pasture to eat grass. The dairy farmer keeps a salt box in the pasture because cows need salt. Cows also need a lot of water. It is important in helping them to digest food and to make milk. Water also helps to keep the cow cool in the summer. She may drink as much as twenty gallons of water a day.

"Educational" coloring books for children, described as "factual story approved by The American Egg Board" and "factual story reviewed by The National Dairy Council and Milk Industry Foundation." Copyright 1975 and copr. 1976, Know-about Publications, Inc., Harrisburg, Pa.

The Story of a Steak

Before you have a steak (whether it's porterhouse or chopped), a cow has to have a calf. This is the story of one particular calf.

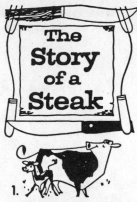

1. This calf was born on a Texas ranch. Several acres of grazing land are required to support each cow and calf.

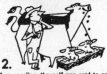

2. As a yearling, the calf was sold to an Iowa farmer for "finishing" in feed lot. Proper feeding of corn and protein supplements adds many extra pounds and a lot of extra eating quality to our beef.

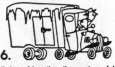

3. After several months in the feed lot, our calf, now a full-grown steer, was sent by rail or truck to the stockyards and consigned to a marketing firm for sale.

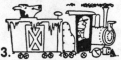

4. Buyers for several local and out-of-town meat packing companies put in bids based on the going consumer price of beef. This steer was one of a carload bought by an Ohio meat packing company.

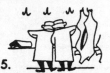

5. At the packing plant, the "beef crew" turned beef on the hoof into meat for the store. Beef was inspected, chilled and graded, prepared for shipment.

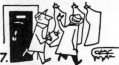

6. Under refrigeration, the quarters of beef were shipped to New York's wholesale meat district — 1500 miles from Texas, where the calf was born.

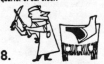

7. Owner of a Brooklyn meat market, after comparing prices and quality, selected a quarter of our steer.

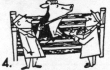

8. In the store, a quarter of beef was turned into steaks, roasts, stew and hamburger; was displayed for customer's selection competing with other meats.

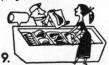

9. Yesterday, a housewife looked over everything in the counter, compared values, decided on steak, porterhouse or chopped, depending on what she wanted to spend.

From *The Story of Beef*
The American Meat
Institute (Chicago).

Proudly, the manager of the Beef Council of California announces:

"We have established ourselves as a responsible and unbiased source of information on beef and the beef industry."

It is amazing to me that the California Beef Council wants us to believe it is "unbiased," given that it is an organization whose sole purpose is to promote the sale of beef. I'd be very surprised, for example, if the Beef Council ever arranged for school children to take a field trip to a factory farm, or a slaughterhouse.

None of these "educational materials" allow a child to ever guess anything resembling the truth about how animals are kept today in the factory farms. Nor would they guess that chickens, pigs and cows are killed by human hands to provide meat. That meat is actually the flesh of an animal is a fact that is systematically overlooked. Words like "killed," or "slaughtered," are not used—words which, while hardly doing justice to the gruesomeness of the actual process, are at least accurate labels for what is done. Instead there appear euphemisms like "dispatched," "processed," "turned beef on the hoof into meat for the store," and "turn the pig into eating meat." Children are taught to overlook the fact that hamburger meat is ground-up cow.

McDonald's, the multi-national hamburger chain, has spent many millions of dollars on an advertising campaign targeted at youngsters that presents a rather unique version of reality. Obviously feeling that little things like the truth are unimportant when talking to children, they have produced a series of commercials in which a lovable clown named Ronald McDonald tells his impressionable young audience that hamburgers grow in hamburger patches.

(Incidentally, the man who played the part of Ronald McDonald, Jeff Juliano, has evidently discovered that hamburgers do not actually grow in hamburger patches. He is now a vegetarian.)

Most children love animals, and those who happen to learn the truth about meat are often abhorred. But they are usually "protected" from such a moment of truth. How can children see through the veil when their teacher passes out a booklet like "Hooray For The Hot Dog," distributed free to schools, as "nutritional education," by Oscar Mayer?

The picture children receive about meat is a sugar-coated lie, only it's not that innocent.

The Oscar Mayer meat company is very proud of its efforts to reach young school children. I remember the fun I had as a child when the Oscar Mayer "Wienermobile" came around. We had a great time and were given bits of sausage and bacon to eat after being entertained. With all the festivities, however, we had no idea we were being indoctrinated. I remember singing the company jingle which I had heard so many times on TV:

"Oh I wish I were an Oscar Mayer wiener,
For that is what I'd really like to be.
For if I were an Oscar Mayer wiener,
Everyone would be in love with me."

This theme song was, for many years, the heart of a campaign of national network television advertising aimed at America's youth. It was sung in the ads by a happy choir of children, and as a child hearing and singing along with the ditty, I, too, felt happy. Of course, I didn't have anything approaching the sophistication to question what was happening, so how could I have known this happy little song had within it an obscene lie? You see, the song produces in its young audience the belief that by eating Oscar Mayer wieners they are actually "loving" the animals who seem to be singing with eagerness to become wieners.

"If we believe absurdities, we shall commit atrocities."

(VOLTAIRE)

Today, Oscar Mayer distributes what they call "nutritional education" materials to schools throughout the country. These include an elaborate presentation of the "I Wish I Were An Oscar Mayer Wiener" song, complete with lyrics, musical notation, and chords. Their suggestion is that school children sing the song at a "march tempo."

In their more recent ads aimed at children, a band of happy youngsters are shown eating bologna and gaily singing, "My Bologna Has a

First Name." Again the effect is produced of delighted animals offering themselves to children as friendly things to eat.

The National Dairy Council distributes a 16 mm sound and color film to schools titled "Uncle Jim's Dairy Farm: A Summer Visit with Aunt Helen and Uncle Jim." It all sounds so sweet and wholesome. The picture children get of a modern dairy farm, however, is far indeed from the reality. It reminds me of a major advertising campaign for a dairy in which a human voice pretending to be a cow says "Us Cows Do Our Best For Jerseymaid." As if the cows were so touched by the loving way they are treated that their milk is a natural expression of their gratitude. In another ad, a deep male voice tells us that a particular company's milk comes from "contented cows." Maybe they are referring to the tranquilizers these most-placid-of-all-animals must sometimes be given.

ANY WAY YOU SLICE IT, IT'S STILL BOLOGNA

From our earliest years in this culture we've been taught a cotton candy version of what happens to food animals. We have been taught to repress the bloody truth. We've worn our blinders for so long that it is hard to see them for what they are, particularly when our parents most likely wore them as well, and the culture as a whole takes such repression completely for granted.

I have seen egg cartons with pictures of smiling hens. The message is that these birds are pleased as punch with the whole situation, and lend their blessings and radiant happiness to our consumption of their eggs. Frankly, I have to wonder how the chickens would feel about this—the real life-birds who are crammed into wire cages, their beaks cut off so they won't kill each other in their panic at being unable to express any of their natural urges.

In front of me right now is an advertisement from a local market which was dropped into my mail box this morning. It shows a cartoon drawing of a bull, winking at me with a big smile on his friendly face. Apparently he is an expert on beef, because he is shown playfully pointing with his tail to certain items of meat, happily beckoning me to try them. This and millions of other such advertisements hammer home the message over and over that bulls are delighted for us to eat bull flesh. I can't help but think that the correct term for this type of thing is "bull shit!"

I've seen ads and I'm sure you have too, in which animals are shown offering themselves to be eaten, virtually begging us to dine upon them. In one television commercial, cartoon hens, looking as happy and playful as the Rockettes, dance the can-can in a chorus line. What, you may wonder, are they so jubilant about? They're singing joyfully about how much we will enjoy their legs.

And how about those ads in which "Charlie the Tuna" is heartbroken because he has **not** been killed and made into canned tuna fish?

It's common in cookbooks to find "cute" little pictures next to the recipes. In one book, accompanying a Mexican chicken dish, there is a picture of a happy chicken lazing about in the sun with a big sombrero on his head. For a chicken-on-toast recipe, we see an enthusiastic chicken surfing on a piece of toast.

In each case, the message is that animals simply love being eaten by us, and are delighted to participate in the whole process.

People will pat their bellies after eating, and say "Yummy, that was a good chicken." But somehow I'm afraid the compliment is lost on the poor bird. You won't often hear someone say what they actually mean: "Yummy, I sure liked the taste of that dead chicken's body."

Only yesterday I was in a market which proudly proclaimed their chickens were "fresh." And here all along I had thought they were selling "dead" chickens. I suggested to the manager that he might be able to clear up any confusion on the matter in the minds of his clientele by changing the sign to read "freshly killed chickens," but he didn't seem overly grateful for my suggestion.

PIERCING THE VEIL

What, then, is it like for someone if, for a moment, he somehow manages to pierce through this veil of repression? Well, it can be downright shocking and can stir up a great deal of confusion and disturbance. Henry S. Salt gives us an account of his experience in his book *Seventy Years Among Savages*:

> *". . . and then I found myself realizing, with an amazement which time has not diminished, that the 'meat' which formed the staple of*

*our diet, and which I was accustomed to regard like bread or fruit,
or vegetables—as a mere commodity of the table—was in truth dead
flesh the actual flesh and blood of oxen, sheep, and swine, and other
animals that were slaughtered in vast numbers."* [4]

Another person recounts:

*"I was shocked speechless. I just sat there staring at my plate. It
was a* **God Damned Turkey** *I was eating! I couldn't believe it!
Those were its legs, right there in front of me, disguised by all the
cranberries and sauce! What did it have to be thankful for on this
great Thanksgiving Day?"*

The meat business depends on our repressing the unpleasant awareness that we are devouring dead bodies. Thus we have refined names
like "sweetbreads" for what really are the innards of baby lambs and
calves. We have names like "Rocky Mountain Oysters" for something
we might not find quite so appealing if we knew what they really
were—pig's testicles.

Our very language becomes an instrument of denial. When we
look at the body of a dead cow, we call it a "side of beef." When we
look at the body of a dead pig, we call it "ham," or "pork." We have
been systematically trained not to see anything from the point of view
of the animal, or even from a point of view which includes the animal's
existence.

In Alexandra Tolstoy's book, *Tolstoy: A Life of My Father*, she tells
of a time her aunt came to dinner, and her father chose to burst the
bubble of repression by which she kept herself isolated from the truth
about her diet:

*"Auntie was fond of food and when she was offered only a
vegetarian diet she was indignant, said she could not eat any old
filth and demanded that they give her meat, chicken. The next time
she came to dinner she was astonished to find a live chicken tied to
her chair and a large knife at her plate.
" 'What's this?' asked Auntie.*

" 'You wanted chicken,' Tolstoy replied, scarcely restraining his
laughter. 'No one of us is willing to kill it. Therefore we prepared
everything so that you could do it yourself.' "

Apparently, Auntie was appalled at the thought of killing the animal
she wished to eat. Like most of us, she did not enjoy being reminded
where meat actually comes from. Most of us are willing to eat the flesh
of animals, but dislike the sight of their blood, and prefer to think of
ourselves, not as killers, but as consumers.

It is all very simple.

1. The whole show is a charade. It is a game based on repression
and untruth.

2. Awareness is bad for the meat business.

3. Conscience is bad for the meat business.

4. Sensitivity to life is bad for the meat business.

5. **Denial, however, the meat business finds indispensable.**

THE GREAT AMERICAN STEAK RELIGION

As the sun dawns across North America every morning, the wave of
slaughter begins. Each day in the United States nine million chickens,
turkeys, pigs, calves and cows meet their deaths at human hands. In
the time it takes you to have your lunch, the number of animals killed
is equal to the entire population of San Francisco.

In our "civilized" society, the slaughter of innocent animals is not
only an accepted practice, it is an established ritual.

We do not usually see ourselves as members of a flesh-eating cult.
But all the signs of a cult are there. Many of us are afraid to even
consider other diet-style choices, afraid to leave the safety of the group,
afraid when there is any evidence that might reveal that the god of
animal protein isn't quite all it's cracked up to be. Members of the
Great American Steak Religion frequently become worried if their
family or friends show any signs of disenchantment. A mother may be
more worried if her son or daughter becomes a vegetarian than if they
take up smoking.

We are deeply conditioned in our attitudes towards meat. We have
been taught to believe that our very health depends on our eating it.

Many of us believe our social status depends on the quality of our meat and the frequency with which we eat it; and we take it for granted that only someone who "can't afford meat" would do without it. Males have been conditioned to associate meat with their masculinity, and quite a few men believe their sexual potency and virility depend on eating meat. Many women have been taught that a "good woman" feeds her man meat.

Our cultural conditioning tells us we must eat meat, and at the same time systematically overlooks the basic realities of meat production. We've been indoctrinated so thoroughly that it has become the ocean in which we swim. Our language is so disempowered by euphemisms and clichés, our shared experience so weakened by repression, our common sense so distorted by ignorance, that we can easily be held prisoner by a point of view beneath the threshold of our awareness.

THE TRUTH

It has often been said that if we had to kill the animals we eat, the number of vegetarians would rise astronomically. To keep us from thinking along such lines, the meat industry does everything it can to help us blank the matter out of our minds.

As a result, most of us know very little about slaughterhouses. If we think about them at all, we probably assume and hope that the animals enjoy a quick and painless death.

But such, regrettably, is not the case. The reality of the slaughterhouse, unfortunately, is as different from the images we tend to have of it as the reality of the factory farms is from the barnyard images most of us still carry.

But the men who actually do the killing for us know what it's like. They finish their shifts, punch the time clock, change out of their blood-splattered clothes, and go home. And something of the slaughterhouse goes home with them:

> *"Barely three months had passed since Yoineh Meir had become a slaughterer, but the time seemed to stretch endlessly. He felt as though he were immersed in blood and lymph. His ears were beset by the squawking of hens, the crowing of roosters, the gobbling of*

geese, the lowing of oxen, the mooing and bleating of calves and goats; wings fluttered, claws tapped on the floor. The bodies refused to know any justification or excuse—every body resisted in its own fashion, tried to escape, and seemed to argue with the Creator to its last breath." [5]

"Meat-packing plants," as slaughterhouses are euphemistically called, are not exactly the most pleasant of working environments. Just being surrounded by death and killing takes an incredible toll on a human being.

The turnover rate among slaughterhouse workers is the highest of any occupation in the country.[6] The Excel Corporation plant in Dodge City, Kansas, for example, had a turnover rate of 43% per month in 1980—the equivalent of a complete turnover of its entire 500 person work force every two and a half months.[7]

Slaughterhouses are particularly difficult to describe because we have been systematically taught not to think about them at all. You probably don't know where a single one is located, so whitewashed have been our minds to their existence. But I can tell you they are not places Walt Disney would want to make a movie about. One writer called them:

". . . infernos of nauseous smells, pools of blood, and screams of terrified animals."

Just about everybody finds the atmosphere of the slaughterhouse uncomfortable. Even the meat producers themselves don't exactly want to spend their vacations there. One meat producer described a typical meat-packing plant atmosphere:

"Earphone-type sound mufflers help mute the deadening cacaphony of high-pressure steam used for cleaning, the clanging of steel on steel as carcasses move down the slaughter line, the whine of the hide and tallow removers and the snarling of a chain saw used to split carcasses into sides of beef here on the killing-room floor.
  "The killing room . . . is filled with animals, minus their hooves, heads, tails and skins, which dangle down from an overhead

track and slowly snake their way past the various stations of the
various slaughterhouse workers like macabre pinatas . . .
   "The animals (have) their throats . . . slit, and then—with
tongues hanging limply out of their mouths—their bodies are
unceremoniously hooked behind the tendons of their rear legs and
are swung up into the air onto the overhead track, which moves
them through the killing room like bags of clothes on a dry cleaner's
motorized rack. Once bled, their hooves are clipped off with a
gigantic pair of hydraulic pincers. They are then beheaded, skinned
. . . and finally eviscerated." [8]

Amidst this carnage, workers in blood-spattered white coats and helmets are in constant motion, removing cattle legs with electric shears, skinning hides with whirring air knives, disemboweling animals with razor-bladed straight knives. The floors are slick with animal grease, and the air is thick with stench.

It is a terribly difficult atmosphere in which to work. According to U. S. Labor Department statistics, the rate of injury in meat-packing houses is the highest of any occupation in the nation. Every year, over 30% of packing-house workers suffer on-the-job injuries requiring medical attention.[9]

It's a few steps removed from anything you'd see at Disneyland.

WE DO IT ALL FOR YOU
But if the slaughterhouse environment is less than ideal for the workers, it falls even shorter of the mark for the billions of terrified veal calves, pigs, chickens and cows who find themselves there.

When they arrive at the slaughterhouse, they are most likely exhausted, sick, and starving. Most likely they were given little food, water, or any other care for their needs on the journey. And now they may not be fed upon arrival, because any food that would be given them would not have time to turn into marketable flesh.

I'm sure most of the workers do their best to be humane, under the circumstances. But these people are under great pressure, in a hurry, and stressed beyond their capacity by the nature of the environment in which they work. It's a tremendous drain on their inner resources to

take continually for granted the constant agonized cries of the animals
being killed. As a result, they often vent their frustrations the only
place they can, on the animals. The men whose job it is to move the
animals along are called "floggers," a term which accurately suggests
that their dealings with the animals are not always considerate. One
industry spokesman pointed his finger at the animals themselves for
the unpleasantries that often occur:

> *"Hogs . . . are slow-moving and considered obstinate. These*
> *characteristics often provoke a handler to the point of undue*
> *violence vented through the toe of a boot, closest club, or even a*
> *rock or piece of concrete."* [10]

The hogs are accused of "provoking" the violence by refusing to do
what is asked of them. But there is a reason the animals resist moving
along; they are, as all animals, more closely tuned in to their environment than man, and they profoundly sense the danger awaiting them.
The industry calls the animals "obstinate," but the truth is they are
terrified for their lives.

EMPTY WORDS
You may have assumed an effort is made in this day and age to spare
the animals unnecessary pain in the killing. That's what I assumed.
Unfortunately, I was wrong.

The Federal Humane Slaughter Act says, in part:

> *"It is therefore declared to be the policy of the United States that*
> *the slaughtering of livestock and the handling of livestock in*
> *connection with slaughter shall be carried out only by humane*
> *methods."*

This sounds lovely, but in practice the Act falls tragically short of
accomplishing its admirable aims. Technically, we now have the means
to render the animals unconscious before they are killed, which would
greatly reduce the pain they must undergo. But often this is not done.
Calves are frequently still butchered in full sight of their mothers.

Chickens are piled in crates on the floor with a bird's eye view of their brethren being butchered. The whole thing is handled with monstrous callousness, and total disregard for the animals' feelings.

The Federal Humane Slaughter Act sounds good, but in practice it is so riddled with loopholes as to be virtually meaningless. Less than 10% of the country's slaughterhouses are inspected for compliance with the Act, and only a very small percentage of even these few plants are under any legal obligation to observe its guidelines anyway. Furthermore, chickens, turkeys, ducks and geese are not considered animals by the Act, and so receive no protection, even in the few cases where the Act does apply.

The vast majority of slaughterhouses today may legally use any method they choose, and are under no obligation whatsoever to take the slightest concern for the animals. With profits being the sole motivation, the result, as you might expect, is not a happy one for these poor creatures.

The same attitudes which determine policies in factory farms govern decisions in slaughterhouses, and these are not attitudes of compassion for the animals. A leading poultry producer discussed the philosophy underlying his endeavors in the trade journal *Poultry World*:

> *"I am in this business for what I can make out of it. If it pays me to do this or that, I do it and so far as I am concerned that is all there is to say about it."* [11]

The industry chooses the cheapest possible methods of killing. They do not purposefully choose to be brutal and sadistic. It just works out that way.

The "captive-bolt pistol" is one of the most effective methods of stunning cow, pigs, and other animals unconscious prior to killing them. Unfortunately, however, the cost of the charges used to fire the thing is enough to deter many slaughterhouses from using it. You may wonder how much money is saved thus, at the cost of forcing the animal to be fully conscious when killed. I've become somewhat accustomed to the industry's callousness, but I was still stunned to learn that the savings amount to approximately a single penny an animal. [12]

WHEN KOSHER ISN'T KOSHER

Now you may think, when you hear a phrase like "ritual slaughter," or "kosher slaughter," that this refers to a better kind of killing. You may think, as I did, that the act is done with respect for the dignity of the animal, and concern that it suffer as little as possible. You may think, as I did, that kosher ways of slaughter are more compassionate than "ordinary" slaughterhouse deaths.

This was, doubtless, the original purpose at the time when this code of slaughter was conceived, and its standards probably produced the most humane and hygienic form of killing then available. But today, to kill the animals this way produces something far removed from the original intent of these laws.

Orthodox Jewish and Moslem dietary laws forbid consumption of meat from animals which are not "healthy and moving" when killed. Religious orthodoxy today interprets this to mean that kosher meat must come from animals who have not been stunned before being killed. They must be fully conscious when it's done. Further, in order to qualify for the kosher stamp of approval, the animal must have its throat slit in a particular way. The consequences of this interpretation of kosher slaughtering are a travesty for the poor creatures involved.

You see, the Pure Food and Drug Act of 1906 requires, for sanitary reasons, that no slaughtered animal may fall in the blood of a previously slaughtered animal. What this means, in practice, is that animals must be killed while suspended from a conveyer belt, rather than while lying on the floor. Stringing up an animal before delivering the final blow doesn't cause it any pain if it has already been rendered unconscious. But when an animal must be conscious when killed, as kosher regulations stipulate, and also must have its throat cut in the particular way kosher law requires, the animal is forced to undergo an enormous amount of extra pain:

> *"Animals being ritually slaughtered in the United States are shackled around a rear leg, hoisted into the air, and then hang, fully conscious, upside down on the conveyer belt for between two and five minutes—and occasionally much longer if something goes wrong on the 'killing line'—before the slaughterer makes his cut."* [13]

It is difficult for us to imagine what these poor animals must suffer. The cows are exhausted and terrified to begin with. A heavy iron chain is clamped around one of their rear legs, then they are jerked off their feet and hung upside down by a single leg. Now cows are by nature as peaceful a creature as you could ever hope to find, but this situation is too much for even these most mellow of animals. They are provoked into hysteria.

> *"The animal, upside down, with ruptured joints and often a broken leg, twists frantically in pain and terror, so that it must be gripped by the neck or have a clamp inserted in its nostrils to enable the slaughterer to kill the animal with a single stroke, as religious law prescribes."* [14]

In actual practice, kosher deaths have become a hideous perversion of the original intent of the dietary laws; the procedure adds incalculably to the agony they must suffer.

You may think that today, because relatively few people "eat kosher," only a very small percentage of animals would be "killed kosher". You may also think that even including the non-religious people who seek out kosher meat, mistakenly believing it to be better, this still wouldn't amount to a significant percentage. And finally you are probably quite sure that if you buy meat that isn't labeled kosher, you are certainly not consuming meat from animals killed in this fashion.

But, I'm sorry to say, you'd be wrong on each account.

You see, for meat to be passed as kosher by Orthodox Rabbis, it is not enough for the animal merely to have been conscious when killed and to have its throat slit in the required way. A kosher Jew is also forbidden to consume the blood of an animal, so the veins and arteries must be cut out of kosher meat. In many parts of a cow, however, removing the blood vessels is very costly, and so the meat packers have resolved this difficulty by removing the blood vessels only from those parts of the animal from which they can be cut out inexpensively. Thus, even though the whole animal was killed kosher, only these parts are then sold as kosher meat. In other words, there's a lot of meat left over. This means that a great deal of the meat in our supermarkets

and restaurants, while not labeled kosher, is in fact from animals
hoisted and slaughtered according to kosher regulations. One authority
states:

> *"It has been estimated that over 90% of the animals slaughtered in*
> *New Jersey—whose slaughterhouses supply New York City as well*
> *as their own state—are slaughtered by the ritual method."* [15]

Another report states:

> *"Although less than 5% of the flesh in the United States is bought*
> *kosher, as much as 50% of the animals are slaughtered as such."* [16]

There is a debate going on now among orthodox Jews as to whether to
allow animals killed by more humane methods to be considered as
kosher. In Sweden, at least, the Orthodox Rabbis have come to allow
animals to be stunned before slaughter. I like to think there is some
possibility that the American Rabbis will follow suit.

NO PICNIC

Though kosher procedures take the cake when it comes to cruelty,
even under the best of conditions slaughtering is no day at the beach.
In the past, much of the killing of animals was done at the farms where
the animals lived. The creatures were not starved, exhausted and disor-
iented from days of travel as they are today. They didn't have to smell
or listen to thousands of their fellow creatures being killed as they
waited their turn. And the people who did the job usually tried to
minimize the animals' pain. But, still, it was a disturbing thing to do.

> *"I never saw our farm manager more upset than the day we were*
> *getting ready to butcher five pigs. He shot one through the nose*
> *rather than through the brain. It ran screaming around the pen*
> *and he almost cried. It took two more bullets to finish the animal*
> *off, and this good man was shaking when he finished. 'I hate that,'*
> *he said to me. 'I hate to have them in pain. Pigs are so damned*
> *hard to kill clean.'"* [17]

The more I've seen of animals being killed, the more I've understood why McDonald's tells little children that hamburgers grow in little hamburger patches. And why the web of repression is so thick that otherwise intelligent people will say: "Don't tell me what happens to the animals. It will spoil my dinner."

The more I've learned about what goes on in slaughterhouses, the more I've understood why these places are deliberately kept from our sight, and why the workers are under strict instructions not to talk to the press. I can see why the meat industry spends so much money feeding our children a cotton candy story of meat.

Animals do not "give" their lives to us, as the sugar-coated lie would have it. No, we take their lives. They struggle and fight to the last breath, just as we would do if we were in their place. The friendly and intelligent pig whose life we take does not simply accept his death as a necessary step in the production of bacon. And he does not line up for his turn at the slaughterhouse singing about how happy he is to be on the way to becoming an Oscar Mayer wiener. Chickens do not approach the knife that will kill them wanting to dance and sing about how much we will enjoy eating their legs. The gentle and patient cow does not surrender docilely to the knife. She twists and bellows for all she's worth, even as she hangs upside down by a leg broken from the strain.

The poet Dylan Thomas once admonished us, "do not go gentle into that dark night." The animals whose lives we methodically take by the millions day in and day out would have understood his meaning. They do not go gently. They go kicking and screaming, bellowing their protest, fighting for their lives, and calling, to the last, to be saved. Calling for somebody, somewhere, to please hear them.

HEARING THEM
The people responsible for today's slaughterhouses do not find any of this disturbing. They are professionals. To them, the whole business is almost ordinary. They have become so locked into denial that they simply go about their work, which just happens to involve coldly butchering millions of innocent animals. Interviewing them, I've seen what Hannah Arendt saw when she probed the minds of the Nazis.

She called it the "banality of evil;" human beings matter-of-factly car-
rying out unspeakable cruelty, then going home and playing with their
children.

I asked one manager if the killing ever bothered him. "No," he
said. "Some of the new guys have problems, but I tell them this is the
way it's done. It's natural."

I did not particularly want to get into an argument with this man,
but neither could I let his remark slide by. So I gestured with my hand
towards the machinery and conveyer belts in the main room, and
shook my head sadly, as if to say, "God help us if this is natural."

"Do you have some kind of problem?" he asked none too kindly,
insinuating that if such were the case I was suffering from a significant
defect in character.

My heart felt heavy as I looked into the face of so much denial.
What could I say?

Later, I went out to my car and cried. My tears were not only for
the animals; they were for this poor man who had become such a
stranger to mercy.

BEYOND DENIAL

It is painful to break the shell of repression. It takes courage to see
what these poor animals endure. It is painful to see how calloused
human beings can become. It can be shattering to see that in our
ignorance we have eaten the products of such a system. It takes courage to keep our eyes open to such tragedy, and our hearts open to our
deepest human responses.

The feelings that arise when we learn what is being done to today's
animals are not signs of weakness. They are proof that there is still
hope for us, that we have not totally succumbed to psychic numbing.
In a culture that takes indifference and denial for granted, we may fear
that our distress at these developments bodes weakness, a signal that
we can't cope, evidence that we have a problem. But the distress we
feel at what is being done is real, valid, and healthy. It speaks of our
commitment to stopping this madness. It is a measure of our humanity.

The pain we feel is not ours alone. Many of us, conditioned to take
seriously only those feelings which pertain to our individual needs and

wants, may not realize that we can suffer on behalf of others. But we can, and we do. We suffer on behalf of the animals when we learn of their plight. We suffer on behalf of the people who in their blindness are the instruments of such cruelty. We suffer on behalf of a society that perpetuates such tragedy. And we suffer on behalf of life itself.

Our pain arises from our kinship with life. We hurt because we are not separate from animals, nor from the people who are the agents of such suffering. We hurt because these animals are our fellow mortals; and because the people administering such cruelty are our fellow human beings. We hurt because we are part, as they are, of the great web of life.

Our pain is not something to fear, for in the heart of our grief we can find our connection to each other, and our power to act. Our power lies in our connection to all life. Our power lies in our deepest human responses. Our power does not lie in looking the other way.

PART

T W O

*"Men dig their Graves with their own Teeth
and die more by those fated
Instruments than the Weapons of
their Enemies."*

-THOMAS MOFFETT
HELTH'S IMPROVEMENT,
1600 A.D.

148

DIFFERENT STROKES FOR DIFFERENT FOLKS

"Sit down before fact like a little child, and be prepared to give up every preconceived notion, follow humbly wherever and to whatever abyss Nature leads, or you shall learn nothing."

(T. H. HUXLEY)

THE WHOLE JUSTIFICATION for the factory farms and slaughter-houses, of course, is that we need their products for our health and happiness.

But do we really?

In the last few decades, there has been a revolution in medicine, a revolution that throws an extremely important light on the significance of our eating habits. As a result of the most exhaustive investigations in medical history of the health consequences of different diet-styles, scientists have now begun to understand for the first time the correlation between human food choices and human health. Very clear guidelines have finally emerged about the relative advantages and disadvantages of eating animal products.

Conventional wisdom has it that animal products constitute two of the four basic food groups, and are essential for human health. But the most rigorous, solid and careful nutritional research on the effects of diet-styles on human health points in a decidedly different direction.

Because the question of what might be the optimum diet is an emotionally charged one for many people, and because many of us have quite a significant emotional investment in believing our opinions and habits to be correct, I want to emphasize that what follows is not merely my own or anyone else's unfounded opinion. It is the result of the most conscientious research, as reported in established and reputable publications such as the *New England Journal of Medicine*, the *British Medical Journal*, the *Journal of the National Cancer Institute*, the *American Journal of Clinical Nutrition*, the *Journal of the American Medical Association*, the *Journal of Pediatrics*, the *Canadian Medical Association Journal*, the *Journal of Immunology*, the *American Journal of Digestive Diseases*, the British medical publication *Lancet*, and other sources of equal stature.

Of course there are many other factors influencing your health besides the food choices you make. Exercise and laughter are health-giving. Smoking and excessive drinking are not. Expressing your feelings is health-giving. Stifling and repressing them is not. And a positive attitude towards life might well be the most important of all.

To paraphrase Mark Braunstein: The person who eats beer and franks with cheer and thanks will probably be healthier than the person who eats sprouts and bread with doubts and dread.

This does not mean, however, that there are not sound nutritional guidelines to assist us in living full and joyful lives. Indeed the findings of modern nutritional scientific research point ever more strongly to the critical role nutrition plays in human welfare and happiness.

IS THERE A DOCTOR IN THE HOUSE?

You might think that your doctor would be a reliable guide to your optimum diet, and would convey to you any emerging truths of sound nutritional research that significantly affect your health. But actually, most doctors don't know very much about nutrition. You'd think they would, but they don't. That's not their department. They have been trained to treat disease with drugs and surgery. They have not been trained to prevent disease through healthy life and diet-styles.

Nutritional education is not just inadequate in contemporary medical schools; in most cases it's nonexistent. At the 69th annual meeting of the American Medical Women's Association, one doctor drew knowing laughs when she told the audience about her lack of nutritional training. Said Dr. Michelle Harrison:

"They had one lecture—on a Saturday morning—and it wasn't compulsory. I don't remember what was in the lecture, because I didn't go."

Only 30 of the nation's 125 medical schools have a single required course in nutrition.[9] A recent Senate investigation revealed that the average physician in the United States received less than **three hours of training in nutrition during four years of medical school.**[10] And few doctors have time for personal research:

"The job of the practicing physician is far from easy. He is constantly being faced with situations in which he must make immediate decisions on the basis of too little evidence. He has neither the leisure nor the facilities to base his diagnoses and prescriptions on his own research. To be effective at all, he must rely on those standards, precepts and procedures that he has been so carefully taught."[11]

Since what today's doctors have been taught makes virtually no mention of the role of nutrition in building health and preventing disease, they can hardly be blamed for not relaying the emerging truths of nutritional research to their waiting patients. Instead, says Roger Williams, doctors are trained to:

". . . wait until deformed and mentally retarded babies are born, then give them loving attention; wait until heart attacks come, then, if the patient is still alive, give him or her the best care possible; wait until mental disease strikes, and give considerate treatment; wait until alcoholism strikes, then turn to the task of rehabilitation; wait until cancer growth becomes apparent, then try to cut it out or burn it out with suitable radiation."[12]

Thirty years ago, when many doctors smoked cigarettes themselves, it would have been pretty hard to elicit sound advice from them on the health consequences of smoking. Many doctors, in fact, recommended smoking to non-smokers, as a way of dealing with social nervousness.

It wasn't that these doctors were evil people, or lackeys for the tobacco industry. It was, rather, that they hadn't been told anything in medical school about the relationship between smoking and major health problems. They lived in the same culture as everyone else, in which smoking was seen as totally legitimate. They saw the same advertisements as everyone else, which sold people on the pleasures and social advantages of smoking. In fact, a famous Camel cigarette commercial loudly trumpeted: "More Doctors Smoke Camels Than Any Other Cigarette," and made a point of linking good healthcare with smoking their brand of cigarette.

Today, a similar situation exists with respect to the health consequences of a meat habit. Today's physician is exposed to the same propaganda promoting meat and dairy product consumption as the rest of us, and he hasn't the nutritional training that would enable him to evaluate these messages any more intelligently than we can. Furthermore, the meat, egg, and dairy industries are particularly keen on "educating" doctors with their biased views of nutrition. The Meat Board, for example, has presented a series of extremely expensive full page color adds in the *Journal of the American Medical Association*,[13] presenting a nutritional slant that one nutritional authority, Dr. Kenneth Buckley, did not find at all impressive. He called it:

"... *slick and deceitful propaganda, coloring and twisting the facts in the most manipulative way.*"[14]

The very presence of these expensive ads in medical journals shows that the meat industry knows it must now fight for the loyalty of a medical profession whose allegiance it once took for granted.

Not so very long ago ads like this would have been unnecessary. Everybody "knew" meat was a healthy food to eat. But 25 years ago everybody "knew" cigarette smoking was harmless.

THREE MILLION HUMAN GUINEA PIGS
The first suspicion by the larger scientific community that traditional assumptions about meat were open to serious doubt came after World War I. At that time, the allied blockade cut Denmark off from all

imports. The Danish government, dreading the possibility of severe food shortages, appointed Dr. Mikkel Hindhede to develop and coordinate a rationing program for the country. Dr. Hindhede's response, which he later reported in the *Journal of the American Medical Association*, was to stop feeding the nation's grain to livestock in order to provide meat, and instead to feed the grain directly to the people.[15] It was a mass experiment in vegetarianism, with over three million subjects.

Scientists were flabbergasted at the results. When they calculated the death rate in Copenhagen from October 1917 to October 1918, the period when food restrictions were the most severe, they found that the overall mortality rate from disease was by far the lowest in recorded history, It was, in fact, a drop of over 34% from the average for the preceding 18 years![16]

It was hard to avoid considering the possibility that there might be a connection between the nation's vegetarian diet, and the greatly-lowered death rate.

Scientists thinking along these lines received more "food for thought" from the Second World War. At that time, Norway was occupied by the Germans, and the Norwegian government was forced to reduce sharply, and in many cases completely eliminate, the availability of meat to its citizens. Once again, scientists were amazed by the results. The death rate from circulatory diseases dropped dramatically. After the war the Norwegians returned to their former diet, and, sure enough, their death rate rose accordingly. Throughout these changing times the correlation between animal fat consumption and deaths from circulatory diseases bordered on true mathematical precision.[17] (See figure on page 153.)

Researchers who stumbled across this correlation wondered if it were a coincidence. So they looked at other countries. They knew that the consumption of meat and other animal products had also been cut significantly in Britain and Switzerland during World War II. Now they found that in these countries there had also been significant improvements in health. In Britain, infant and post-natal deaths dropped to their lowest rate ever, and instances of anemia dropped markedly. Children's growth rates and dental health were demonstrably better

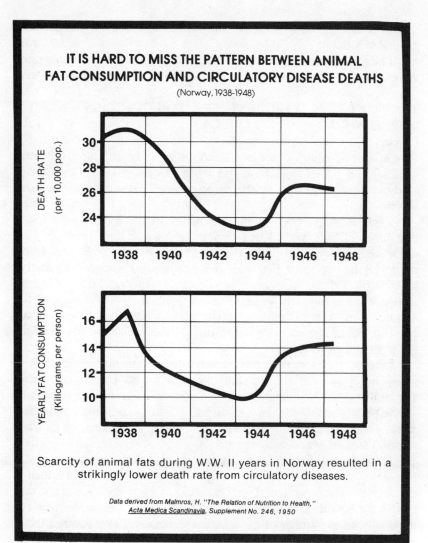

IT IS HARD TO MISS THE PATTERN BETWEEN ANIMAL FAT CONSUMPTION AND CIRCULATORY DISEASE DEATHS

(Norway, 1938-1948)

Scarcity of animal fats during W.W. II years in Norway resulted in a strikingly lower death rate from circulatory diseases.

Data derived from Malmros, H. "The Relation of Nutrition to Health,"
Acta Medica Scandinavia, Supplement No. 246, 1950

than ever before, and there were many other signs of greatly improved general health. [18]

The possibility that a vegetarian diet might have something to recommend it was becoming increasingly difficult to dismiss.

THE LOWEST AND HIGHEST LIFE EXPECTANCIES IN THE WORLD

Of course, medical researchers knew these wartime "experiments in vegetarianism" didn't constitute scientific proof of anything. But the results were indeed suggestive and many researchers were moved to study comprehensively the effects of different diet-styles on human health.

This had never really been done before in anything like the scale that occurred after World War II. For 99.999% of history, mankind has eaten whatever it could find, or grow, or kill, or raise. Issues of what might be the optimum diet, and what the health consequences might be of various diets, were never studied in any depth. Such thoughts were a luxury to which we had not yet attained.

But after World War II, scientists began for the first time to compile comprehensive statistics correlating the diet-styles and health of all the populations in the world.

One fact that emerged consistently was the strong correlation between heavy flesh-eating and short life expectancy. The Eskimos, the Laplanders, the Greenlanders, and the Russian Kurgi tribes stood out as the populations with the highest animal flesh consumption in the world—and also as among the populations with the lowest life expectancies, often only about 30 years.[19]

It was found, further, that this was not due to the severity of their climates alone. Other peoples, living in harsh conditions, but subsisting with little or no animal flesh, had some of the highest life expectancies in the world. World health statistics found, for example, that an unusually large number of the Russian Caucasians, the Yucatan Indians, the East Indian Todas and the Pakistan Hunzakuts have life expectancies of 90 to 100 years.[20]

The United States has the most sophisticated medical technology in the world, and one of the most temperate of climates. One of the highest consumers of meat and animal products in the world, it also has one of the lowest life expectancies of industrialized nations.

The cultures with the very longest life spans in the world are the Vilcambas, who reside in the Andes of Ecuador, the Abkhasians, who live on the Black Sea in the USSR, and the Hunzas, who live in the Himalayas of Northern Pakistan.[21] Researchers discovered a "striking similarity" in the diets of these groups, scattered though they are in different parts of the planet. All three are either totally vegetarian or close to it.[22] The Hunzas, who are the largest of the three groups, eat almost no animal products. Meat and dairy products combined account for only 1 1/2% of their total calories.[23]

Particularly striking to researchers who have visited these cultures is that the people not only live so long, but that they enjoy full, active lives throughout their many years, and show no signs of the many degenerative diseases that afflict the elderly in our culture.

> *"They work and play at 80 and beyond; most of those who reach their 100th birthday continue to be active, and retirement is unheard of. The absence of (excess protein) in their diets engenders slower growth and slim, compact body frames. With age, wisdom accumulates, but physical degeneration is limited so the senior citizens of these remote societies have something unique to contribute to the lives of others. They are revered."*[24]

ONE OF THE WORLD'S GREATEST LABOR-SAVING DEVICES

Ignoring the growing weight of worldwide evidence to the contrary, the Beef Council tells us in massive multi-million dollar advertising campaigns that "beef gives strength." But since I have seen the results of rigorous scientific research on the subject, I can't help but be reminded of Laurence Peter's wonderful remark:

> *"Prejudice is one of the world's greatest labor-saving devices; it enables you to form an opinion without having to dig up the facts."*

It is not, of course, a coincidence that the Beef Council and other meat promoters have fostered the common prejudice that meat-eating brings

strength. The meat industry profits in direct proportion to the degree
this idea flourishes. As a result, it has conscientiously spent millions of
dollars to get us to believe that if we are so foolhardy as to "risk" not
eating meat, then we are well on our way to ending up looking like the
starving masses of India.

So widely held is the prejudice that meat-eaters as a group are
stronger and more fit than vegetarians, that this proposition is not
generally recognized for what it is. But then again, prejudices have a
way of seeming like truth when enough people agree upon them.

The belief that vegetarians are risking their health by not eating
meat is deeply ingrained in our collective psyche. It's as if each would-
be vegetarian, as he or she considers or begins to embark upon the
adventure, must listen to an incessant droning in the back of the
mind—"meat gives strength, you are weakening yourself, meat gives
strength, you are weakening yourself . . ."

Even long-standing and well informed vegetarians are not immune
from the force of this collective thought-form, and can become prickly,
snobby and defensive in the face of the prevailing cultural assumptions. They may feel they are in a constant battle to justify their diet
style against the of assumptions of this collective agreement even when
they are not spoken aloud. It can be like a nagging and constant under-
tow, pulling in a different direction from which they are going, and
against which they feel they must defend themselves.

But what happens if we consult the scientific studies that have not
relied on "the labor-saving device" of prejudice, but have actually
worked to dig up the facts of the matter?

Numerous studies, published in the most reputable scientific and
medical journals, have compared the strength and stamina of people
eating different diet-styles. According to these studies, all of them rigorous, the common prejudice that meat gives strength and endurance,
though plastered on thousands of billboards, and drummed into us
since childhood, has absolutely no foundation in fact.

THE LAB RESULTS SPEAK
At Yale, Professor Irving Fisher designed a series of tests to compare
the stamina and strength of meat-eaters against that of vegetarians. He

selected men from three groups: meat-eating athletes, vegetarian athletes, and vegetarian sedentary subjects. Fisher reported the results of his study in the *Yale Medical Journal*.[25] His findings do not seem to lend a great deal of credibility to the popular prejudices that hold meat to be a builder of strength.

> *"Of the three groups compared, the . . . flesh-eaters showed far less endurance than the abstainers (vegetarians), even when the latter were leading a sedentary life."*[26]

Overall, the average score of the vegetarians was over double the average score of the meat-eaters, even though half of the vegetarians were sedentary people, while all of the meat-eaters tested were athletes. After analyzing all the factors that might have been involved in the results, Fisher concluded that:

> *". . . the difference in endurance between the flesh-eaters and the abstainers (was due) entirely to the difference in their diet . . . There is strong evidence that a . . . non-flesh . . . diet is conducive to endurance."*[27]

A comparable study was done by Dr. J. Ioteyko of the Academie de Medicine of Paris.[28] Dr. Ioteyko compared the endurance of vegetarians and meat-eaters from all walks of life in a variety of tests. The vegetarians averaged two to three times more stamina than the meat-eaters. Even more remarkably, they took only one-fifth the time to recover from exhaustion compared to their meat-eating rivals.

In 1968, a Danish team of researchers tested a group of men on a variety of diets, using a stationary bicycle to measure their strength and endurance. The men were fed a mixed diet of meat and vegetables for a period of time, and then tested on the bicycle. The average time they could pedal before muscle failure was 114 minutes. These same men at a later date were fed a diet high in meat, milk and eggs for a similar period and then re-tested on the bicycles. On the high meat diet, their pedaling time before muscle failure dropped dramatically—to an average of only 57 minutes. Later, these same men were switched to a strictly vegetarian diet, composed of grains, vegetables and fruits, and then tested on the bicycles. The lack of animal products didn't seem to hurt their performance—they peddled an average of 167 minutes.[29]

Wherever and whenever tests of this nature have been done, the results have been similar. This does not lend a lot of support to the supposed association of meat with strength and stamina.

Doctors in Belgium systematically compared the number of times vegetarians and meat-eaters could squeeze a grip-meter. The vegetarians won handily with an average of 69, whilst the meat-eaters averaged only 38. As in all other studies which have measured muscle recovery time, here, too, the vegetarians bounced back from fatigue far more rapidly than did the meat-eaters.[30]

I know of many other studies in the medical literature which report similar findings. But I know of not a single one that has arrived at different results. As a result, I confess, it has gotten rather difficult for me to listen seriously to the meat industry proudly proclaiming "meat gives strength" in the face of overwhelming evidence to the contrary.

WORLD RECORDS
On the athletic field, as in the laboratory, the endurance and accomplishments of vegetarians makes me question whether we need animal products for fitness. The achievements of vegetarian athletes are particularly noteworthy considering the relatively small percentage of vegetarian entrants. Athletes after all, are not immune from the cultural conditioning that meat alone gives the required strength and stamina. Yet some have adopted vegetarian diets and the results invite scrutiny.

Dave Scott, of Davis, California is a scholar-athlete who is well acquainted with the scientific literature on diet and health. He is also universally recognized as the greatest triathlete in the world. He has won Hawaii's legendary Ironman Triathlon a record four times, including three years in a row, while no one else has ever won it more than once. In three successive years, Dave has broken his own world's record for the event, which consists, in succession, of a 2.4 mile ocean swim, a 112 mile cycle, and then a 26.2 mile run. Dave's college major was exercise physiology, and he says he keeps up on the latest developments in the field by reading "an incredible amount" of books and journals. He calls the idea that people, and especially athletes, need animal protein a "ridiculous fallacy." There are many people who consider Dave Scott the fittest man who ever lived. Dave Scott is a vegetarian.

I don't know how you might determine the world's fittest man. But if it isn't Dave Scott it might well be Sixto Linares. This remarkable fellow tells of the time:

> ". . . when I became a vegetarian in high school, my parents were very very upset that I wouldn't eat meat . . . After fourteen years, they are finally accepting that it's good for me. They know it's not going to kill me."

During the fourteen years that Sixto's parents begrudgingly came to accept that his diet wasn't killing him, they watched their son set the world's record for the longest single day triathlon, and display his astounding endurance, speed and strength in benefits for the American Heart Association, United Way, the Special Children's Charity, the Leukemia Society of America, and the Muscular Dystrophy Association. So deeply ingrained, however, is the prejudice against vegetarianism that even as their son was showing himself possibly to be the fittest human being alive, his parents only reluctantly came to accept his diet. Sixto says he experimented for awhile with a lacto-ovo vegetarian diet (no meat, but some dairy products and eggs), but now eats no eggs or dairy products and feels better for it.

It doesn't seem to be weakening him too much. In June, 1985, at a benefit for the Muscular Dystrophy Association, Sixto broke the world record for the one day triathlon by swimming 4.8 miles, cycling 185 miles, and then running 52.4 miles.

Robert Sweetgall, of Newark, Delaware, is another fellow who doesn't just sit around all day. He is the world's premier ultra-distance walker. In the last three years, Robert has walked a distance greater than the 24,900 mile equatorial circumference of the earth. He says he is a:

> ". . . vegetarian for moral reasons; there's enough food on earth for us not to have to kill animals to eat."

Though not chosen for its health value alone, Sweetgall's vegetarian diet doesn't seem to put him at too much of a disadvantage. After walking a 10,600 mile perimeter around the United States, he set out on a loop that would take him, via about 20 million footsteps, through parts of all 50 states within the next year.

Then there is Edwin Moses. No man in sports history has ever dominated an event as Edwin Moses has dominated the 400 meter hurdles. The Olympic Gold Medalist went eight years without losing a race, and when *Sports Illustrate* gave him their 1984 "Sportsman of the Year" award, the magazine said:

"No athlete in any sport is so respected by his peers as Moses is in track and field."

Edwin Moses is a vegetarian.

Paavo Nurmi, the "Flying Finn," set twenty world records in distance running, and won nine Olympic medals. He was a vegetarian.

Bill Pickering of Great Britain set the world record for swimming the English Channel, but that performance of his pales beside the fact that at the age of 48 he set a new world record for swimming the Bristol Channel. Bill Pickering is a vegetarian.

Murray Rose was only 17 when he won three gold medals in the 1956 Olympic Games in Melbourne, Australia. Four years later, at the 1960 Olympiad, he became the first man in history to retain his 400 meter freestyle title, and he later broke both his 400 meter and 1500 meter freestyle world records. Considered by many to be the greatest swimmer of all time, Rose has been a vegetarian since he was two.

You might not expect to find a vegetarian in world championship body-building competitions. But Andreas Cahling, the Swedish body builder who won the 1980 Mr. International title, is a vegetarian, and has been for over ten years of highest level international competition. One magazine reported that Cahling's:

". . . showings at the 'Mr. Universe' competitions, and at the professional body-building world championships, give insiders the feeling he may be the next Arnold Schwarzenegger."

Another fellow who is not exactly a weakling is Stan Price. He holds the world record for the bench press in his weight class. Stan Price is a vegetarian. Roy Hilligan is another gentlemen in whose face you probably wouldn't want to kick sand. Among his many titles is the coveted "Mr. America" crown. Roy Hilligan is a vegetarian.

Pierreo Verot holds the world's record for downhill endurance skiing. He is a vegetarian.

Estelle Gray and Cheryl Marek hold the world's record for cross-country tandem cycling. They are complete vegetarians, not even consuming eggs or dairy products.

The world's record for distance butterfly stroke swimming is held jointly by James and Jonathan deDonato. They are both vegetarians.

If you wanted to be an evangelist for the "meat gives strength" cult, and were looking for a 97-pound vegetarian weakling to pick on, you'd probably be better off staying away from Ridgely Abele. He recently won the United States Karate Association World Championship, taking both the Master Division Title for fifth degree black belt, and the overall Grand Championship. Abele, who has won eight national championships, is a complete vegetarian, who eats no meat, eggs, or dairy products.

The list goes on and on. Toronto, Canada, is the home of a national fitness institute that tests all the top athletes in that country. For a number of years tennis pro Peter Burwash consistently ranked between 50th and 60th. Then as an experiment, he switched to a vegetarian diet, though he thought at the time that vegetarians were emaciated, unhealthy creatures. Now, however, he knows better. One year after making the switch, Peter Burwash was tested at the institute and found to have the highest fitness index of any athlete in any sport in the entire country of Canada.

Another man you might have a hard time convincing that a meat diet-style yields superior physical performance is Marine Captain Alan Jones of Quantico, Virginia. I would never have believed that one could be a vegetarian Marine, but Jones is managing to do it, and his health doesn't seem to be suffering too much for his efforts.

Although crippled by polio when he was five years old, Jones is another candidate for world's fittest man and has amassed a record of physical accomplishments unmatched by any human being that ever lived. Not only does he hold the world record for continuous situps (17,003), but in one particular 15-month period he accomplished possibly the most remarkably array of physical achievements ever attained by a human being:

September, 1974—Lifted a 75-pound barbell over his head 1,600 times in 19 hours
February, 1975—Made 3,802 basketball free throws in 12 hours, including 96 out of 100
June, 1975—Swam 500 miles in 11 days through the Snake and Columbia Rivers, from Lewiston, Idaho to the Pacific Ocean
September, 1975—Skipped rope 43,000 times in five hours
October, 1975—Skipped rope 100,000 times in 23 hours
November, 1975—Swam over 68 miles in the University of Oregon swimming pool, without a sleeping break
December, 1975—Swam one-half mile in 32° F (0° C) water, without a wet suit, in the Missouri River near Sioux City, Iowa
January, 1976—Performed 51,000 sit-ups in 76 hours

Meanwhile, across the Pacific Ocean, the Japanese are every bit as serious and fanatic about baseball as are Americans. So, in October 1981, when Tatsuro Hirooka took over as manager of a professional team who had finished in last place the previous season, he knew some changes had to be made. But the changes he made were not the ones most of us would expect. He told the players on the Siebu Lions that meat and other animal foods increase athletes' susceptibility to injury, and decrease their ability to perform. Therefore, said the new manager, like it or not, they were all going on a vegetarian diet.

The Lions took quite a ribbing during the 1982 season. One rival manager sneered they were "only eating weeds," and made some rather derogatory remarks about their masculinity. But the sneerer had to eat his words when the Lions beat his team for the Pacific League Championship, and then went on to defeat the Chunichi Dragons in the equivalent of our World Series. Lest anyone think this was a fluke, the vegetarian Lions came back the next year, and once again trounced the opposition, winning again both the League and National Championship.

Please note that I have not provided this listing of athletic accomplishments of some vegetarians because I think this in itself proves the vegetarian diet superior. It doesn't. It proves only that for these given individuals, with their specific biochemical individualities, a vegetarian diet worked superbly at a particular time.

But when we couple the experiences of Dave Scott, Edwin Moses, Murray Rose, Alan Jones and all the rest, with the data from systematic laboratory research published in reputable scientific journals, then, perhaps, we might have serious grounds to doubt the widely held prejudice that assumes greater weakness as an inevitable consequence of a vegetarian diet.

A SELF-FULFILLING PROPHECY

Although studies show that a vast majority (over 95%) of former meat-eaters report that a switch to a vegetarian diet increases their energy, vitality, and overall feeling of well-being, there are a few exceptions. Some don't. How are we to account for people who report experiencing greater strength when eating meat? Might these cases show there is something to the "meat gives strength" view after all?

First off, assessing the health consequences of any diet, we must not forget the principle of biochemical individuality. We have different concentrations of gastric juices; our stomachs are shaped and function differently; we metabolize our food according to patterns which are unique to each of us; our digestive processes are as individualized as snowflakes. So, when someone tells me he or she feels better as a meat-eater, I take that seriously.

One possible explanation is that they have made the switch away from meat too abruptly for their particular systems, and not allowed enough time for the adjustment. Different people require different transition times. Some can go "cold turkey," and get along fine. Others gradually have to shed red meat, then chicken, and work their way along slowly.

Another possibility is that the people who report they feel better with meat in their diet have been eating a nutritionally inadequate vegetarian diet. There are many kinds of vegetarian diets. Some are excellent, but others leave plenty to be desired. Just because a diet is vegetarian doesn't guarantee that it's healthier. Vegetarian diets that include too many "empty calories" (calories which supply no nutrients) can be nutritionally deficient. Such foods as white flour products, sugar, refined and processed foods, alcohol, and foods high in fat, fill us up and may give us something to burn temporarily, but give us little nurturance. Fruit Loops, Twinkies and Coca-Cola are all vegetarian foods, but they don't provide anyone, no matter what his biochemical individuality, with what he needs to be healthy. Some people will show the deficiency sooner than others, but empty calories will eventually take their toll on everyone.

There is yet another little-known but significant way for a vegetarian diet to fall short nutritionally, producing a craving for meat and a sense of strength when it is eaten. Surprisingly, if you consume too many dairy products, be they in the form of milk, cheese, yogurt, butter, ice cream, or whatever, there is a real possibility of iron deficiency. The best sources of iron are most vegetables. Calorie for calorie, kale has 14 times as much iron as a typical sirloin steak. Furthermore, vitamin C in fresh fruits and vegetables greatly increases the body's ability to absorb and utilize iron.[31] But if you consume a lot of dairy products when you give up meat (perhaps haunted by the nagging cultural fear—"are you getting enough protein?"), then the dairy products tend to crowd out some of the needed grains, vegetables and fruits from your diet. Cow's milk is so low in iron that you'd have to drink 50 gallons to get the iron available from a single bowl of spinach (See Figure, page 165.)

There is another important reason why you can become iron deficient if you overdo milk products. They not only provide no iron, they also block its absorption. Breast fed babies, for example, have a much higher rate of iron absorption than those fed cow's formulas, even if the formulas are especially fortified with extra iron.[32]

Although they do not provide as much iron as many vegetables, most meats do provide some. And meats are the iron sources most of us depended on as we grew up. Consequently, iron-deficient vegetarians may well feel an attraction to meat—the well-remembered source of iron—and feel better when they eat it.

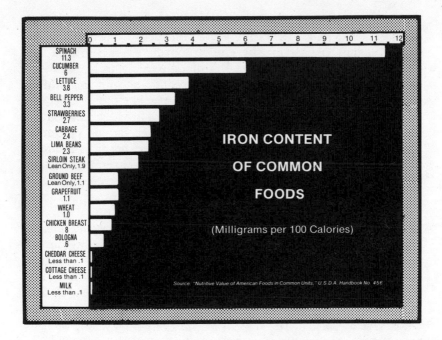

IRON CONTENT

OF COMMON

FOODS

(Milligrams per 100 Calories)

Source: "Nutritive Value of American Foods in Common Units," U.S.D.A. Handbook No. 456

SPINACH 11.3
CUCUMBER 6
LETTUCE 3.8
BELL PEPPER 3.3
STRAWBERRIES 2.7
CABBAGE 2.4
LIMA BEANS 2.3
SIRLOIN STEAK Lean Only, 1.9
GROUND BEEF Lean Only, 1.1
GRAPEFRUIT 1.1
WHEAT 1.0
CHICKEN BREAST 8
BOLOGNA .6
CHEDDAR CHEESE Less than .1
COTTAGE CHEESE Less than .1
MILK Less than .1

Such people are not very likely to consider that the source of the problem might be the over-consumption of dairy products. They don't know the "nutritional education" materials used in the school systems of the United States—the ones telling us to "drink three glasses of milk a day," urging us to drink lots of milk "for your health's sake," and humbly calling milk "nature's most perfect food"—were provided to the schools by the National Dairy Council.

Vegetarians who have therefore become convinced that only animal products provide strength sometimes consume more dairy products than their particular biochemical individualities can handle. As a result they do in fact end up weakened and desirous of meat. Should they then replace some of the dairy with meat they may well feel stronger, since they will be adding more iron to their potentially deficient system. Ironically, their belief in the strength-giving attribute of meat has now become a self-fulfilling prophecy.

For many people, almost any dairy products can be too much. At about the age of four, a surprisingly large percentage of people begin to lose the ability to digest lactose, the carbohydrate found in milk, because they no longer synthesize the digestive enzyme lactase. This condition, known as lactose intolerance, results in symptoms of diarrhea, gas, and stomach cramps. Different people have different degrees of lactose intolerance, but it is especially high in adult Blacks and Asians, occurring in as many as 90% of these genetic populations. If lactose-intolerant individuals switch to a vegetarian diet and try to substitute dairy products for meat, they may not understand that it is the added dairy products, not the lack of meat, causing the problems.

THE POWER OF BELIEF

Alexander Pope once said, "All looks yellow to the jaundiced eye." He was referring, of course, to the power of prejudice to color our perceptions of reality.

> *"In Rhodesia, a white truck driver passed a group of idle natives and muttered, 'They're lazy brutes!' A few hours later he saw natives heaving 200-pound sacks of grain onto a truck, singing in rhythm to their work. 'Savages!' he grumbled. 'What do you expect?' "*

(GORDON ALLPORT)

Recent medical history provides a particularly striking example of how potently an erroneous belief can color people's experience. Surgeons tend to look for surgical answers to disease; it's how they make their living. And sometimes, in their zeal to provide new surgical procedures, they may employ new techniques a bit prematurely, before determining, through appropriate experimentation, just exactly what value or lack of value the new techniques may have.

In the early 1950's, physicians were hard pressed to come up with an effective treatment for the pains of angina pectoris.[33] But then surgeons hit on a surgical procedure which they thought might solve the problem. The surgery consisted of opening the chest and tying off the internal mammary artery, which supplies blood to the muscles of the inner chest wall. A branch of this vessel brings blood to the pericardum, the sac enclosing the heart. Theoretically, it was supposed that tying off the artery below the branch might increase the blood flow to the heart. (The chest walls, it was known, could find alternative supplies.) And, in fact, a large number of patients who underwent this surgery reported a decrease of angina pain after recovering from the severe trauma of the operation.

The surgeons thought they had come up with a dandy of an operation, and it became the fashionable treatment for angina. However, in 1960, there appeared in the *American Journal of Cardiology* a remarkable report that shed a completely different light on the reasons why angina sufferers who underwent the surgery experienced decreased pain.[34] It seems that a number of surgeons, aware that this particular procedure had never been adequately tested, and also aware that angina is notoriously responsive to placebo treatment, had begun to consider the possibility that the patients experienced a decrease in pain only because they "believed" in the surgery—in other words, that this major operation was, in fact, totally worthless.

Doctors have known for centuries of the "placebo effect." You can give patients pills specifically designed to be devoid of any conceivable medical efficacy, and some of these patients, because they believe they are receiving substances with genuine medical value, will report improvement. Now doctors were beginning to consider the staggering possibility that the reported benefits from the angina surgery were the result of a placebo effect.

How were they to find out? It's relatively easy to test pills for a placebo effect. You simply do a double-blind study, giving some patients the "real thing," others placebos, and see what happens. But it's not so easy to put surgery to the test. The ethics of performing sham surgical operations are sticky, to say the least. In this case, however, the doctors were sure enough of their hunch that they did, in fact, eventually perform a number of sham, or placebo, operations. They then reported the results in the *American Journal of Cardiology*.[35]

Amazingly, the patients who underwent the sham surgery reported the same degree of angina relief as those undergoing the "real" surgery!

The verdict was unavoidable. The fashionable operation had derived its efficacy entirely from the placebo effect.

Surgeons now realized that this operation was no longer ethically justifiable. But they were not so easily to be deprived of a chance to operate on angina sufferers. They conceived an even more intrusive procedure—internal mammary artery implant. This involved poking a hole in the heart muscle, cutting the artery, and then inserting the cut end of the artery into the heart, hoping it would sprout new branches, thus supplementing the coronary arteries and bringing more blood to the heart. Again patients who underwent the surgery reported decreases in angina pain after recovering from the surgical trauma, and again the surgeons trumpeted their success.

No one ever put this procedure to the test of comparison with sham surgery. However, autopsies later done on patients who received this surgery showed that the implanted arteries had not sprouted new branches, nor provided any new blood supplies to the heart, as had been hoped. In short, any success this massive intervention had was due, again, to the placebo response.

So great had been the faith of the patients in surgery as a healing modality, that even though they underwent traumatic surgery that was in fact physically worthless, many of them reported symptomatic relief.

It seems we haven't even begun to scratch the surface of understanding how profound and powerful a thing faith is.

Is it any wonder, then, given the "faith" we have all been continuously programmed to have in meat, that some people report they feel better when meat is part of their diet? To me, given the extent of our meat habit programming, the amazing thing is that such a great majority of meat-eaters who switch to a vegetarian diet-style actually report more energy, greater vitality, new feelings of lightness and ease in their bodies, and increased well-being. When I see the very high percentage of former meat-eaters who are delighted with the switch in diet-style, in spite of massive cultural conditioning to the contrary, I have to wonder whether those who report they feel stronger eating meat might possibly be a bit more under the influence of the prevailing cultural assumptions than they realize.

That would be understandable. Prejudices are hard to uproot when they are not recognized as such, and even more so when they are still being repeatedly reinforced within the culture at large.

But what would happen if we were simply to **consider the possibility** that our longstanding belief in meat as the best dietary source of health and fitness might not be the whole story?

Perhaps then it would be time for a new journey to begin.

THE RISE AND FALL OF THE PROTEIN EMPIRE

> *"Think of the fierce energy concentrated in an acorn! You bury it in the ground, and it explodes into a giant oak! Bury a sheep, and nothing happens but decay!"*
>
> (GEORGE BERNARD SHAW)

> *"You put a baby in a crib with an apple and a rabbit. If it eats the rabbit and plays with the apple, I'll buy you a new car."*
>
> (HARVEY DIAMOND)

AM SITTING in elementary school. The teacher is bringing out a nice colored chart and telling all us kids how important it is to eat meat and drink our milk and get lots of protein. I'm listening to her, and looking at the chart which makes it all seem so simple. I believe my teacher, because I sense that she, herself, believes what she is saying. She is sincere. She is a grown-up. Besides, the chart is decorated and fun to look at. It must be true.

Protein, I hear, that's what's important. Protein. Lots of it. And you can only get good quality protein from meat and eggs and dairy products. That's why they make up two of the four "basic food groups" on the chart.

That day at lunch I feel like doing something good for myself and the world, so I spend the ten cents I have left of my weekly allowance for another carton of milk.

Now I am an adult, and looking back, I know my teacher had all she could handle to keep control of the classroom and teach a few basics. When teaching aids were given to her that helped get the class's attention, and helped ease her burden, she was grateful. Not for a moment did it occur to her to wonder about the political dynamics that lead to the development of those aids. Neither she nor any of us little kids could have imagined that the pretty chart was actually the outcome of extensive political lobbying by the huge meat and dairy conglomerates.[1] Nor could we have imagined the many millions of dollars which had been poured into the campaigns that produced those pretty charts. My teacher believed what she taught us, and never for a moment suspected she was being used to relay industrial propaganda.

Our innocent and captive little minds soaked it all up like sponges. And most of us, as planned, have been willing and unquestioning consumers of vast amounts of meat and dairy products ever since. Even those few of us who have come to experiment with vegetarian dietstyles are often still haunted by the voices of our teachers and the lessons of those charts. When things aren't going well, a voice in the back of our minds whispers: "Maybe you aren't getting enough protein . . ."

STEP RIGHT UP, STEP RIGHT UP

Of course, just because the concept of the "basic four" food groups was promoted by the National Egg Board, the National Dairy Council, and the National Livestock and Meat Board, doesn't mean it is necessarily false. Just because there were hucksters in our classrooms doesn't mean the hucksters lied.

But it does mean their motives were a little less pure than we thought, and their "concern" for our education a little more self-interested than we knew. It might cast a shadow upon the wisdom of unquestioningly accepting the "truths" we were taught. It might mean, for example, that we should consult sources of information less biased than the Egg Board, or the Meat Board, or the others who applied so much political and economic pressure to get those nice pretty charts to say what they wanted them to say.

Since I've discovered that the National Dairy Council is the foremost supplier of "nutritional education" materials to classrooms in the United States, and seen in a thousand other ways how heavily organizations specifically trying to promote the sale of animal products influence our "nutritional education," I've had to wonder whether we

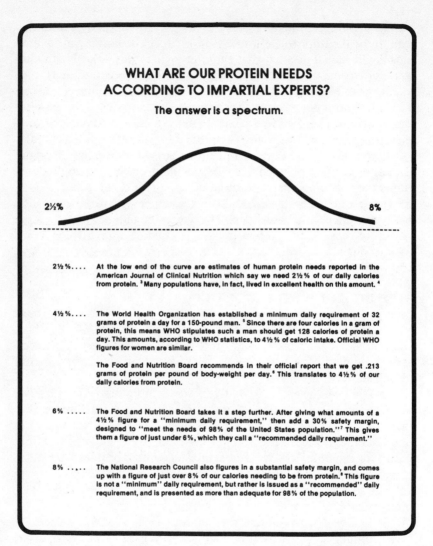

WHAT ARE OUR PROTEIN NEEDS ACCORDING TO IMPARTIAL EXPERTS?

The answer is a spectrum.

2½%   8%

2½%.... At the low end of the curve are estimates of human protein needs reported in the American Journal of Clinical Nutrition which say we need 2½% of our daily calories from protein. [3] Many populations have, in fact, lived in excellent health on this amount. [4]

4½%.... The World Health Organization has established a minimum daily requirement of 32 grams of protein a day for a 150-pound man. [5] Since there are four calories in a gram of protein, this means WHO stipulates such a man should get 128 calories of protein a day. This amounts, according to WHO statistics, to 4½% of caloric intake. Official WHO figures for women are similar.

The Food and Nutrition Board recommends in their official report that we get .213 grams of protein per pound of body-weight per day. [6] This translates to 4½% of our daily calories from protein.

6% ..... The Food and Nutrition Board takes it a step further. After giving what amounts of a 4½% figure for a "minimum daily requirement," then add a 30% safety margin, designed to "meet the needs of 98% of the United States population." [7] This gives them a figure of just under 6%, which they call a "recommended daily requirement."

8% ..... The National Research Council also figures in a substantial safety margin, and comes up with a figure of just over 8% of our calories needing to be from protein. [8] This figure is not a "minimum" daily requirement, but rather is issued as a "recommended" daily requirement, and is presented as more than adequate for 98% of the population.

might have been misled about our protein needs. Feeling a little unsure, I've turned to the light of recent unbiased scientific research, to get a better understanding of what our protein needs might actually be. These are studies produced by groups without a product to sell.

I've found that not all authorities agree on a precise figure for our daily needs of protein, but their calculations do fall within a specific range. It is a range that runs from a low estimate of **two and a half percent** of our total daily calories up to a high estimate of over **eight percent**.[2] The figures at the high end include built-in safety margins, and are not "minimum" allowances, but rather "recommended" allowances.

Interestingly, I have found there is a great deal of controversy in the scientific community about the wisdom of including such safety margins. Not everyone thinks it's necessary. One passionate nutritional commentator, Dr. David Reuben, spoke for many informed scientists when he was asked who it is who needs the extra 30% allowance of protein. He answered:

> *"The people who sell meat, fish, cheese, eggs, chicken, and all the other high prestige and expensive sources of protein. Raising the amount of protein you eat by 30% raises their income by 30%. It also increases the amount of protein in the sewers and septic tanks of your neighborhood 30% as you merrily urinate away everything that you can't use that very day. It also deprives the starving children of the world the protein that would save their lives. Incidentally, it makes you pay 30% of your already bloated food bill for protein that you will never use. If you are an average American family, it will cost you about $40 a month to unnecessarily pump up your protein intake. That puts another $36 billion a year into the pockets of the protein producers."*[9]

Other authorities hold the view that the 30% safety margin is important to protect those few individuals whose protein needs are unusually high. But there needn't be any conflict if we bear biochemical individuality in mind. Clearly, some people, owing to their biochemical individualities, will need the extra 30%. But just as clearly, others will need 30% less than the norm. Fortunately, we do not have to arrive at a single figure that would ostensibly be best for everyone.

Roger Williams, the biochemist and nutrient researcher who has probably contributed more to our understanding of biochemical individuality than any scientist alive, suggests that the range of protein needs among people may vary as much as four fold.[10] Interestingly, a four fold range is just the span covered by the extremes of current scientific thinking. For if we top off the highest figures to make room for the extra protein needs of the most extreme cases, we have a spectrum ranging from **two and a half** percent at the low end up to **ten percent** at the top. Science tells us that the protein needs of the vast majority of people would be easily met within that range.

Nature, it seems, would agree totally. Human mother's milk provides five percent of its calories from protein. Nature seems to be telling us that little babies, whose bodies are growing the fastest they will ever grow in their life, and whose protein needs are therefore at a maximum, are best served by the very modest level of 5% protein.

WHAT IF WE NEED A WHOLE LOT?
But what if we happen to be one of those people whose biochemical individualities are such that we need a whole lot of protein? What if we are at the high end of the spectrum? Don't we need to eat meat in order to get enough? And if not meat, don't we then need eggs or dairy products?

The answers to those questions are shown quite graphically in the chart on page 176 which shows the percentage of calories from protein in various non-meat, non-dairy foods.

Even in fact, were we at the very top end of the spectrum in terms of our protein needs, needing to derive a full **ten percent** of our calories from protein, unless we are trying to live only on fruits and sweet potatoes, vegetarian foodstuffs easily provide for our protein needs. If we ate only brown rice, and if our biochemical individualities required the maximum of protein, then, of course, we would fall a little short. But if we do nothing more than include beans or fresh vegetables to complement the rice, then our protein needs are easily and well

COMPARISON OF THE MILKS
OF DIFFERENT SPECIES

	Percent of Calories As Protein	Time Required to Double Birth-weight (days)
Human	5%	180days
Mare	11%	60 days
Cow	15%	47 days
Goat	17%	19 days
Dog	30%	8 days
Cat	40%	7 days
Rat	49%	4 days

Data derived from: Bell, G., Textbook of Physiology and Biochemistry, 4th ed., Williams and Wilkins, Balentine, 1954, pgs. 167-170. Adapted in McDougall, J., The McDougall Plan, New Century Publishers, 1983, pg. 101

satisfied without recourse to any animal products. This is true even in the most extreme case, where our protein needs are at the very highest end of the spectrum.

If we ate nothing but wheat (which is 17% protein), or oatmeal (15%), or pumpkin (15%), we would easily have more than enough protein. If we ate nothing but cabbage (22%), we'd have over double the maximum we might need.

In fact, if we ate nothing but the lowly potato (11% protein) we would still be getting enough protein. This fact does not mean potatoes are a particularly high protein source. They are not. Almost all plant foods provide more. What it does show, however, is just how low our protein needs really are.

There have been occasions in which people have been forced to satisfy their entire nutritional needs with potatoes and water alone. I wouldn't recommend the idea to anyone, but under deprived circumstances it has been done. Individuals who have lived for lengthy periods of time under those conditions showed no signs whatsoever of protein deficiency, though other vitamin deficiencies have occurred.[12]

LEARNING TO SHOUT HOORAY FOR MEAT AND MILK

I am back in my elementary school again. The teacher is telling us kids that animal protein is superior to vegetable protein. It's the only "complete" protein. That sounds good. I have learned to root for the "good guys" on television shows, and now I learn that "good" protein comes only from meat and dairy products. Inside I shout "Hooray!" for meat and milk. At lunch I wish my mother had put more bologna on my sandwich, so I could be stronger and better at football.

Since then I have learned that the belief in animal protein as superior to vegetable protein goes back to 1914, when Osborn and Mendel did some of the earliest laboratory research on protein requirements. They were studying rats, and (in studies I do not ethically condone) found the rats grew faster on animal protein than they did when the source of protein in their diet was plants.[13]

It wasn't long before investigators began to classify meat, eggs, and dairy foods as "Class A" proteins, and to classify plant origin proteins as "Class B."

PERCENTAGE OF CALORIES
FROM PROTEIN

LEGUMES

Soybean sprouts	54%
Mungbean sprouts	43%
Soybean curd (tofu)	43%
Soy flour	35%
Soybeans	35%
Soy sauce	33%
Broad beans	32%
Lentils	29%
Split peas	28%
Kidney beans	26%
Navy beans	26%
Lima beans	26%
Garbanzo beans	23%

GRAINS

Wheat germ	31%
Rye	20%
Wheat, hard red	17%
Wild rice	16%
Buckwheat	15%
Oatmeal	15%
Rye	14%
Millet	12%
Barley	11%
Brown Rice	8%

FRUITS

Lemons	16%
Honeydew melon	10%
Cantaloupe	9%
Strawberry	8%
Orange	8%
Blackberry	8%
Cherry	8%
Apricot	8%
Grape	8%
Watermelon	8%
Tangerine	7%
Papaya	6%
Peach	6%
Pear	5%
Banana	5%
Grapefruit	5%
Pineapple	3%
Apple	1%

VEGETABLES

Spinach	49%
New Zealand spinach	47%
Watercress	46%
Kale	45%
Broccoli	45%
Brussels sprouts	44%
Turnip greens	43%
Collards	43%
Cauliflower	40%
Mustard greens	39%
Mushrooms	38%
Chinese cabbage	34%
Parsley	34%
Lettuce	34%
Green peas	30%
Zucchini	28%
Green beans	26%
Cucumbers	24%
Dandelion greens	24%
Green pepper	22%
Artichokes	22%
Cabbage	22%
Celery	21%
Eggplant	21%
Tomatoes	18%
Onions	16%
Beets	15%
Pumpkin	12%
Potatoes	11%
Yams	8%
Sweet potatoes	6%

NUTS AND SEEDS

Pumpkin seeds	21%
Peanuts	18%
Sunflower seeds	17%
Walnuts, black	13%
Sesame seeds	13%
Almonds	12%
Cashews	12%
Filberts	8%

Data obtained from "Nutritive Value
of American Foods in Common Units,"
U.S.D.A. Agriculture Handbook No. 456

Studies in the 1940's clarified the matter further when researchers found the ten particular amino acids which are essential to the growth of rats. If any of these particular substances were removed from the rats' diet, they found the rats' growth was impaired. By laborious experiments, the optimum proportion of amino acids which produced the fastest growth was determined and the amino acid pattern that emerged was similar to that found in animal protein, particularly to that found in eggs.[14]

There was no way to duplicate these experiments on human subjects. So while we now knew the optimum amino acid pattern for rat growth, we had no equivalent information for human beings.[15]

Based on what we knew for rats, however, it was assumed by some investigators that the proportion of essential amino acids, which promoted the most rapid growth in rats, would be the best for human beings as well. No serious investigator took this to be more than a working hypothesis, but it did at least give us something to go on.[16] Meanwhile, with less than uncompromising respect for the truth, the National Egg Board took the opportunity to begin actively promoting the idea that eggs were the ideal protein food.

It wasn't only the Egg Board that saw a chance to jump on the band wagon. The Dairy Council, the Livestock and Meat Board, and virtually all the other organizations (whose purpose it was to promote the sale of animal products) joined the campaign, and none of them seemed overly concerned with minor details, such as the fact that the data was known only for rats.

Through their well-funded efforts, the idea that animal protein was superior to vegetable protein became virtually the Official Nutrition Doctrine of the United States. Anyone who thought otherwise came to be seen as some kind of crank, zealot, or nut.

DIET FOR A SMALL PLANET

Then, in the late 1960's, a woman named Frances Moore Lappe wrote an influential book entitled *Diet for a Small Planet*.[17] She accepted the hypothesis that the pattern of amino acids found in animal protein was superior for human nutrition than that found in vegetable protein. And she accepted the pattern of amino acids found in eggs as the ultimate standard against which to measure all other proteins. But then she showed that when plant foods are mixed in certain ways, the result is that the amino acids in the "inferior" vegetable proteins combine to produce proteins which more closely approximate the ideal egg standard. In fact, she showed that in many cases, thanks to the synergistic effect of protein complementarity, mixed vegetable proteins actually outrank meat in their value to the body.

Lappe was delighted to discover that almost all the traditional societies had independently evolved diets that combined vegetable proteins in a way that brought their combined amino acid patterns closer to that of the egg. And since she accepted the egg as the ideal pattern, she saw the workings of a deep inherent wisdom in these traditional diet-styles.

In Latin America, it was corn tortillas with beans, or rice with beans. In the Middle East, it was bulgar wheat with garbanzo beans (chickpeas), or pita bread with hummus (made from garbanzo beans and sesame seeds). In India, it was rice or wheat chapatis with dahl (lentils). In southern China, Japan, and much of Indonesia, it was soy products with rice. In northern China, it was soy products with wheat or millet. In Korea it was soy foods with barley.

Lappe's enthusiasm for protein combining was contagious. Her book was beautifully written, and contained charts and tables that gave the details of how complementary vegetable proteins increased each other's nutritional value, by bringing each other up towards the egg standard. Furthermore, Lappe tapped a deep and powerful spring in the psyche of the times when she showed the terrible waste of a meat-centered diet and how it is part of a pattern of consumption that deprives millions of people the essentials of life. Her book sold over three million copies.

Many people, whose "nutritional education" had hitherto been overseen by the National Dairy Council and the Meat Board, now saw, for the first time, scientific evidence that they did not have to eat meat in order to get the "best quality" protein. Numerous individuals were freed from thinking only animal proteins could meet their dietary needs.

Lappe did not, however, really question the position of the egg at the top of the protein ladder. She was evidently not aware that its placement there derived only from experiments with rats, not human beings. However, Nathan Pritikin, whose Longevity Centers featured diet-style counseling as the basis for dramatic success in treating and preventing heart disease, was one of the many nutritionists who spotted this flaw in Lappe's work. He could not agree that eggs were the ideal, having seen far too much clinical evidence to the contrary.

Although applauding the spirit in which Lappe had written *Diet for a Small Planet*, many experts felt, with Pritikin, that because she had proceeded from a wrong premise her conclusions were misleading. In her enthusiasm for protein complementarity, they felt she had unintentionally cast regular old "uncomplemented" vegetable protein in a less favorable light than the truth warranted. Pritikin said:

> *"Unfortunately, the book is one of the most misleading documents in the last few years because everybody now thinks food balancing is essential. (The book) gives the impression that vegetable proteins don't have sufficient percentages of amino acids."* [19]

Actually, Lappe never really said it was necessary to combine vegetable proteins to get enough. She only said that if you did they came much closer to the level of eggs, and usually surpassed meats. It is clear she never meant to cast a shadow over uncombined vegetable proteins. She wrote *Diet for a Small Planet* specifically to show how wasteful meat habits are, and to show that animal protein isn't necessary.

But ironically, the very popularity of her work served to reinforce the idea that animal protein was superior, though it was now understood by many that with careful combining, vegetable proteins could be made quite competitive.

Many of her readers inferred that if you don't eat animal protein, than you need a doctorate in chemistry, and had better keep a slide rule in your kitchen. Many felt obligated to check amino-acid tables and food-combining charts before preparing a meal.

Meanwhile, Lappe herself was learning more, and revising her judgments about the value of uncomplemented vegetable protein. She became convinced that her emphasis in *Diet for a Small Planet* on protein complementarity had been misplaced. So she re-wrote *Diet For a Small Planet*, and in 1981, reissued an almost completely new tenth anniversary edition.[20] Now she said:

> *"In 1971 I stressed protein complementarity because I assumed that the only way to get enough protein . . . was to create a protein as usable by the body as animal protein. In combating the myth that meat is the only way to get high-quality protein, I reinforced another myth. I gave the impression that in order to get enough protein without meat, considerable care was needed in choosing foods. Actually, it is much easier than I thought . . . (I) helped create a new myth—that to get the protein you need without meat you have to conscientiously combine nonmeat sources . . . With a healthy, varied diet, concern about protein complementarity is not necessary for most of us."* [21]

It is very rare when well-known figures are willing to reverse themselves publicly, especially when the issue is the very one which made them famous. I can't help but admire this kind of integrity. And obviously, Frances Moore Lappe is convinced that her earlier emphasis on protein combining was unwarranted. In the original 1971 edition of *Diet for a Small Planet*, over 200 of the 280 pages dealt specifically with the ins and outs of protein combining. In the 1981 edition, only about 60 of the 455 pages deal with the matter, and much of this is an explanation of how her thinking has changed. The details of protein complementarity, which comprised the bulk of the original book, are relegated in her revised edition to a short appendix, at the back of the book.

In the new *Diet for a Small Planet*, the woman who brought the concept of complementing vegetable proteins to the world goes out of her way to show it isn't necessary. She writes:

> *"If people are getting enough calories, they are virtually certain of getting enough protein . . . The simplest way to prove the overall point is to propose a diet which most people would consider protein-deprived, and ask, does its protein content add up to the allowance recommended by the National Academy of Sciences?"* [22]

CAN YOU EASILY GET ENOUGH PROTEIN WITHOUT EGGS OR DAIRY PRODUCTS?

YES! WITHOUT EVEN TRYING

HYPOTHETICAL ALL-PLANT FOOD DIET

From Revised Edition of *DIET FOR A SMALL PLANET*

	Calories	Total Protein (grams)
Breakfast		
1 cup orange juice	111	1.7
1 cup cooked oatmeal	148	5.4
½ oz. sunflower seeds	80	3.5
1 T. brown sugar	52	0
3 T. raisins	87	0.9
Lunch		
2 T. peanut butter	172	7.8
2 slices whole wheat bread	112	4.8
1 T. honey	64	0.1
1 apple	87	0.3
2 carrots, small	42	1.1
Dinner		
1 cup cooked beans	236	15.6
1 cup cooked brown rice	178	3.8
3 stalks broccoli (1½ c.)	52	6.2
4 mushrooms	28	2.7
2 T. oil	248	0
1 cup apple juice	109	0.3
½ banana	64	0.8
Snack		
1½ cup popcorn, with oil	123	2.7
Total	**1,993**	**57.7**
National Academy of Sciences Recommended allowance for a 128-pound woman	2,000	44.0

She then puts together a day's menu, with no meat, no dairy products, no eggs, and no protein supplements, and comments:

> *"Even without accounting for improved protein usability due to combining complementary proteins, this diet has adequate protein without exceeding calorie limits."* [23]

Lappe's hypothetical menu is for a 128-pound woman. It contains 57.7 grams of protein, far more than the 44 grams recommended by the National Academy of Sciences for a woman that size. She points out that even if we were to assume the superiority of animal protein, and completely ignore any conceivable benefits that might be gained from vegetable protein combining, her hypothetical menu would still exceed the allowance with ease.

Men might wonder whether they would get enough protein in this fashion. They would indeed, since caloric needs and protein needs rise hand in hand. What matters is the **percentage** of the total caloric intake derived from protein. Men, eating proportionately more calories than Lappe's 128-pound woman, would get proportionately more protein, and be covered. We saw earlier that a spectrum of **two-and-a-half percent** to **ten percent** would be adequate for just about everybody. Without meats, eggs or dairy products, Lappe's hypothetical menu still derives over **eleven-and-a-half percent** of its calories from protein.

THE INCREDIBLE OVERSOLD EGG

It is not only Frances Moore Lappe whose mind is changing as new evidence comes in from protein research; the most rigorous scientific journals are likewise convinced. An editorial in the medical journal *Lancet* reports:

> *"Formerly, vegetable proteins were classified as second-class, and regarded as inferior to first-class proteins of animal origin, but this distinction has now been generally discarded."* [24]

What are we to make of this turnaround? Is it possible that even if we accept the dubious hypothesis that the egg is the ultimate protein standard for humans, we still do not need meat, eggs or dairy products in order to get adequate protein? Could it be that the whole issue of "getting enough protein" is actually just a figment of our collective imaginations, with nothing behind it except for the propaganda of the meat, dairy and egg industries?

That, remarkably, seems to be the case.[25] The Food and Nutrition Board of the National Academy of Sciences, hardly a bastion of nutritional radicalism, spoke of people who consume no dairy products, meats, or eggs:

> *"Pure vegetarians from many populations of the world have maintained . . . excellent health."* [26]

A team of Harvard researchers, investigating the effects of a strictly plant food diet, found:

> *"It is difficult to obtain a mixed vegetable diet which will produce an appreciable loss of body protein without resorting to high levels of sugar, jams and jellies, and other essentially protein-free foods."* [27]

A clinical study reported in the *Journal of the American Dietetic Association* compared the intake of the essential amino acids for meat-eaters, lacto-ovo vegetarians (those consuming dairy products and eggs), and pure vegetarians (no eggs or dairy products).[28] This study raised the protein requirements for each amino acid to a height that would cover even the needs of pregnant women and growing adolescents. They found that not only were all three diet-styles sufficient, they were all **well above sufficient**:

> *"Each group exceeded twice its requirement for every essential amino acid and surpassed this amount by large amounts for most of them."* [29]

At an annual meeting of the American Association for the Advancement of Science, the eminent nutritionist Dr. John Scharffenberg gave a major presentation which was later made into a book. He did not seem to feel that "getting enough protein" was a major worry:

"Let me emphasize, it is difficult to design a reasonable experimental diet that provides an active adult with adequate calories that is deficient in protein." [30]

Many consider Nathan Pritikin the foremost expert on nutrition in modern times. Thousands of people came to his Longevity Centers. Some came in wheelchairs, or preparing for coronary bypass operations. Many went jogging home a month later. Most improved tremendously. The heart of Pritikin's program was his diet. He said:

"Vegetarians always ask about getting enough protein. But I don't know any nutrition expert that can plan a diet of natural foods resulting in a protein deficiency, so long as you're not deficient in calories. You need only six percent of total calories in protein . . . and it's practically impossible to get below nine percent in ordinary diets." [31]

It seems Nature must have wanted us to have enough protein. For simply following the instinct of hunger and eating enough natural food of whatever kind, it is almost impossible to be deficient in this vital nutrient.

And it doesn't matter very much whether or not we hold one form of protein to be superior. Either way, and whatever the demands of our biological individuality, the evidence forces us to conclude that we will get enough protein, even without dairy products, eggs, or protein complementarity.

I admit that I have sometimes had a hard time accepting these truths. I have been powerfully programmed, and have become emotionally attached to the old ideas about protein. But dispassionate appraisal of the evidence virtually forces me to conclude that the "problem" of where vegetarians will get their protein, even those who forego dairy products and eggs, is in actuality a "nonproblem." [32]

In fact, researchers who purposefully want to design diets deficient in protein often have a devil of a time. It is possible, but it's far from easy. By the same token, it is possible for a vegetarian to be deficient in protein, but it takes some doing. Here's how it can be done:

THE NONPROTEIN DIET

1) By eating excessive junk food. Such "food"—which includes fatty, highly refined and processed foods, most sweets, and excess alcohol— give us only "empty" calories. These are calories which provide momentary fuel, but do not nourish our cells or organs. They provide little in the way of vitamins, minerals, protein or fiber. A diet with a lot of fat, candy, soda pop, white bread, pastries and/or fried foods will probably lead to protein deficiency, as well as a deficiency in every other nutrient we need.

2) By trying to live on fruit alone. Of course, most of us wouldn't consider fruit as a staple for any length of time, and so needn't worry about this. But there are some who try to be "fruitarians." Usually, their reasons are more spiritual than nutritional, and it is a good thing, because from a nutritional point of view, a fruitarian diet may lack adequate protein.

3) By eating only those few crops whose protein content is unusually low. This would be nearly impossible in the United States. But there are parts of West Africa where the staple food is the cassava root, which provides only about two percent of its calories as protein. Sadly, people there sometimes have little else to eat. Some of them, as a result, encounter protein deficiency.[33]

4) If an infant were to be fed just grains and vegetables, it might have difficulty absorbing enough protein due to the immaturity of its digestive system. Studies have shown potatoes can supply 100% of an infant's protein needs, but grains may fall short. Of course, if an infant is breastfed, then there is nothing to worry about.[34]

5) The only other way vegetarians could fail to fulfill their protein needs, would be by starving. If you don't get enough food, then you aren't going to get enough protein. Of course, you aren't going to get enough carbohydrates or vitamins or fiber or minerals or anything else either. This condition, which tragically occurs among the very poorest of the world, is known as kwashiorkor. But we hardly need a fancy name for someone who is starving to death.[35]

GROWING UP BIG AND STRONG

I'm back in the classroom again. My teacher is telling us kids that if we want to be big and strong we had better eat lots of protein. And when we work hard and play hard then we need even more protein. I'm thinking of my Superman comic books, and remembering the pictures of Charles Atlas on the back, with his huge muscles and rippling vitality. Squinting my eyes a little, I resolve to bite the bullet and ignore my intense dislike for meatloaf. Some things are more important than whether they taste good or not.

Most of us, naturally, still believe what our teachers taught us. But one man who doesn't quite go along with all this, and who would appear to know what he's talking about, is a man who might be capable of kicking sand in even Charles Atlas's face. I'm speaking of Arnold Schwarzenegger, the virtual symbol of male muscular development. In his book, *Arnold's Body Building for Men*, Schwarzenegger writes:

> *"Kids nowadays . . . tend to go overboard when they discover body building and eat diets consisting of 50 to 70% protein—something I believe to be totally unnecessary . . . (In) my formula for basic good eating: eat about one gram of protein for every two pounds of body weight."* [36]

This formula is in keeping with the range we have already discovered. To meet Arnold Schwarzenegger's suggested protein quota, you'd do fine without meat, eggs, or dairy products. If you ate only broccoli, I'd probably wonder whether you had lost your marbles, but you'd get more than four times Schwarzenegger's suggested requirement.

When it comes to the relationship between protein and physical work, it turns out that once again my teacher, bless her heart, didn't quite hit the nail on the head. True, we need protein to replace enzymes, rebuild blood cells, grow hair, produce antibodies, and to fulfill certain other specific tasks. But there is virtually no greater demand for any of these functions from hard physical work. If we are working or playing hard, it is not more protein we need, but rather we require more carbohydrates to burn, because it is carbohydrates that provide our fuel.

Study after study has found that protein combustion is no higher during heavy exercise than under resting conditions. This is why Dave Scott can set world records for the triathlon without consuming lots of protein. And why Sixto Lenares can swim 4.8 miles, cycle 185 miles, and run 52.4 miles in a single day without meat, dairy products, eggs, or any kind of protein supplement in his diet.

The popular idea that we need extra protein if we are working hard turns out to be simply another part of the whole mythology of protein, the "beef gives strength" conditioning foisted upon us by those who profit from our meat habit. Such thoughts have been planted in our minds since we were little children, and have, for many of us, become so much a part of our psychic landscape that we simply "know" they are true. We have come to take them for granted as given facts, much as people once took for granted that the world was flat.

But today, even the conservative National Academy of Science, an organization hardly renowned for going out on a limb and taking controversial positions, says:

> *"There is little evidence that muscular activity increases the need for protein."* [37]

Modern nutritional science tells us clearly that our protein needs are easily met without any fuss. And yet many of us are haunted, somewhere in the back of our minds, by the fear that if we do not eat enough protein we may end up looking like one of the people on a CARE poster. Because we absorbed this fear when we were very young, it has become part of the very foundations of our psyche. We have become living examples of the old German proverb,

"An old error is always more popular than a new truth."

We have become protein obsessed, and we pay an incalculable price for it. We feed an enormous amount of grain to livestock which could otherwise be fed to the world's hungry. We cause a great deal of needless suffering to animals. And finally, we seriously compromise our health.

Though we know that most anything in excess can be harmful, be it aspirin or alcohol, sex, food or sunshine, we rarely apply this understanding to our protein consumption. We have for the most part been so afraid of not getting enough protein that we have ignored the growing body of scientific research that points to the serious health consequences of ingesting too much.

OSTEOPOROSIS AND THE PROTEIN CONNECTION

By now, if my grade school teacher is still alive, she is probably gray-haired and in her sixties. If she is like most other women of that age in the United States, her "old bones" are probably not quite what they used to be. She may be a little stooped over with age; and she may well have lost significant height from the days when she towered over a classroom of youngsters who looked up to her every word.

Actually, if she is like most women that age in the United States, her "old bones" are far indeed from what they once were. They have lost significant amounts of minerals, especially calcium, and as a result are springy, fragile, and weak. It is not at all uncommon for the bone mineral losses in post-menopausal women to cause them chronic back pain, while at the same time making them susceptible to frequent fractures. Often they lose height, and find themselves increasingly stooped over, for the weakened vertebrae just cannot support the body load. Unfortunately, this crumpling of the body posture is not just an aesthetic misfortune. Increased pressure is put on the inner organs, and they are unable to function as they should.[38]

I remember my teacher fondly, and wouldn't wish this on her for all the world. But in fully twenty-five percent of sixty-five year old women in the United States, bone mineral losses (called "bone resorption") are so severe the condition is given the clinical name "osteoporosis."[39] For a person technically to qualify for this label, it means she has lost fifty to seventy-five percent of the original bone material from her skeleton. Fully one out of every four women sixty five years old in our culture has lost over half her bone density.[40] Today, more deaths are caused by osteoporosis than cancer of the breast and cervix combined.

Unfortunately, the loss of calcium and other minerals from the bones is a gradual process which goes on steadily for a long time before it becomes evident. There is no flashing red light to warn us that our bodies are losing calcium. And it is usually not apparent until loose teeth, receding gums, or a fractured hip show how brittle and chalky the bones have become. The end result of the skeletal structure's gradual erosion is calcium-deficient bones that may break with the slightest provocation. Even a mere sneeze may crack a rib.

One of the reasons the decreasing bone density is hard to detect until it reaches such an unfortunate stage is that even in extreme cases

THE RAVAGES OF OSTEOPOROSIS

On the standard American diet, almost all females suffer significant loss
of bone density as they age.

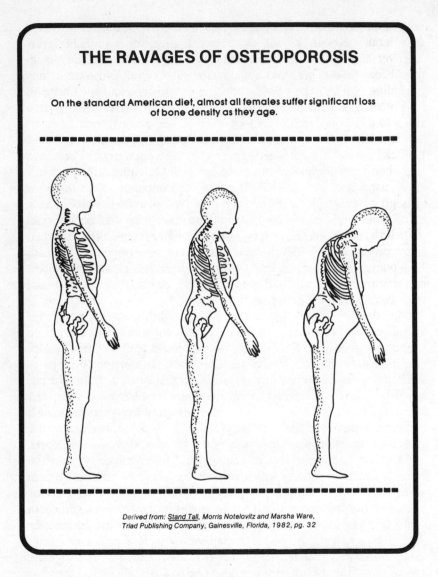

Derived from: <u>Stand Tall</u>, Morris Notelovitz and Marsha Ware,
Triad Publishing Company, Gainesville, Florida, 1982, pg. 32

of osteoporosis, the calcium level of the blood is usually normal. In the body's ranking of needs, the blood level of calcium takes definite priority over the bone level of calcium. The body needs calcium in the blood for vital operations, such as controlling muscular contractions, including the heart, blood clotting, transmission of nerve impulses, and other utterly essential tasks. When the body needs to supply calcium to the blood for any reason, it acts as if the bones were a "bank" of stored calcium, and through a series of biochemical reactions a "check" is drawn on the calcium bank. Your body draws calcium from your bones to supply calcium to your blood.

I used to believe that bones lost calcium only if there were not enough calcium in our diets. The National Dairy Council is the foremost spokesman for this point of view, and the solution they propose, not all that surprisingly, is for us all to drink more milk and eat more dairy products. In fact, the dairy industry has of late spent a great deal of money promoting this point of view; and it does seem logical. But modern nutritional research clearly indicates a major flaw in this perspective.[41] Osteoporosis is, in fact, a disease caused by a number of things, the most important of which is excess dietary protein![42]

The correspondence between excess protein intake and bone resorption is direct and consistent. Even with very high calcium intakes, the more excess protein in the diet the greater the incidence of negative calcium balance, and the greater the loss of calcium from the bones.[43]

The figure on page 192 shows the results of the independent work of five different research teams studying the effect of low and high protein diets on calcium balance. On the chart, a positive calcium balance means the bones are not losing calcium, while a negative calcium balance means they are, and osteoporosis is developing.

One long-term study found that with as little as 75 grams of daily protein (less than three-quarters of what the average meat-eating American consumes) more calcium is lost in the urine than is absorbed by the body from the diet—a negative calcium balance. In every study the same correspondence was found: the more protein that is taken in, the more calcium that is lost.[44] This is true even if the dietary calcium intake is as high as 1400 milligrams per day, far higher than the standard American diet.

IS OSTEOPOROSIS
DUE TO CALCIUM DEFICIENCY
OR EXCESS PROTEIN?

STUDY No.	CALCIUM INTAKE -milligrams-	CHANGE IN CALCIUM BALANCE WITH A LOW-PROTEIN DIET	CHANGE IN CALCIUM BALANCE WITH A HIGH-PROTEIN DIET
1	500	+ 31	-120
2	500	+ 24	-116
3	800	+ 12	-85
4	1400	+ 10	-84
5	1400	+ 20	-65
AVERAGE	920	+ 19	-94

Study No. 1 . . .   **Anad, C., "Effect of Protein Intake on Calcium Balance of Young Men Given 500 Mg Calcium Daily," <u>Journal of Nutrition</u>, 104:695, 1974**

Study No. 2 . . .   **Hegsted, M., "Urinary Calcium and Calcium Balance in Young Men as Affected by Level of Protein and Phosphorous Intake," <u>Journal of Nutrition</u>, 111:53, 1981**

Study No. 3 . . .   **Walker, R., "Calcium Retnetion in the Adult Human Male As Affected By Protein Intake," <u>Journal of Nutrition</u>, 102:1297, 1972**

Study No. 4 . . .   **Johnson, N., "Effect of Level of Protein Intake on Urinary and Fecal Calcium and Calcium Retention of Young Adult Males," <u>Journal of Nutrition</u>, 100:1425, 1970**

Study No. 5 . . .   **Linkswiler, H., "Calcium Retention of Young Adult Males As Affected by Level of Protein and of Calcium Intake," <u>Trans New York Academy of Science</u>, 36:333, 1974**

Data as per McDougall, Dr. John, <u>McDougall's Medicine,</u>
New Century Publishers, New York, 1985

In other words, the more protein in our diet, the more calcium we lose, regardless of how much calcium we take in. The result is that high-protein diets in general, and meat-based diets in particular, lead to a gradual but inexorable decrease in bone density, and produce the ongoing development of osteoporosis.[45]

Summarizing the medical research on osteoporosis, one of the nation's leading medical authorities on dietary associations with disease, Dr. John McDougall, says:

> *"I would like to emphasize that the calcium-losing effect of protein on the human body is not an area of controversy in scientific circles. The many studies performed during the past 55 years consistently show that the most important dietary change that we can make if we want to create a positive calcium balance that will keep our bones solid is to decrease the amount of proteins we eat each day. The important change is not to increase the amount of calcium we take in."*[46]

The National Dairy Council has spent tens of millions of dollars to make us think that osteoporosis can be prevented by drinking more milk and eating more dairy products. But the only research that even begins to suggest that the consumption of dairy products might be helpful has been paid for by the National Dairy Council itself.

OSTEOPOROSIS AROUND THE WORLD

Throughout the world, the incidence of osteoporosis correlates directly with protein intake. In any given population, the greater the intake of protein, the more common and more severe will be the osteoporosis.[47] In fact, world health statistics show that osteoporosis is most common in exactly those countries where dairy products are consumed in the largest quantities—the United States, Finland, Sweden, and the United Kingdom.[48]

Nathan Pritikin studied the medical research on osteoporosis, and found no basis at all for the Dairy Council viewpoint:

> *"African Bantu women take in only 350 mg. of calcium per day. They bear nine children during their lifetime and breast feed them*

for two years. They never have calcium deficiency, seldom break a bone, rarely lose a tooth. Their children grow up nice and strong. How can they do that on 350 mg. of calcium a day when the (National Dairy Council) recommendation is 1200 mg.? It's very simple. They're on a low-protein diet that doesn't kick the calcium out of the body . . . In our country, those who can afford it are eating 20% of their total calories in protein, which guarantees negative mineral balance, not only of calcium, but of magnesium, zinc, and iron. It's all directly related to the amount of protein you eat. "[49]

The Bantus consume much less calcium than do Americans. Yet, even their oldest women are essentially free of osteoporosis,[50] while the disease is epidemic in older American women. The dairy industry has said that the Bantus' far higher bone densities on much lower calcium intakes may be due to genetic factors. But genetic relatives of the Bantus living in the United States, and eating the standard American diet-style, have levels of osteoporosis that equal those of their white neighbors.[51] Therefore the only sensible conclusion, in light of all the research, is that the Bantus' far lower protein consumption has kept their bones healthier.[52]

At the other end of the scale from the Bantus are the native Eskimos. If osteoporosis were a calcium deficiency disease it would be unheard of among these people. They have the highest dietary calcium intake of any people in the world—more than 2,000 mg. a day from fish bones.[53] On the other hand, if osteoporosis is caused by excess protein in the diet, they would suffer greatly from the disease, because their diet is also the very highest in the world in protein—250 to 400 grams a day from fish, walrus, and whale.[54] As it happens, unfortunately, the native Eskimo people have one of the very highest rates of osteoporosis in the world.[55]

Studies comparing the bone densities of people with different diet-styles show a pattern completely opposed to the dairy industry's declarations. The research invariably reveals greater bone resorption and development of osteoporosis with a greater intake of meat and dairy products,[56] not the other way around.

On August 22, 1984 the *Medical Tribune* reported a major study of bone densities in the United States. The conclusion was typical of the many such studies: vegetarians were found to have "significantly stronger bones."

In March, 1983, the *Journal of Clinical Nutrition* reported the results of the largest study of this kind ever undertaken.[57] Researchers at Michigan State and other major universities found that, by the age of 65 in the United States:

***Male vegetarians had an average measurable bone loss of 3%.*
***Male meat-eaters had an average measurable bone loss of 7%.*
***Female vegetarians had an average measurable bone loss of 18%.*
***Female meat-eaters had an average measurable bone loss of 35%.*

By the time she reaches the age of sixty-five, the average meat-eating woman in the United States has lost over a third of her skeletal structure. In contrast, older vegetarian women tend to remain active, maintain erect postures, and are less likely to fracture or break bones even with their increased physical activity. If their bones do break or fracture, they heal faster and more completely.[58]

WHY ARE VEGETARIANS PROTECTED?
You may wonder, since osteoporosis seems to be caused by excessive dietary protein, why vegetarians seem so protected from its ravages. Isn't it possible to overdose on vegetarian proteins? A United States Department of Agriculture survey found that American vegetarians consume, on the average, 150% of their actual protein requirements. The biggest overdose is found among children aged three to eight. These youngsters, many of whom are told to "drink three glasses of milk a day," consume, on the average, 209% of their actual protein needs.[59]

I suspect that many of the parents of these vegetarian children, who are no doubt vegetarians themselves, are afraid their children won't get enough protein. Attempting to appease the protein tyrant in their own minds, they make doubly sure their kids eat lots of milk and cheese and yogurt and eggs, thinking they are doing them a good turn.

The kids end up eating far more protein than they actually need, even with all their growing requirements taken into account.

Even haunted by the protein myth, however, vegetarians tend not to over-consume protein to the extent that meat-eaters do, and this is one reason they do not suffer nearly as much osteoporosis. But even if a vegetarian were to consume as much excess protein as a meat-eater, he or she would still have stronger bones because meat, eggs, dairy products and fish contribute to osteoporosis in yet other ways.

KEEPING PHIT

Keeping our blood at an essentially neutral pH is a top priority for the body. If our blood were to become too acidic we would die. Accordingly, if the diet contains a lot of acid forming foods, then the body, in its wisdom, withdraws calcium from the bones and uses this alkaline mineral to balance the pH of the blood. As we can see from the figure on page 197, meat, eggs and fish are the most acid-forming of foods, and hence the ones that cause calcium to be drawn from the bones to restore the pH balance. Most fruits and vegetables, on the other hand, generally yield an alkaline ash, and so require no depletion of calcium stores from the bones to maintain the neutrality of the blood.[60]

There is yet another reason why vegetarians are relatively immune to osteoporosis, even though the Dairy Council keeps telling us that calcium intake is the answer to this disease. What they neglect to mention is that the body's ability to absorb and utilize calcium depends directly on the amount of phosphorous in the diet.[61]

In one study, young women maintained a positive calcium balance when their diets provided 1500 mg of calcium and 800 mg of phosphorous, per day. But when phosphorous intake was raised to 1400 mg a day, the women went into negative calcium balance, even though their calcium intake had not been reduced.[62] More important, apparently, than the amount of calcium taken in is the calcium/phosphorous ratio. The lower this ratio, the greater the loss of bone density, and the greater the development of osteoporosis. The higher the calcium/phosphorous ratio, the less bone loss takes place, and the stronger the skeleton, assuming the intake of protein is not excessive.

The foods whose calcium is least available, because their calcium/phosphorous ratio is low, are liver, chicken, beef, pork and fish, in that

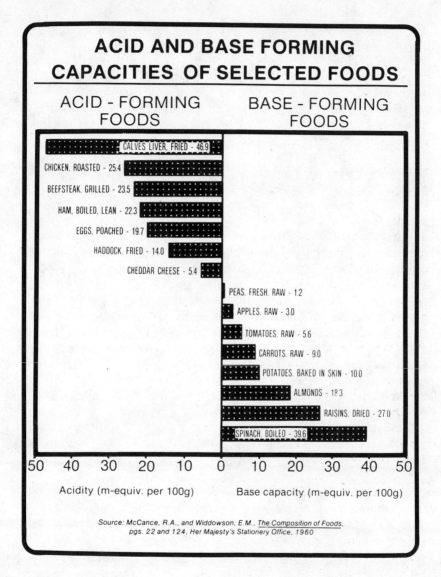

ACID AND BASE FORMING CAPACITIES OF SELECTED FOODS

ACID - FORMING FOODS

BASE - FORMING FOODS

CALVES LIVER, FRIED - 46.9
CHICKEN, ROASTED - 25.4
BEEFSTEAK, GRILLED - 23.5
HAM, BOILED, LEAN - 22.3
EGGS, POACHED - 19.7
HADDOCK, FRIED - 14.0
CHEDDAR CHEESE - 5.4

PEAS, FRESH, RAW - 1.2
APPLES, RAW - 3.0
TOMATOES, RAW - 5.6
CARROTS, RAW - 9.0
POTATOES, BAKED IN SKIN - 10.0
ALMONDS - 18.3
RAISINS, DRIED - 27.0
SPINACH, BOILED - 39.6

50 40 30 20 10 0 10 20 30 40 50

Acidity (m-equiv. per 100g)   Base capacity (m-equiv. per 100g)

Source: McCance, R.A., and Widdowson, E.M., The Composition of Foods,
pgs. 22 and 124, Her Majesty's Stationery Office, 1960

order. The calcium in vegetables and fruits, in sharp contrast, is much more available, due to their higher calcium/phosphorous ratios. Lettuce, for example, is not particularly high in calcium, but its calcium is readily utilized by the body because its ratio of calcium to phosphorous is comparatively high—70 times higher than that of liver, and 23 times higher than beef or pork. The foods whose calcium is best utilized are those with the highest calcium/phosphorous ratios, such as the green leafy vegetables. The calcium in these foods is dramatically more available than that found in animal products. If the calcium/phosphorous ratio for mustard greens, for example, were to be represented by a towering skyscraper, the equivalent ratio for chicken would barely amount to a small doghouse.[63]

FUDGING THE TRUTH

The claims of the dairy industry are based on the idea that bone loss is due solely to a diminished intake of dietary calcium. So drink your milk. But the only studies in the medical literature to support this contention were sponsored by the National Dairy Council itself.

Remarkably, even those studies funded by the National Dairy Council for the express purpose of showing the benefits of milk for women susceptible to osteoporosis have, in fact, ended up showing something quite different. In one Dairy Council sponsored study, women who drank an extra three eight-ounce glasses of low fat milk every day for a year showed no significant increase in calcium balance. Even with all the extra mild-derived calcium, they were still in negative calcium balance after a full year of the regime. The scientists who conducted the test knew why. They said the women continued to have a negative calcium balance, and continued to develop osteoporosis, due to:

". . . the average thirty percent increase in protein intake during milk supplementation."[64]

The additional protein load from the milk tended to wash calcium and other minerals out of the subjects' bodies, and thus throw them into negative calcium balance.

Not surprisingly, the Dairy Council is not keen to have the public know the results of this and the many similar studies.

In 1984, the *British Medical Journal* published a report indicating that calcium intake is, in fact, completely irrelevant to bone loss. The researchers enlisted post-menopausal women, who agreed to take 500 mg of supplemental calcium every day for two years. They were divided into three groups: 1) those whose diets contained less than 550 mg of calcium, 2) those who consumed between 550 mg and 1100 mg of calcium daily, and 3) those whose diet provided more than 1100 mg. At the end of two years, there was no difference in bone demineralization among the three groups. In fact, their bone losses were virtually the same as those found in women taking no calcium supplements at all, and whose diets contained less than the recommended daily allowance of calcium. This was true even though some of the women in the test were taking huge amounts of calcium from food and supplemental sources—in some cases, over 2,000 mg a day.[65]

Even the most conservative medical investigators no longer deny the connection between excess protein and osteoporosis. In a report published in *Lancet*, Drs. Aaron Watchman and Daniel Bernstein commented on work sponsored by the United States Department of Health and Harvard University. They called the association of meat-based diets with the increasing incidence of osteoporosis "inescapable."[66]

There are, of course, other factors besides "getting lots of protein" that contribute to osteoporosis. Small, light-skinned Caucasian women are more susceptible, as are women who bear no children and those who've had their ovaries removed. Lack of exercise is a factor, as is the consumption of soft drinks (they are very high in phosphorous), junk food, excess salt, and acid-forming foods. Smoking increases risk, as do certain anti-culvulsant medications. Yet though there are a number of factors that can contribute to osteoporosis, excess protein consumption clearly towers above them all as the chief causative influence.

Quite frankly, the more I've studied the conclusions of the hundreds of studies in the medical literature, the harder it has gotten for me to abide the National Dairy Council's promotion of milk "for strong bones." In spite of its high calcium content, milk, due to its high protein content, appears actually to **contribute** to the accelerating development of osteoporosis. The occurrence of this disease in the United States has reached truly epidemic proportions, and the promotion of dairy products as an "answer" to the suffering of millions seems, not only self-serving, but absolutely immoral and downright dishonest.

ENOUGH IS ENOUGH

As if osteoporosis weren't enough, it turns out there are other problems derived from too much protein, particularly too much animal protein. One such problem is kidney stones.

The calcium lost from our bones due to excess protein has to go somewhere after it has served its purpose in our bloodstream. And so does the calcium we have ingested but have not been able to absorb due to high phosphorous/calcium ratios. It all ends up in our urine, producing very high levels of calcium in the kidney system, and all-too-often crystallizing into kidney stones. This is why kidney stones, the most painful of all medical emergencies, occur far more frequently in meat-eaters than in vegetarians.[67]

Additionally, there is a great deal of evidence implicating excessive protein consumption in the destruction of kidney tissue and the progressive deterioration of kidney function.[68] Extra protein doesn't just trickle out of the body. It takes hard work on the part of the kidneys to get rid of the excess. Many animal studies have shown that the higher the protein in the diet, the greater the incidence and the more severe the cases of kidney hypertrophy and inflammation.[69]

The same things happen to human kidneys if we over-consume protein. People who have suffered kidney damage or loss are usually able to preserve their remaining kidney function only if they are put on a protein restricted diet.[70] Those kidney patients whose protein intake is not restricted, and particularly those who continue to eat meat, show rapid deterioration of their kidneys to the point where many become dependent on kidney dialysis machines.[71]

It is important to stress that the link between kidney disease and excess protein consumption, like the link between osteoporosis and excess protein consumption, is no longer considered merely probable within the informed medical community. Too many tests by too many researchers under too wide a variety of conditions have been too consistent in their implications. It is now considered certain.

As the evidence against too much protein mounts, you may shake your head and wonder just how our protein obsession ever got started in the first place.

Almost all the early nutritional research was done on livestock, at the behest of people raising animals for meat and milk. Their objective was to produce the biggest animals in the shortest length of time. The idea that rapid growth and large size are inherently desirable was implicit in the undertaking. Nutritional research was therefore geared to finding what diets would accomplish this aim.

Early experiments which found that rats grew faster when fed animal protein led to the hypothesis that animal protein was superior. Further research has validated that rats so fed do indeed grow faster. But the "bigger is better" mentality has been dealt quite a blow by other discoveries. It has been found that rats fed animal protein also die sooner, plus suffer from a multitude of diseases vegetarian rats do not.[72]

A report aptly titled "Rapid Growth—Shorter Life" appeared in the *Journal of the American Medical Association*. It showed that high animal-protein diets measureably shortened the life spans of a number of different animals.[73] These findings corroborate the world health statistics that show human meat-eating populations do not, as a rule, live as long as vegetarian populations.

It has also been discovered that meat-eaters have higher rates of cancer than do vegetarians. Just how excess protein may be linked to cancer is not yet understood, but there is growing evidence they are indeed linked. The meat and dairy industries like to question the credentials of anyone who suggests their products might not promote optimum health. But it would be hard to doubt the credentials of T. Colin Campbell, a professor in the division of Nutritional Sciences at Cornell University, and the senior science advisor to the American Institute for Cancer Research. He said recently that there is:

> ". . . a strong correlation between dietary protein intake and cancer of the breast, prostate, pancreas, and colon."[74]

Other authorities with equally impeccable credentials agree. Myron Winick, director of Columbia University's Institute of Human Nutrition, says the data indicates:

> ". . . a relationship between high-protein diets and cancer of the colon." [75]

It just goes on and on . . .

NOW WHAT?

I'm back in my grade school classroom. The teacher is telling all us little kids about the importance of eating lots of meat, and drinking lots of milk. She is pointing to a colorfully decorated chart, which makes it all seem so simple. She is telling us about the importance of getting enough protein, and making it clear that animal protein is the only "complete" protein. Her voice rings with authority, because she believes every word she is saying.

I'm listening, but not completely. I'm thinking about my pet kitten, about how furry and cuddly and playful he is, and about a neighbor's dog who recently had puppies.

My teacher's voice drifts over me and slides away. I look outside the window and see a bird who seems to feel my attention, because as I look she begins to sing.

That day at lunch I feel like doing something good for myself and the world. I decide to save my milk money, and give it to people who do not have enough to eat.

FOOD FOR THE CARING HEART

"People often say that humans have always eaten animals, as if this is a justification for continuing the practice. According to this logic, we should not try to prevent people from murdering other people, since this has also been done since the earliest of times."

(ISAAC SINGER)

THE HUMAN HEART doesn't actually look very much like a valentine, but it is nevertheless a wondrous and beautiful muscle. About the size of a clenched fist, it begins to beat only a few weeks after conception, and thereafter pumps forth the rhythm of our lives through every moment of our uterine and earthly existence. Only at the moment of our death does it cease.

This beating has a definite purpose: to pump blood to all parts of the body. The life of our very cells depends on the oxygen and nutrition brought to them by the flow of our blood. If for some reason any muscle did not receive a fresh flow of blood it would quickly die.

Since the heart is also a muscle, it, too, must continuously receive a fresh flow of blood, and you might think that receiving a blood supply would never be a problem for the heart, since its chambers are always full of blood. But the heart is not able to directly use any of the blood contained within its pumping chambers, any more than a stereo amplifier can plug into itself. Instead, the heart muscle feeds from the blood supplied to it through two specific vessels, called the coronary arteries.

In a healthy person, the blood flows freely and easily through the coronary arteries, and the well fed heart keeps pumping away as it should. But if one of the coronary arteries, or one of its branches, should become blocked off, and so be unable to supply the heart with blood, then even though the heart's chambers are full of blood, that part of the heart dependent on the blocked-off artery will die.

In medical terminology, this is called a "myocardial infarction." Most of us know it by another name—a heart attack. Heart attacks are by far the largest cause of death in the United States today. Every 25 seconds another person is stricken. Every 45 seconds another person dies.

If a heart attack victim is fortunate, and the part of the heart that dies is small, he will survive, and the dead tissue will come gradually to be replaced by scar tissue. But if a larger part of the heart is deprived of blood, there really isn't very much that can be done to save his life. Many heart attack victims die within minutes of the unexpected seizure.

Heart attack victims often never have the slightest warning anything is wrong. There are no bodily symptoms to signal the oncoming disaster. They may have only that morning heard their physician pronounce them fit as a fiddle. But, then, suddenly, the victims feel a sudden, severe crushing pain in their chests. Often the pain shoots down the arm, and sometimes it flares up the neck, particularly on the left side. There may be cold sweating, nausea, vomiting and shortness of breath. The symptoms are accompanied by a feeling of being overwhelmed by enormous terror and dread.

Though heart attacks strike suddenly, and often without forewarning, they do not just happen. A heart attack is the inexorable final step of a slow and lengthy process. You can put cold water in a pot, put the pot on the stove, and turn on the heat. For a while nothing much will seem to change as you watch. But if the heat is high enough, at a certain point bubbles will appear on the surface of the water. You will see very little change all the while the water heats from 32° towards 212°. But then, suddenly, just as it approaches the threshold of 212°, there are dramatic visible changes, and the water boils.

Similarly, the apparent suddenness of a coronary artery closing off and the consequent heart attack is actually quite misleading. In reality, for this final step to occur, our arteries must have been approaching "the boiling point" for some time.

The slow and steady process which takes place in our arteries and inexorably increases our heart attack susceptibility has a name. This process, which is in fact the deeper cause of almost all heart attacks, is called "atherosclerosis."

Atherosclerosis is often referred to in common speech as "hardening of the arteries," and although this is not an entirely inaccurate way of describing what happens, "narrowing of the arteries" would be a better catchphrase, though this, too, would be less than exact.

Atherosclerosis is the process by which arteries gradually accumulate fatty and waxy deposits on their inner walls—thus reducing the size of the openings through which the blood can flow. The foreign deposits which adhere to the inner walls of the arteries are called "atheromas," or "plaques."

When these plaques become advanced enough, the fatty contents of the deposits will rupture into the artery and form a clot. These clots may clog up the already reduced arterial opening, and thus entirely prevent the flow of blood through the artery.

If a clot forms in one of the two coronary arteries that supply the heart with its only source of life-giving blood, and the coronary artery becomes blocked by the clot, the heart is deprived of its supply of life-giving blood, and the result is a heart attack.

There could be no heart attack unless the coronary arteries had already become partially closed and irritated by atherosclerotic deposits. Atherosclerosis, the real culprit, is what must be eliminated to prevent heart attacks.

There is another part of the body particularly vulnerable to having its blood supply cut off by an obstructed artery. It is the part of the body whose functioning, or lack of it, has often been the source of wit:

> *"The brain is a wonderful organ; it starts working the moment you get up in the morning, and does not stop until you get into the office."*

In truth, however, the physical failure of the brain to function is far from a laughing matter. Strokes, like heart attacks, often occur with no

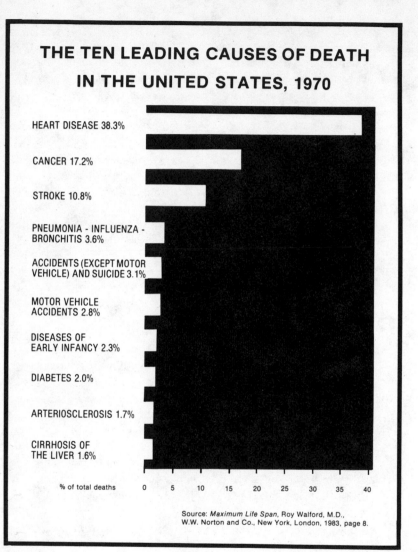

THE TEN LEADING CAUSES OF DEATH
IN THE UNITED STATES, 1970

HEART DISEASE 38.3%

CANCER 17.2%

STROKE 10.8%

PNEUMONIA - INFLUENZA -
BRONCHITIS 3.6%

ACCIDENTS (EXCEPT MOTOR
VEHICLE) AND SUICIDE 3.1%

MOTOR VEHICLE
ACCIDENTS 2.8%

DISEASES OF
EARLY INFANCY 2.3%

DIABETES 2.0%

ARTERIOSCLEROSIS 1.7%

CIRRHOSIS OF
THE LIVER 1.6%

% of total deaths   0   5   10   15   20   25   30   35   40

Source: *Maximum Life Span*, Roy Walford, M.D.,
W.W. Norton and Co., New York, London, 1983, page 8.

prior warning, and, like heart attacks, they often kill. Strokes account for more deaths in the United States today than any other cause except heart attacks and cancer.

In fact, strokes are very similar events to heart attacks, except that they take place in different bodily locations. For just as atherosclerotic deposits in the arteries feeding the heart set the stage for heart attacks, atherosclerotic deposits in the arteries feeding the brain set the stage for strokes. And just as the affected part of the heart dies when its blood supply becomes blocked off, so the affected part of the brain dies when its blood supply is compromised by arterial blockage. As with the heart, this can only occur when the arteries have become hardened, narrowed and encrusted with atherosclerosis.

If we add up the deaths caused by heart attacks, strokes, and other consequences of atherosclerosis, we get a figure larger than all other causes of death in the United States combined. Statistically, you and I each have better than a 50-50 chance of dying from a disease directly caused by the clogging up of our arteries.

HOPE

For years it was thought that heart disease and strokes were simply misfortunes we had to somehow learn to accept. But over the last thirty years, this has changed. The most comprehensive research in medical history has discovered something of marvelous and far-reaching consequence: we are not helpless victims of atherosclerosis. It is a disease which, knowingly or unknowingly, we bring upon ourselves, and by the same token, can prevent.

I am reminded of one of Aesop's Fables:

The Eagle and the Arrow
An eagle sat on a lofty rock, watching the movements of a hare whom he sought to make his prey. An archer, who saw the eagle from a place of concealment, took an accurate aim and wounded him mortally. The eagle gave one look at the arrow that had entered his heart, and saw in that single glance that its feathers had been furnished by himself.

"It is a double grief to me," he exclaimed woefully, "that I should perish by an arrow feathered from my own wings."

The most advanced medical knowledge in history is telling us that heart attack and stroke victims—50% of us—perish from a disease nurtured by our own hands.

The growth in the medical understanding of heart disease that has taken place in the last thirty years is one of the great stories in medical history. With each passing year, more and more of the most respected medical organizations in the world have come to the same conclusion: Diets high in saturated fat and cholesterol raise the level of cholesterol in the blood, produce atherosclerosis, and lead directly to heart disease and strokes. Diets low in saturated fat and cholesterol lower the level of cholesterol in the blood, decrease atherosclerosis, and lower the likelihood of heart disease and strokes.[1]

The medical statistics are clear. We can virtually stab ourselves in the heart with our forks by eating a diet that promotes atherosclerosis. Or we can overwhelmingly reduce our potential for heart disease by eating a diet that supports the health of our cardiovascular system.

Many a deeply inspiring story has emerged from the dedicated medical researchers working day in and day out for year after year to discover what has been learned. At the same time, however, there are other stories which are anything but inspiring. There are powerful interests who profit from the sale of foods high in saturated fat and cholesterol who recognize that the advances in medical understanding are not to their financial advantage. And though they have not been able to impede the growth of medical knowledge, they have been remarkably successful in preventing the public from having the full benefit of what has been learned, employing ruse after ruse in their efforts to keep our nation hooked on foods high in saturated fat and cholesterol. What the tobacco industry is for lung cancer, these industries have become for the heart attack.

THE FIRST EVIDENCE
Some of the first evidence indicating that atherosclerosis was not simply a consequence of "growing old," but was rooted in our dietary intake of saturated fat and cholesterol, came inadvertently from the Korean War. Soldiers who had been killed were autopsied, and medical researchers were stunned by what they found. More than 77% of the

American soldiers had blood vessels which were already narrowed by atherosclerotic deposits, while the arteries of the equally young soldiers of the opposing forces showed no similar damage.[2]

At the time, it was thought that the pronounced differences in the conditions of the soldiers' arteries might be more a consequence of genetic predisposition than of their differing diet-styles. But this idea became quickly untenable when a large group of Korean soldiers were put on the U.S. Army diet. They rapidly developed significant increases in their blood cholesterol levels, an unmistakable sign of developing atherosclerosis.[3]

Traditional nutritionists had thought highly of meat, dairy products and eggs ever since the early animal experiments which showed rats grew faster on animal protein. As well, the first vitamin ever discovered, Vitamin A, had originally been isolated from butterfat, which also added to the aura of supremacy these foods enjoyed.

But as a result of the autopsies, the possibility that dairy products, meat and eggs might be seriously involved in heart disease now had to be taken seriously for the first time. Meat, dairy products and eggs are the chief source of dietary saturated fat. Along with fish, they are the **only** sources of dietary cholesterol.

Stirred by the results of the Korean War autopsies, medical researchers undertook a major effort to learn more. From 1963 to 1965, a worldwide study of heart disease and stroke patterns was done, called the International Atherosclerotic Project. This truly mammoth undertaking involved examining the arteries of over 20,000 autopsied bodies throughout the world.[4] The findings revealed an unmistakable pattern: people who lived in areas where consumption of saturated fat and cholesterol were high had markedly more atherosclerosis, more heart attacks, and more strokes.[5]

It took a while for medical researchers to grasp the full implications of what was being learned, because the emerging truth required them to do a complete about-face from their well-entrenched assumptions.

The meat, dairy and egg industries, meanwhile, were not exactly eager to support the researchers' new findings. They financed numerous studies which attempted to vindicate their products and discredit

what they called the saturated fat and cholesterol "theory" of atherosclerosis. Some pointed out that animal foods were not the only products high in saturated fat, and attempted to point an accusing finger at
plant sources. Directing attention to coconuts, palm kernel oil, and
chocolate, which are all high in saturated fat, they loudly proclaimed
that meat, dairy products and eggs should not be singled out and found
guilty as the sole suppliers of saturated fats in our diets. But scientists
who were not on the payroll of these industries, and who were perhaps
a bit more impartial in their motivation, pointed out that coconuts,
palm kernel oil and chocolate are the **only** plant foods significantly
high in saturated fat. They also suggested that meat, eggs and dairy
products probably make up a larger percentage of most people's diets
than do coconuts, palm kernel oil, and chocolate.

Further, they pointed out that cholesterol cannot be found in any
plant food. As the figure on page 211 shows, our entire intake of cholesterol is necessarily derived from meat, fish, dairy products and eggs.

THE MOUNTING CONSENSUS
With each new study the evidence was becoming harder and harder to
brush aside. The industries who foresaw their profits seriously threatened by the advancing knowledge, however, managed to overlook
much that was being learned, and to insist that hereditary influences
were more important than one's intake of saturated fat and cholesterol.
To find out if there could be any truth to this, Dr. M. G. Marmot and
his co-workers at the University of California, Berkeley, undertook a
major study of the heart disease rates of men of Japanese descent who
lived in different parts of the world and ate according to the various
local diet-styles. The results stunned a medical world still finding it
hard to believe meat, dairy products and eggs were suspect. The study
found an almost exact statistical correlation for all groups between
consumption of saturated fat and cholesterol, and deaths due to coronary heart disease.[6]

With each passing year the evidence mounted. In 1970, Dr. Ancel
Keys of the University of Minnesota School of Public Health published the results of a massive seven-country study analyzing the role of
diet in heart disease.[7] The study involved over 12,000 men in Finland,

CHOLESTEROL CONTENT
OF COMMON FOODS

ANIMAL FOOD		PLANT FOOD	
Cholesterol Content (in Milligrams per 100 Gram Portion)		*Cholesterol Content (in Milligrams per 100 Gram Portion)*	
Egg, whole	550		
Kidney, beef	375		
Liver, beef	300	All grains	0
Butter	250	All vegetables	0
Oysters	200	All nuts	0
Cream cheese	120	All seeds	0
Lard	95	All fruits	0
Beefsteak	70	All legumes	0
Lamb	70	All vegetable oils	0
Pork	70		
Chicken	60		
Ice cream	45		

Source: Pennington, J., _Food Values of Portions Commonly Used_,
Harper and Row, 14th ed., New York 1985

Greece, Italy, Japan, the Netherlands, the United States, and Yugoslavia. It found telling correlations between the amount of saturated fat
and cholesterol in a people's diet, the levels of cholesterol in their
blood, and their death rate from heart disease. Of these nations, the
United States and Finland had the highest consumption of animal
products, the highest consumption of saturated fat, the highest consumption of cholesterol—and the highest death rate from heart disease.[8]

It was becoming increasingly difficult to deny the evidence implicating saturated fat and cholesterol, though the industries whose products were being incriminated were trying diligently. Unable to counter
the accumulating evidence, they ignored it, continuing to insist hereditary factors were primary.

Dr. Keys' massive study, and others like it, however, indicated
otherwise. It was common knowledge that different groups of the men
under study such as clerks, miners, mechanics, farmers and doctors
tend to have their own diet-styles, with their corresponding levels of
saturated fat intake. And it was also common knowledge that Japanese
who lived in the West had diet-styles different from those in Japan. But
when the levels of saturated fat in the diets of each of these various
groups were compared to their blood cholesterol counts, the results
were spectacular. As the figure on page 213 shows, the correlation
between saturated fat consumption and blood cholesterol levels could
hardly have been more exact.

Even those researchers most attached to traditional ideas were
coming to conclude that the more saturated fat and cholesterol in a
person's diet, the more cholesterol would be in his blood, the worse
shape his arteries would be in, and the more likely a candidate he
would be for a heart attack or a stroke.

The meat, dairy and egg industries were far from pleased with the
way things were going.

INCREASING CLARITY

The evidence implicating the traditional mainstays of the Western diet
was not accepted overnight. Because firmly established beliefs were
being so seriously threatened, it was subjected to the most rigorous

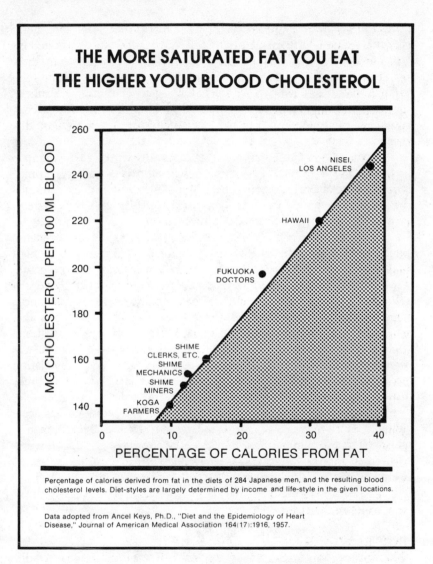

**THE MORE SATURATED FAT YOU EAT
THE HIGHER YOUR BLOOD CHOLESTEROL**

Percentage of calories derived from fat in the diets of 284 Japanese men, and the resulting blood cholesterol levels. Diet-styles are largely determined by income and life-style in the given locations.

Data adopted from Ancel Keys, Ph.D., "Diet and the Epidemiology of Heart Disease," Journal of American Medical Association 164(17):1916, 1957.

testing in medical history. Though I do not ethically condone most laboratory experiments on animals, the results of such tests were another nail in the coffin for conventional dietary wisdom. At the University of Chicago, Dr. Robert Wissler and his co-workers fed a standard American diet to rhesus monkeys. To a second group of monkeys they fed a diet different only in that it was lower in saturated fat, cholesterol and calories. After a time, they killed the monkeys and examined their arteries. The monkeys fed the standard American diet had six times as much atherosclerosis as the other monkeys.[9]

Scientists were not only finding they could produce atherosclerosis in animals by feeding them diets with saturated fat and cholesterol, they were also finding that they could then unclog the arteries of the animals by reducing their intake of these particular substances. At the University of Iowa, Dr. Mark Armstrong and his colleagues fed a group of monkeys a diet rich in egg yolk, one of the leading suppliers of saturated fat and cholesterol in the American diet. The coronary arteries of these monkeys rapidly became encrusted with atherosclerosis. After the arteries of the monkeys had become over half closed, the researchers markedly reduced the amount of saturated fat and cholesterol that the monkeys consumed. A year and a half later, the atherosclerosis in the monkeys' arteries was less than one-third what it had become on the diet high in saturated fat and cholesterol.[10] Spokesmen for the meat, dairy and egg industries tried to discount the experiments; but researchers were increasingly impressed because these and similar experiments were repeated with a variety of different animals and the findings were consistent. The only animals able to handle saturated fat and cholesterol without developing substantial atherosclerosis were the natural carnivores. Dr. William S. Collins wrote of these studies in *Medical Counterpoint*:

> "*Recent studies, many of them in my laboratory at the Maiominides Medical Center, appear to indicate that the carnivorous animal has almost unlimited capacity to handle saturated fats and cholesterol, whereas the vegetarian and herbivorous animals have a very restricted capacity to handle these food components. It is virtually impossible to produce atherosclerosis in the dog, for example, even when 120 grams (1/2 pound) of butter*

fat are added to his meat ration . . . On the other hand, adding only two grams of cholesterol daily to a rabbit's chow for two months produces striking fatty changes in its arterial wall. [11]

With each passing year and new set of studies, it was becoming increasingly clear that, like the primates who are closest to us biologically, human beings are among the animals unable to handle saturated fat and cholesterol. The more of these we eat, the more we develop atherosclerosis, and the more likely we are to die of heart disease.

MORE EVIDENCE

In 1964, the heart specialist Dr. Paul Dudley White, renowned for his treatment of President Eisenhower's heart attack, went to visit the Hunzas of Kashmir, to see for himself whether the claims were true that these people lived to exceedingly old ages without any heart disease. He did blood pressure, blood cholesterol, and electrocardiogram studies, yet found not a trace of coronary heart disease, even in the 25 men he studied who were over the age of 90. In his report, published in the *American Heart Journal*, Dr. White suggested a causative correlation between the Hunza's diet-style, which was almost pure vegetarian, and their astounding lack of heart disease.

Scientists began to reason that if meat, eggs and dairy products were in fact the culprits they were becoming to appear, then it would be expected that lacto-ovo vegetarians, who do not eat meat, would have lower heart attack rates and lower heart disease mortality than meat-eaters. If this theory were correct, pure vegetarians, who consume no eggs, dairy products, or meat, would have even lower rates.

Numerous studies were undertaken to find out if this might be the case. One of the largest studies of this kind was conducted at Loma Linda University in California, and involved no less than 24,000 people. Reported in the *American Journal of Clinical Nutrition*, this study found the heart disease mortality rates for lacto-ovo vegetarians to be only one-third that of meat-eaters. Pure vegetarians truly impressive figures—only one-tenth the heart disease death rate of meat-eaters. [12]

Other studies verified these findings. Lacto-ovo vegetarians suffer much less heart disease than do meat-eaters. And pure vegetarians suffer much less than do lacto-ovo vegetarians. [13]

The meat, dairy and egg industries were beginning to panic now, and grasping for straws, suggested that other life-style factors, such as smoking, were to blame.

The staff of the Medical Research Center in Cardiff, Wales, took this possibility seriously and decided to check it out. Their major study statistically eliminated other lifestyle factors, including smoking, as variables. The mortality rate from heart disease was still found to be far less for vegetarians than for non-vegetarians.

Even *Time* Magazine got into the act. Never particularly known for taking controversial stands on dietary issues, *Time* did a cover story on the latest medical findings regarding cholesterol and heart disease and noted:

> *"In regions where . . . meat is scarce, cardiovascular disease is unknown."* [14]

The medical consensus linking meat, dairy products and eggs to heart disease was becoming virtually unanimous. An article by cardiologist Dr. Kaare Norum, published in the *Journal of the Norwegian Medical Association* left no doubt about the universality of the growing consensus. Dr. Norum polled a large international cross-section of scientists who were "actively engaged in arteriosclerosis problems." Ninety-nine percent of the heart disease researchers affirmed the link between diet and heart disease. The dietary culprits they cited were too many calories, too much saturated fat, and too much cholesterol. [15]

It was getting to the point where a medical researcher would just about have to bury his head in the sand to avoid seeing the pattern.

SMOKE SCREEN

The growing certainty that saturated fat and cholesterol promote heart disease and strokes was a foreboding omen for the meat, dairy and egg industries. They found themselves increasingly on the defensive, in a position as embarrassing as the one occupied in recent years by the tobacco industry.

The medical evidence regarding the tragic health consequences of smoking is utterly overwhelming. [16] But the tobacco industry does what

THE MOUNTING CONSENSUS

With each passing year more and more expert organizations publicly affirmed the role of saturated fat and cholesterol in heart disease.

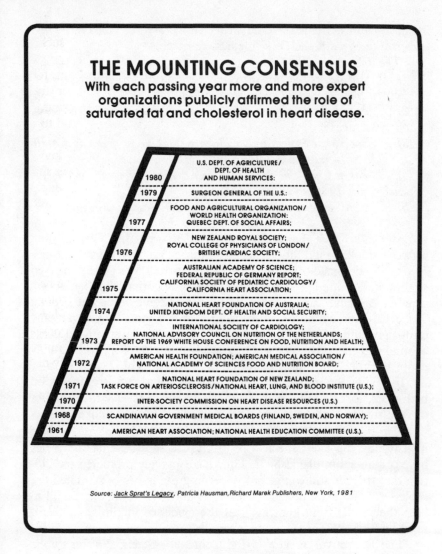

1980	U.S. DEPT. OF AGRICULTURE / DEPT. OF HEALTH AND HUMAN SERVICES:
1979	SURGEON GENERAL OF THE U.S.:
1977	FOOD AND AGRICULTURAL ORGANIZATION / WORLD HEALTH ORGANIZATION: QUEBEC DEPT. OF SOCIAL AFFAIRS;
1976	NEW ZEALAND ROYAL SOCIETY; ROYAL COLLEGE OF PHYSICIANS OF LONDON / BRITISH CARDIAC SOCIETY;
1975	AUSTRALIAN ACADEMY OF SCIENCE; FEDERAL REPUBLIC OF GERMANY REPORT; CALIFORNIA SOCIETY OF PEDIATRIC CARDIOLOGY / CALIFORNIA HEART ASSOCIATION;
1974	NATIONAL HEART FOUNDATION OF AUSTRALIA; UNITED KINGDOM DEPT. OF HEALTH AND SOCIAL SECURITY;
1973	INTERNATIONAL SOCIETY OF CARDIOLOGY; NATIONAL ADVISORY COUNCIL ON NUTRITION OF THE NETHERLANDS; REPORT OF THE 1969 WHITE HOUSE CONFERENCE ON FOOD, NUTRITION AND HEALTH;
1972	AMERICAN HEALTH FOUNDATION; AMERICAN MEDICAL ASSOCIATION / NATIONAL ACADEMY OF SCIENCES FOOD AND NUTRITION BOARD;
1971	NATIONAL HEART FOUNDATION OF NEW ZEALAND; TASK FORCE ON ARTERIOSCLEROSIS / NATIONAL HEART, LUNG, AND BLOOD INSTITUTE (U.S.);
1970	INTER-SOCIETY COMMISSION ON HEART DISEASE RESOURCES (U.S.)
1968	SCANDINAVIAN GOVERNMENT MEDICAL BOARDS (FINLAND, SWEDEN, AND NORWAY);
1961	AMERICAN HEART ASSOCIATION; NATIONAL HEALTH EDUCATION COMMITTEE (U.S.).

Source: Jack Sprat's Legacy, Patricia Hausman, Richard Marek Publishers, New York, 1981 it can to confuse the issue. One writer caricatured the tobacco industry's stance towards the latest medical research:

"The Tobacco Industry . . .

1) . . . still insists that the three main causes of lung cancer are flat feet, backgammon, and gargling with Top Job.

2) . . . considers a scientific test to be inconclusive unless it kills everyone who takes it.

3) . . . hopes that enough kids will start smoking to make up for all the older smokers who are dropping dead.

4) . . . has warned the Surgeon General that telling everything he knows may be hazardous to his health.

5) . . . won't even concede that inhaling water causes drowning."[17]

In order to say that the final word isn't yet in on the "alleged" link between smoking and lung cancer, the tobacco industry funds studies specifically designed to confuse the issues. It then uses these contrived studies in its attempt to convince the public that the "question" whether smoking causes cancer is still unanswered. A recent Federal Trade Commission survey discovered that the industry's advertising campaign calling for an "open debate" on the "unsubstantiated perils of smoking" is apparently working. Half of all smokers still actually doubt whether smoking is dangerous to their health.

In giving the impression that there are legitimate arguments on both sides, and that the issues have not yet been resolved, you might say the tobacco industry has succeeded in creating a smoke screen.

Placed in an increasingly parallel position to that of the tobacco industry by the latest medical research, the saturated fat industries have responded in like fashion. They have actively promoted the illusion that there is still confusion concerning the issues of saturated fat, cholesterol and heart disease. They have done whatever they could to keep the public from knowing that the evidence incriminating saturated fat and cholesterol is now overwhelming.

The Executive Director of the Center for Science in the Public Interest, Michael Jacobson, is aware of the tactics of these industries. Says Jacobson:

"Despite the massive amount of scientific evidence linking fat to heart disease, a relative handful of researchers has created in many minds the illusion that great controversy surrounds the 'theory'. . . For instance, in June 1980, a committee of the National Academy of Sciences issued a report defending the current fatty diet. The main authors of the report were professors who had for many years received grants from or were paid consultants to the National Dairy Council, the National Livestock and Meat Board, the American Egg Board . . . and other industries whose profits depend on Americans' pathogenic diet. One such professor was quoted in the press as being surprised that people thought the $250,000.00 he received as a consultant to the egg and other industries would cloud his objectivity regarding the nutritional value of eggs . . .

"Dietary fat and cholesterol . . . speed the development of some of the most dreaded diseases and contribute to hundreds of thousands of deaths a year. These diseases include coronary heart disease, peripheral arteriosclerosis, gangrene, hearing loss, cancers of the breast and colon, and cerebral hemorrhage . . .

"While doctors have developed methods to prevent or cure most infectious diseases, they have found the chronic diseases much tougher to eradicate. The bacteria and other microbes that cause infectious diseases have no friends or allies to defend their interests, and can be treated mercilessly as the health menaces they are. However . . . some of the agents that cause degenerative diseases have powerful allies in the industrial world . . .

"Over the years, the 'fat lobby'—the meat, dairy and egg industries, and their academic and political allies—has not only influenced our nation's food and nutrition policies, it has **determined** *those policies."* [18]

THE BATTLEFIELD

You might think that with the growing wave of evidence indicating saturated fat and cholesterol as killers of more Americans than all the wars in our nation's history combined, the meat, dairy and egg industries would be hard-pressed to maintain control over our food and nutrition policies. But the cards are stacked. They may not have inter-

ests of public health on their side, but their lobbying groups and political action committees are well financed, battle-hardened veterans of
political in-fighting. Opposing them are scientists and medical researchers whose skills don't lie in the political sphere, and who have
little financial backing compared to what the industries provide their
representatives. The fight is far from fair.

> *"As a rule, scientists and medical researchers make poor players in
> the complex game of special-interest politics, although they often
> think otherwise. They are not well endowed with the stamina,
> patience, and shrewdness that this game requires, and deep down
> they view it as an anti-intellectual activity beneath their scholarly
> dignity. Even when organized into illustrious professional groups
> they shrink from combat and bloodletting. This is more a reflection
> of the unsuitedness of their training and temperament to the
> political arena than it is a mark of weakness of conviction."* [19]

On one side of the battlefield stands a formidable and experienced
alliance of meat, egg, and dairy producers, with their purchased political and scientific allies. On the other side stands a relatively unorgan-
ized collection of independent medical researchers, underfinanced
public interest and consumer groups, and the handful of political leaders who are willing to endure the sizable risk of an unpopular stance.

In this battle, the industries who sell us foods high in saturated fat
and cholesterol have produced multi-million dollar public relations
campaigns, telling us brightly of the "incredible, edible egg," repeat-
ing that beef is "nutrition you can sink your teeth into," and reassuring
us that "milk does a body good." They do not mention that these foods
clog our arteries, and promote heart disease and strokes.

Of course no advertising mentions the disadvantages of the products it promotes. But time and time again these industries have drawn
the ire of consumer groups, the courts, and medical researchers for
their flagrant disregard of fact.

In 1985, the Beef Council had the dubious distinction of being a
repeat winner of the Harlan Page Hubbard Memorial Award for the
year's most deceptive and misleading advertising.[20] The award, named

for a famous charlatan who glowingly advertised a worthless patent medicine, is given by a collection of consumer groups who are used to the distortions and exaggerations that typify Madison Avenue. But even to their weathered eyes the "beef gives strength" campaign took the cake for implying that beef is low in fat. The servings shown in the ads were only three ounces, when, according to USDA data, the average beef steak serving is double that. By not explaining that the serving shown in the ad is only half the size most people eat, the industry conveyed the impression that servings of beef are much lower in fat than they actually are. In announcing the award, Bonnie Liebman of the Center for Science in the Public Interest also pointed out that the technicians who did the laboratory analysis which produced the calorie and fat counts referred to in the ads used scalpels to remove every possible bit of fat from the meat samples. Thus the fat and calorie levels reported were not only for a serving size much smaller than viewers understood it to be, but also for a serving which had been trimmed of fat with a meticulousness no homemaker could possibly match.[21] The industry ads also did not mention that cholesterol is found mostly in lean tissues, not in fat, and so no matter how meticulously you trim away the fat you cannot significantly reduce the level of cholesterol.

The industry ads have to go to such great lengths to give the impression their products are healthy because the truth is so incriminating.

Meanwhile, the California Milk Producers presented a series of expensive television ads in which celebrities such as columnist Abigail Van Buren ("Dear Abby"), swimmer Mark Spitz, baseball player Vida Blue, and dancer Ray Bolger proclaimed that "Everybody Needs Milk." The Federal Trade Commission, however, didn't agree. It took legal steps towards prosecuting the milk producers and their advertising agency, calling the advertising "false, misleading and deceptive."[22] The dairymen quickly changed their tune, and came up with a new slogan—"Milk Has Something for Everybody."

One medical researcher familiar with the matter laughed when he saw their latest deception. Said Dr. Kevin McGrady, "Milk has something for everybody all right—higher blood cholesterol, and increased risk of heart disease and strokes."

EGG ON THEIR FACE

The meat and dairy industries are not alone in their misleading presentations to the public. The egg industry has also produced advertising campaigns designed to deny the saturated fat and cholesterol problems arising from consumption of their product. Of all foods, eggs are the highest in cholesterol, but the egg industry has not been one to stand by and let a fact like that take a bite out of its profits.

In 1971, after the American Heart Association took its stand on dietary cholesterol and heart disease, the egg producers countered by forming the National Commission on Egg Nutrition for the specific purpose of fighting the American Heart Association viewpoint. To accomplish this purpose, the newly formed commission presented a series of expensive ads in the Wall Street Journal and elsewhere. These ads attacked what they called the "theory" that saturated fat and cholesterol promote heart disease. A typical ad stated:

"There is absolutely no scientific evidence that eating eggs, even in quantity, will increase the risk of a heart attack." [23]

On seeing these ads, the American Heart Association immediately asked the Federal Trade Commission to prohibit this "false, deceptive and misleading advertising."[24] The Federal Trade Commission considered both sides of the matter, and then filed a formal complaint against the National Commission on Egg Nutrition, and its advertising agency, Richard Weiner, Inc.[25] Understandably dismayed by this turn of events, the egg industry hired the best legal counsel it could find. The attorneys studied the matter in depth, then turned around and told the egg industry that its "chances of beating the lawsuit on scientific grounds are almost nil."[26]

There followed a lengthy court battle, in which the egg producers tried, among other rationalizations, to defend their ad campaign under the First Amendment guarantee of free speech.[27] But the judge wasn't convinced; in his 101 page decision, he called the statements made by the National Commission on Egg Nutrition:

". . . false, misleading, deceptive and unfair." [28]

Ruled Judge Ernest G. Barnes:

> *"There exists a substantial body of competent and reliable scientific evidence that eating eggs increases the risk of heart attacks or heart disease . . . This evidence is systematic, consistent, strong and congruent."* [29]

The ruling also chastised the egg industry for deceptively camouflaging their intentions by naming their organization the National Commission on Egg Nutrition:

> *"(The name) National Commission on Egg Nutrition implies an impartial, independent, quasi-governmental health commission, when in fact it is an association of persons engaged in the egg industry."* [30]

The National Commission on Egg Nutrition was unable to convince the Federal Trade Commission, the Court, and even its own attorneys that eggs do not raise blood cholesterol and promote heart disease. But this did not prevent the egg industry from trying to make the American public believe eggs were not a danger.

In its efforts to scramble the public mind, the egg industry designed and paid for numerous studies they hoped would give the appearance that the cholesterol in eggs is harmless. [31] An authority on clinical nutrition research, Dr. John McDougall, studied the medical literature, and noticed something interesting:

> *"Of the six studies in the medical literature that fail to demonstrate a significant rise in blood cholesterol level with the consumption of whole eggs, three were paid for by the American Egg Board, one by the Missouri Egg Merchandising Council, and one by the Egg Program of the California Department of Agriculture. Support for the sixth paper was not identified . . .*
>
> *"The trick is in knowing how to design your experiment so you will get the results you are looking for. To get little or no increase in cholesterol results, you first saturate your subjects with cholesterol*

*from other sources, because studies show that once people consume
more than 400 to 800 milligrams of cholesterol per day, additional
cholesterol has only a minor effect on blood cholesterol levels . . .
Well designed studies by investigators, independent of the food
industry, clearly demonstrate the detrimental effects of eggs on blood
cholesterol levels.* [32]

The studies financed by the egg industry seemed to exonerate eggs.
But independent investigators consistently got very different results.[33]
At the University of Minnesota, scientists found that a diet with 380
mg of egg yolk cholesterol per day caused an average blood cholesterol
level 16 mg higher than a diet with only 50 mg cholesterol.[34] At the
Harvard School of Public Health, Dr. Mark Hegstead achieved similar
results, finding that each 100 mg of egg yolk cholesterol raised blood
cholesterol levels in adult men an average of four to five mg.[35]

Still, the egg industry continued to insist that egg consumption did
not raise blood cholesterol, and to claim their studies were valid. In
1984, yet another impartial study was undertaken to resolve the issue.
This study, published in the British medical journal *Lancet*, sought to
test the effects of egg consumption on blood cholesterol with as much
objectivity as humanly possible.

The experiment was imaginative. A group of subjects was fed an
egg daily, disguised in a dessert. Another group of subjects was fed an
identical dessert, without the egg. Otherwise their diets were identical,
and contained no eggs or other high-cholesterol foods. In order to in-
sure the test's objectivity, the whole thing was done double-blind: neither the researchers nor the subjects knew who had eaten the eggs until
the test was completed. The results were convincing and the egg industry's position was dealt quite a blow when, after only three weeks,
the subjects whose desserts contained the egg showed a 12% rise in
their blood cholesterol levels; the other group showed no such rise.[36] It
is hard to overestimate the significance of this information. A 12% rise
in blood cholesterol levels amounts to a 24% rise in heart attack risk.

The egg industry, however, was not dismayed. They realized that
in any struggle there are bound to be obstacles that must be sur-
mounted. Resolutely, they continued to deny the link between eggs
and heart disease.

When the Senate Select Committee on Nutrition and Human Needs, under the chairmanship of Senator George McGovern, met to establish guidelines for the nation's food choices, the egg industry presented five different research studies which they claimed exonerated eggs. These reports, however, were so confusing that McGovern asked the National Heart, Lung and Blood Institute for an expert opinion on their validity.

The Institute carefully examined each of the five studies, then reported to Congress that the studies seemed deliberately designed to distort the facts. The Institute's impartial appraisal was that the studies were "seriously flawed, . . . meaningless and should be discarded."[37]

Undaunted, the egg industry did the only thing it could. It hired an advertising agency and began a massive publicity campaign based on the very studies that had been so thoroughly discredited. Fliers were inserted into many millions of egg cartons reassuring egg consumers that "eggs don't raise cholesterol."[38]

Through it all the egg industry has remained as dedicated as they could be. They evidently figure that if two wrongs don't make a right, perhaps three or four might do the trick.

MORE SHENANIGANS

The shenanigans continue to this day. The industries profiting from our consumption of saturated fat and cholesterol have had to search desperately for a means to defend their products, but they have been willing to do so. You may have heard that cholesterol is necessary for bodily functioning. This was one of the key features of the National Commission on Egg Nutrition's advertising campaign that was ruled "false, misleading, deceptive and unfair." The ads headlined the fact that cholesterol plays an essential role in the body's biochemistry. Featuring "facts about cholesterol," the ads proclaimed the many bodily functions which are dependent on cholesterol for their operation.

The courts put a stop to this false advertising. But to this day "educational materials" supplied to our nation's schools by the meat, dairy and egg industries continue to assert that cholesterol is indispensable to human life processes. At one level, the claims are correct. Cholesterol does play an essential role in the body's biochemistry. However, the implication is strongly made that there is therefore a value in consuming cholesterol in our diets—an implication with absolutely no basis in fact.

In reviewing the egg industry's defense of dietary cholesterol on these grounds, the court heard testimony from many of the nation's top medical researchers. The egg industry, of course, brought in its own experts. After considering all the presentations and arguments, the court found that there is not a single case on record of anyone ever suffering from a deficiency of dietary cholesterol.

> *"As far as we can determine, all of us would do just as well if we had no cholesterol in our diet. Cholesterol can be made by all of the cells in the body so we don't need to take in any." (Dr. Robert Levy, Director of the National Heart, Lung and Blood Institute)*[39]
> *"There is no known evidence that low-cholesterol diets are harmful, or that dietary cholesterol is an essential nutrient in any human condition." (Task Force to the American Society of Clinical Nutrition)*[40]

Under court order, the egg industry finally had to stop running ads that represented cholesterol as an essential dietary nutrient. And the court told them once again to stop denying the link between cholesterol and heart disease.

Undaunted, however, the egg industry simply reversed its field and carried on its campaign to muddle the issues. It began now to join the meat and dairy industries in their protestations that the body tends to produce less cholesterol as more is consumed in the diet. They implied, therefore, that dietary cholesterol is harmless. We can eat as much as we want, they said, because our bodies will compensate.

To support this, the meat, dairy and egg industries have repeatedly referred to some of the earliest cholesterol experiments, undismayed by the fact that the results have been retracted by the very people who performed them.[41] These early studies were done before it was discovered that the body can absorb cholesterol only if it is accompanied by fat. Not knowing this, the researchers used pure cholesterol crystals. We know now that it was only because the cholesterol was given in crystalline form that blood cholesterol levels didn't rise in these early experiments.[42] The industries that profit from our cholesterol consumption still refer to these early studies, using them as "proof" our bodies compensate for cholesterol intake by producing proportionately less. They have chosen to disregard the public statements made by the researchers themselves, that these early experiments have no bearing whatsoever on the health consequences of cholesterol consumption, because, unlike cholesterol crystals, cholesterol in food is always accompanied by sufficient fat to be absorbed by the body.

The industries wanting to keep us hooked on cholesterol have to resort to such shenanigans because current medical research gives them no other place to stand. It is true that as we eat more cholesterol, we produce a bit less. But the decrease in body production is nowhere near equal to the amount consumed. Until we reach dangerous saturation points, every milligram of dietary cholesterol tends to elevate the amount of cholesterol in our blood, cause atherosclerosis, and open the door to heart attacks and strokes.[43]

The *American Journal of Clinical Nutrition* reported an impartial study designed to measure the effect of different amounts of dietary cholesterol on blood cholesterol levels. A number of men were put on cholesterol-free diets for 21 days, and their blood cholesterol levels carefully monitored. Then the men were divided into four groups. For the next 42 days, each group was fed a diet with a specific cholesterol level. Then their blood was measured to see how they had fared. The results, shown in the figure on page 228, lived up to the egg industry's worst fears. The more cholesterol the subjects consumed, the more rapidly and the higher their blood cholesterol counts rose.[44]

Literally dozens of independent studies have shown the same thing. But the meat, egg and dairy industries, in their efforts to make the whole thing appear controversial, have managed to ignore them all. They have not always been able to avoid stumbling over the truth, but they seem always to manage to pick themselves up and carry on as if nothing had happened.

HUCKSTERS IN THE CLASSROOM
Perhaps the most insidious weapon of the saturated fat industries is the deep credibility and legitimacy they have in the public mind. They can

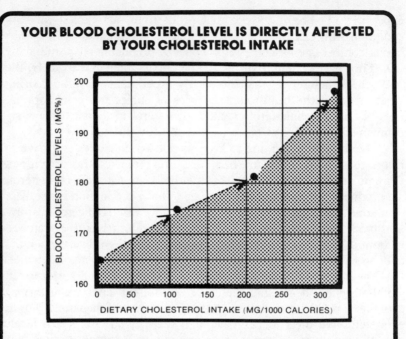

YOUR BLOOD CHOLESTEROL LEVEL IS DIRECTLY AFFECTED BY YOUR CHOLESTEROL INTAKE

A study was done to measure the effect of dietary cholesterol on blood cholesterol. 56 men were put on a cholesterol-free diet for 21 days. They were then divided into 4 groups. Each group was given a diet with a fixed cholesterol intake for the next 42 days. Then their blood cholesterol levels were measured. The results:

Number of Men	Dietary Cholesterol Intake (mg/1000 ca.)	Blood Cholesterol Levels (mg%)	Net Changes
18	0	164.7	3.4
11	106	174.7	13.0
13	212	181.4	23.8
14	317	198.4	40.5

Source: Mattson, F. "Effect of Dietary Cholesterol on Serum Cholesterol in Man," Amer. Journ. Clin. Nutr. 25:589, 1972

count on our loyalty because for decades they have provided schools with much of the materials used for "nutritional education."

Dr. Pascal Imperato, former Commissioner of Health for New York City, and Chairman of the Department of Medicine at New York's Downstate Medical Center, notes:

> *"The National Dairy Council, with the government's permission, (is still) the largest and most important provider of nutrition education in the country . . . That the Dairy Council can still convincingly promote saturated fat and cholesterol-rich diets reflects . . . the credibility it built in the days before the link between these elements and atherosclerosis was known."* [45]

Most of us grew up thinking of the National Dairy Council as a benign organization whose purpose was wholesome and pure. Just as the "National Commission on Egg Nutrition" sounds like an independent health organization concerned with our well-being, the name "National Dairy Council" seems to imply an impartial group of elders who have come together to provide us their wisdom and council. When they told us milk was "nature's most perfect food," we believed them. When they told us to drink a glass of milk with every meal, we did as we were told. Little did we know this was an organization especially organized to sell the American public as much milk, and particularly as much milk fat, as possible.

The trade magazine, *Dairyman,* understands that the Dairy Council's job is to promote the sale of milk. As they explained:

> *"It's important to understand the unique role the Dairy Council plays in promoting milk. The Dairy Council does no paid consumer advertising. That noncommerical status is important. As a highly respected education entity its programs give the dairy industry entry into areas difficult to penetrate with straight product promotion, especially the schools and medical-dental professions."* [46]

The Dairy Council "penetrates" the school with a nutritional message that is far from unbiased, though they present it as if it were. They do not mention that the research they use to support their position is usually research they have themselves funded. But in a self-profile titled "Milk Still Makes a Difference," the Dairy Council says of such research:

> *"Research supported through the National Dairy Council's grant-in-aid program seeks to set the record straight about the influence of diet on heart disease. We cannot rest until our product is completely vindicated and put into proper perspective."* [47]

Frankly, I wonder what sort of objectivity can be found in research sponsored by a National Dairy Council grant given specifically to "vindicate" their product.

The Center for Science in the Public Interest is not overly taken with the scientific rigor behind the Dairy Council's message. Says the Center's Executive Director, Michael Jacobson:

> *"In virtually every school district in the country, the minds of two generations of children have been fed the self-serving pap served up in generous portions by the National Dairy Council."* [48]

With active chapters in 128 U.S. cities, the National Dairy Council has over $14 million to invest each year for the sole purpose of getting the public to spend its money on dairy products. And because milk products are priced by federal law according to a pricing structure that provides the dairymen more profit on higher-fat products, the Dairy Council particularly pushes those dairy products with the highest percentage of fat. It apparently does not concern itself with the fact that these are precisely the dairy products which make the greatest contribution to heart disease and strokes.

A child may be only three or four years old when he or she first gets a taste of National Dairy Council materials, such as "Little Ideas," a set of food pictures ostensibly designed to help preschoolers identify foods. It starts out with butter and continues on with 16 other milk products, most of which are high in saturated fat. [49]

As the child progresses, he or she unknowingly continues to receive the Dairy Council message. The Dairy Council provides a se-

quence of curriculum packages to nursery, elementary, junior and senior high schools, called, ironically, "Food: Your Choice."[50] These
materials, which are specifically designed to "help" youngsters choose
dairy products, have been the chief source of nutritional information
for countless American children.

The package designed for "three-to-five-year-old children," called
"Food: Early Choices," cheerfully provides hand puppets, playing
cards, posters, puzzles, and records—along with a message that makes
high-saturated fat milk products sound enticingly attractive.[51]

The package designed for first graders, called "Food: Your Choice,
Level One," is a large box filled with colorful materials, including
bright posters about making milk shakes and pancakes. The recipes
call for ice cream and butter. When yogurt and milk are indicated, it is
never the low-fat versions that are mentioned. The kit also includes
mimeograph supplies to enable the teacher to give handouts to the
children. Of the many handouts available, none features lowfat dairy
products. Instead, cream cheese, ice cream, whole milk and butter are
pictured and happily recommended.[52] These are, of all dairy products,
the very highest in saturated fat.

You may never have thought of ice cream as a health food, but in
"Ice Cream for You and Me," the Dairy Council advises its captive
subjects that:

> *"Ice cream is a healthful food made from milk and cream along
> with other good foods."*[53]

Included in the National Dairy Council's idea of the "healthful milk
group," along with ice cream, is another food you might not have
realized is a health food—chocolate pudding.[54]

The National Dairy Council demonstrates its devotion to milk fat
and its unique version of a balanced diet by telling the children they
should:

> *"Drink milk at every meal and have some in foods like these:
> cheese, ice cream, baked custard, bowl of cream of tomato soup,
> with a pat of butter on top."*[55]

The Dairy Council likes to reach children when they are youngest and most impressionable, and then to reinforce their ideas of "basic four" nutrition at every age level. All the way up through elementary, junior and senior high schools, youngsters are bombarded with the Dairy Council message.

Teenagers are the target for the Dairy Council's helpful little publications: "A Boy And His Physique," and "A Girl And Her Figure."[56] What do you imagine overweight teenagers receive as their first suggestion from the Dairy Council?

"(Drink) whole milk most of the time, skim milk part of the time, if you need to lose weight."[57]

Also highly recommended are "stay-slim sundaes," comprised of ice cream with fruit instead of chocolate sauce for a topping.[58] Perhaps the most remarkable suggestions offered by the Dairy Council to overweight teenagers are the items listed in the "lower calorie section." One bright idea for youngsters with a weight problem is cream cheese, softened with cream, molded into balls, rolled in peanuts and served with fruit![59] Honest! I'm not making this up! Another helpful "low calorie" item is angelfood cake and ice cream.[60]

Given these outrageous recommendations, it is hard to avoid the conclusion that the Dairy Council is more concerned with getting youngsters hooked on a lifetime pattern of high-fat dairy product consumption than with providing sound nutritional education.

HOW TO LIE WITH STATISTICS

Quantifying the amount of fat in a given food is another sensitive area, since there are several ways the fat content of food can be measured. The method generally recognized as the most accurate and reliable is to measure the percentage of calories in a given food which are provided as fat.[61] A second method, useful in certain specific cases, is to measure the grams of fat in a serving of a given food. By both these methods, meat, eggs, and almost all dairy products are seen as what they are—high fat foods.

The industries who profit from our consumption of saturated fat, however, realize that widespread understanding of this fact would

PERCENTAGE OF CALORIES AS FAT

MEATS

Sirloin steak, hipbone, lean w/fat	83%
Pork sausage	83%
T-bone steak, lean w/fat	82%
Porterhouse steak, lean w/fat.	82%
Bacon, lean.	82%
Rib roast, lean w/fat	81%
Bologna.	81%
Country-style sausage	81%
Spareribs	80%
Frankfurters	80%
Lamb rib chops, lean w/fat	79%
Duck meat, w/skin.	76%
Salami	76%
Liverwurst	75%
Rump roast, lean w/fat	71%
Ham, lean w/ fat.	69%
Stewing beef, lean w/fat	66%
Goose meat, w/skin	65%
Ground beef, fairly lean	64%
Veal breast, lean w/fat.	64%
Leg of lamb, lean w/fat	61%
Chicken, dark meat w/skin, roasted	56%
Round steak, lean w/fat.	53%
Chuck rib roast, lean only	50%
Chuck steak, lean only	50%
Chicken, light meat w/skin, roasted	44%
Turkey, dark meat w/skin	47%
Lamb rib chops, lean only	45%
Sirloin steak, hipbone, lean only	47%

VEGETABLES

Mustard greens	13%
Kale	13%
Beet greens	12%
Lettuce	12%
Turnip greens	11%
Mushrooms.	8%
Cabbage	7%
Cauliflower.	7%
Eggplant	7%
Asparagus	6%
Green beans	6%
Celery	6%
Cucumber	6%
Turnip	6%
Zucchini	6%
Carrots.	4%
Green peas	4%
Artichokes.	3%
Onions.	3%
Beets	2%
Chives	1%
Potatoes	1%

FISH

Tuna, chunk, oil-packed	63%
Herring, Pacific.	59%
Anchovies	54%
Bass, black sea	53%
Perch, ocean	53%
Caviar, sturgeon	52%
Mackerel, Pacific	50%
Sardines, Atlantic, in oil, drained	49%
Salmon, sockeye (red).	49%

LEGUMES

Tofu.	49%
Soybean	37%
Soybean sprouts	28%
Garbanzo bean	11%
Kidney bean	4%
Lima bean	4%
Mungbean sprouts.	4%
Lentil	3%
Broad bean	3%
Mung bean	3%

Source: "Nutrititive Value of American Foods in Common Units,"
U.S.D.A. Handbook No. 456

PERCENTAGE OF CALORIES AS FAT

DAIRY PRODUCTS

Butter. 100%
Cream, light whipping 92%
Cream cheese. 90%
Cream, light or coffee 85%
Egg Yolks. 80%
Half and half. 79%
Blue cheese 73%
Brick cheese. 72%
Cheddar cheese. 71%
Swiss cheese. 66%
Ricotta cheese, whole-milk type. 66%
Eggs, whole. 65%
Ice Cream, 16% 64%
Mozarella cheese, part skim type 55%
Goat's milk 54%
Cow's milk 49%
Yogurt, plain. 49%
Ice cream, regular 48%
Cottage cheese 35%
Low fat milk (2%) 31%
Low fat yogurt (2%) 31%
Ice milk 29%
Non-fat cottage cheese (1%). 22%

MEAT AND FISH PRODUCTS

Hormel Spam luncheon meat 77%
Mrs. Paul's Buttered Fish Filets. 75%
Del Monte Bonito 67%
Morton Beef Tenderloin. 64%
Mrs. Paul's Fried Shrimp 58%
Mrs. Paul's Clam Crepes 55%
Hormel Dinty Moore Corned Beef. 53%
Swanson Salisbury Steak. 52%
Nabisco Chicken in a Biskit 51%
Morton House Beef Stew 49%
Mrs. Paul's Flounder. 48%
Swanson Veal Parmigiana 48%
Swanson Fried Chicken 46%
Hormel Dinty Moore Beef Stew 45%
Morton Beef Pot Pie 45%
Mrs. Paul's Fish Au Gratin 43%
Morton Chicken Croquettes. 40%

FRUITS

Olive 91%
Avocado. 82%
Grape 11%
Strawberry. 11%
Apple. 8%
Blueberry. 7%
Lemon 7%
Pear 5%
Apricot. 4%
Orange 4%
Cherry 4%
Banana 4%
Cantaloupe. 3%
Pineapple. 3%
Grapefruit. 2%
Papaya 2%
Peach 2%
Prune 1%

GRAINS

Oatmeal 16%
Buckwheat, dark 7%
Rye, dark. 7%
Whole wheat 5%
Brown rice. 5%
Corn flour 5%
Bulgar 4%
Barley. 3%
Buckwheat, light 3%
Rye, light. 2%
Wild rice 2%

NUTS AND SEEDS

Coconut 85%
Walnut 79%
Sesame. 76%
Almond 76%
Sunflower. 71%
Pumpkin seeds 71%
Cashew. 70%
Peanut. 69%
Chestnut 7%

Source: "Nutritive Value of American Foods in Common Units,"
U.S.D.A. Handbook No. 456

erode their profits. In a classic example of the art of lying with statistics, they have come up with a method of measuring fat which disguises the high-fat levels of meats, dairy products and eggs: they measure fat as a percentage of weight. Patricia Hausman of the Center for Science in the Public Interest notes:

> *"The method of measuring . . . the percentage of fat by weight . . . has been abused as a clever way of deceiving consumers about the fat content of food. When expressed as a percentage of a food's weight, the fat content of most foods will sound deceptively low. Whole milk, for example, contains only 3 to 3.7 percent fat by weight, simply because milk, like most foods, contains large amounts of water. By weight, whole milk is 87% water.* **Fat supplies half the calories in milk.***"* [62]

The National Livestock and Meat Board has produced extremely expensive advertising campaigns, announcing that hot dogs are "calorie conscious," and contain only "30 percent fat." Nowhere in the ads does it mention that this "30 percent" figure is calculated by a method specially chosen for its ability to create a misleadingly low number. Similarly, Oscar Mayer uses the "30 percent" figure in the "nutritional education" materials it supplies free of charge to schools, telling its young audience it is a "myth" that:

> *". . . sausage products, including wieners and cold cuts, are 'fatty.'* *"*[63]

Oscar Mayer then proceeds to make its products seem like a veritable dream come true, when it comes to fat, by comparing them with foods which are the very highest in fat to be found anywhere—margarine, mayonnaise, salad dressing and cream cheese.[64] Similarly, they have found a way for their meats to come out looking absolutely fabulous on their cholesterol charts—they simply compare them to eggs, the highest of all foods in cholesterol.[65] In another instance they proudly compare the nutritional value of their wieners to a food item that doesn't exactly provide the stiffest competition—"a 12 oz. can of Coke."[66] In fact, the Oscar Mayer company has made an art of making their fatty, unhealthy products look nutritionally attractive to children by comparing them to a competition that couldn't have been better chosen for the task.

The degree to which meat and dairy products are actually health-giving was recently clarified when the Center for Science in the Public Interest officially renamed Wendy's Triple Cheeseburger: "The Coronary Bypass Special." Tongue in cheek, perhaps, but definitely right on target.

SAFE AND SENSIBLE

One Dairy Council publication is called "The Basic Four Ways to Safe and Sensible Weight Control." Words like "safe" and "sensible" and "basic" portray the feeling most of us grew up having about the Dairy Council, its message and its products. But this publication turns out, like other Dairy Council materials, to represent something far removed from an objective understanding of weight control. It prescribes a glass of whole milk and a pat of butter at every meal to the dieter. Heading its list of "lower caloried" snacks is a product you probably never realized was such a boon to the overweight—ice cream.

It is hard for us to imagine how immense a role the National Dairy Council has played in making us feel we are well fed only when we consume the foods its industry produces. We have been made to feel that to do without these foods would be a severe deprivation and in the back of most of our minds there lives the belief, planted there unbeknownst to us by the Dairy Council, that milk is "nature's most perfect food." In fact, milk is nature's most perfect food for a baby calf, an animal who, with its four stomachs, will double its weight in 47 days.

Even vegetarians continue to be heavily influenced by the hidden persuasions of the Dairy Council. In fact, vegetarians are often especially vulnerable to the pull of its message. Having to some extent defied the prevailing cultural norms by giving up meat, they can easily feel attracted to dairy products as a way of paying their dues to the "basic four" concepts. They may not follow the Dairy Council's specific commandment to "drink three glasses of milk a day," but there lingers in their minds a residue that makes cheese, yogurt, and sometimes even ice cream seem desirable, safe, and even necessary for a wholesome diet.

This is not an accident. The Dairy Council has spent enormous amounts of money to create these feelings in you and me and the rest of the American public. Their staff provides workshops in most major cities to train teachers in the Dairy Council's brand of nutrition. In 1977, Congress began the "National Nutritional Education Training Program," designed to educate children, teachers, and school cafeteria personnel about good nutrition. So accustomed have most states become to the National Dairy Council as the source of their nutritional education materials, that over half the states simply used the additional federal money to buy more Dairy Council supplies.[67]

As I have uncovered the grip which the Dairy Council holds over our schools, I have had to wonder how they ever got such a position within an educational system that is supposed to be noncommercial. The answer is that they have been getting away with it for so long that hardly anyone thinks to question the matter. It was back in 1915 that the dairy farmers founded the National Dairy Council, for the expressed purpose of "educating the public about the importance of drinking milk and consuming dairy products."[68] At that time, nutritionists and teachers knew the Dairy Council had a vested interest in getting children to "drink their milk," but they didn't mind. Nothing was known back then, in the early infancy of nutritional science, to contraindicate the use of dairy products, and the teachers were glad to have the materials. The result was that the Dairy Council became the nation's de facto nutrition educator.

Over the years, the Dairy Council has been able continually to strengthen its foothold in our school systems because it would be impossible at this point for any private company to compete with them in supplying educational materials. Their prices are extremely low because they receive many millions of dollars a year in subsidies from the milk producers who profit from our continued consumption of dairy products, particularly those high in fat.

The dairy industry is also one of the nation's largest advertisers, producing TV commercials and putting up billboards across the country promoting milk, cheese, and butter consumption. Using catchy slogans like "Milk, The Fresher Refresher," and "Every Body Needs Milk," it spends many millions of dollars every year on an advertising budget whose purpose is the same as any other advertising budget—to get us to buy their products. The only difference is that when we see an ad for Marlboro cigarettes, we know the Marlboro company paid a lot of money for the chance to grab our attention and sway our habits. But because we were educated by National Dairy Council materials, and because their programming has gone so deeply into our psyches as to seem like the given truth, when we see ads for milk and dairy products we tend to think we are seeing a public service message. The dairy industry is not terribly unhappy about this, and in fact has been known to end their "messages" with an announcement, in a sincere and sober voice, that the "preceding announcement has been brought to you as a public service by the National Dairy Council."

KEEPING US HOOKED

In its battle to keep Americans consuming high levels of saturated fat and cholesterol, the dairy industry has many friends. McDonald's donates a "Nutrition Action Pack" to classrooms across the country. The material comes complete with the golden arches trademark at the bottom of each page, and is something less than the unbiased nutritional presentation it pretends to be. The coverage of the four basic food groups represents the "Bread and Cereal" group with hamburger buns.

On September 21, 1983, McDonald's ran a 16 page color insert in the *Chicago Tribune* which extolled the virtues of what it called a "properly balanced diet." It was an interesting version of a "properly balanced diet," in that it basically amounted to Big Macs, fries, and shakes. Extra copies of the insert were then distributed in the schools through the Chicago Board of Education. It was, in the words of the Aaron Cushman Public Relations Agency, "a combination textbook and advertisement."

Another organization devoted to keeping us hooked on saturated fat and cholesterol is the National Livestock and Meat Board. After the American Heart Association came on record publicly indicting saturated fat and cholesterol as agents of heart disease, the Meat Board promptly began an extensive advertising campaign designed to discredit the American Heart Association. They actually tried to make it seem as if the vast majority of reputable scientists had never even heard of this "supposed" connection between saturated fat, cholesterol and heart disease. As Patricia Hausman of the Center for Science in the Public Interest noted:

> *"To anyone who relied on the Meat Board for information, it looked like the American Heart Association had a few maniacs running its show, while the vast majority of scientists thought the diet-heart connection was hopelessly off base."* [69]

In its ongoing effort to discredit the "theory" that saturated fat and cholesterol promote heart disease, the Meat Board has come up with one argument that has been particularly effective because it actually sounds eminently reasonable. You are supposed to believe that there is no reason to be concerned about your intake of saturated fat and cholesterol as long as your blood cholesterol count is normal.

But what is a "normal" blood cholesterol level? And furthermore, what is the advantage of being "normal" if that means an average that is already too high?

You see, if you go to a physician to have your blood cholesterol level tested, he or she will send a sample of your blood to a lab. The lab will then send the results back to your doctor. Your blood cholesterol level, usually called "serum cholesterol," or "plasma cholesterol," will be expressed in units of milligrams per 100 milliliters (mg/ml), which is commonly called "milligram percent" (mg%). Usually, along with the actual figures, the lab will mark in the right hand column whether each specific blood parameter for which they tested was found to be "normal" or "abnormal." Most busy doctors simply run down the right hand column looking for abnormalities. Many labs consider values up to 330 mg% to be "normal," while other labs may set the cutoff point as low as 290 mg%. [70]

The problem, however, is that though a man with a blood cholesterol count of 290 mg% will often be considered "normal," he has *more than ten times* the likelihood of dying from a heart attack than a man of similar age with a count of 190% mg! [71] Even smaller differences are of tremendous importance. A person with a blood cholesterol level of 260 mg% is at least five times more likely to die from a heart attack than a person with a level of 200 mg%.[72]

The problem with being "normal" is that the "normal" population of our country is suffering from severe atherosclerosis that is getting worse with every passing meal. As one authority put it:

> *"The average male in (our) society has a greater than 50 percent chance of dying from a heart attack. Under these circumstances, no consolation should be gained from being average."* [73]

Nathan Pritikin, who probably knew as much about preventing heart disease as any man who ever lived, dismissed the myth of "normal" blood cholesterol levels:

> *"If your blood cholesterol level is more than 100 plus your age, up to a maximum of 160, you have closed arteries. (But) anyone with cholesterol below 160 is considered 'abnormal' or 'subnormal' in our country. 'Normal' cholesterol levels are 160-330 . . .*
>
> *"Every so-called 'normal' level in our country is guaranteed to close arteries. 'Normal' in our country simply means that you can walk from one room to another. Our cholesterol levels are **not** normal. They are averages for asymptomatic people, but the next day those people could drop dead from a heart attack."* [74]

The meat, dairy and egg industries tell us not to worry unless our blood cholesterol levels are "abnormal." But people with "normal" levels are dying, literally by the millions, from the high levels of saturated fat and cholesterol in the meat, dairy products and eggs they eat.[75]

THE BATTLE CONTINUES
In its ongoing struggle to convince us that "normal" cholesterol counts are fine and dandy, the industry has resorted to all sorts of chicanery. When the *British Journal of Nutrition* reported a study which measured the blood cholesterol levels of a group of men known for high consumption of saturated fat, the Meat Board triumphantly announced to the public that these men's:

". . . serum cholesterol levels were within reasonable limits."[76]

It depends on what you call reasonable. The blood cholesterol counts of the studied group were high enough to give them ten times the probability of suffering a fatal heart attack compared to what would otherwise be expected.[77]

Recently, in an effort to confuse you even more, the saturated fat sellers have begun to talk a great deal about high-density lipoproteins and low-density lipoproteins. They are eager to point out that in cases where most of the cholesterol in the blood is carried by high-density lipoproteins, the risk of heart disease is much less than when it is carried by low-density lipoproteins. This, they imply, is the key factor, not blood cholesterol levels. They are not so eager to point out that less than ten percent of people with high blood cholesterol fall into the fortunate high-density lipoprotein category.[78] Nor do they seem all that enthusiastic about informing the public that low-fiber diets lower high-density lipoprotein levels, thereby raising the risk of heart attacks. Perhaps their lack of enthusiasm has something to do with the fact that meat, dairy products, and eggs provide no fiber, and so the more of these we eat, the less likely we are to be one of the lucky few protected by high-density lipoproteins.

In their ongoing campaign to make their products look good no matter what, the meat, dairy and egg industries have often pointed out that people sometimes die of heart attacks even after they have lowered their blood cholesterol counts. It is true that lowering your blood cholesterol after a lifetime of high levels cannot guarantee freedom from a heart attack. But studies have shown that atherosclerosis can definitely be reversed, and a great many heart attacks and strokes prevented, when a lowered blood cholesterol level is maintained over a period of time.[79] Researchers at the University of California studied subjects ranging in age from 29 to 65. Those who dropped their blood cholesterol levels by an average of 65 mg%, and maintained the lower figures through reduced intake of saturated fat and cholesterol, showed marked decreases in atherosclerotic deposits.[80]

Even in the most advanced cases of atherosclerosis, diet-style changes can be of enormous benefit. In a major study in Montclair,

New Jersey, 100 patients with confirmed coronary artery disease who had suffered previous heart attacks were put on a diet low in saturated fat and cholesterol. Over a ten year period, 16 of them suffered fatal heart attacks. In a control group of 100 other men in similar conditions, whose diet was not reduced in saturated fat and cholesterol, 28 men died from heart attacks.[81]

Other studies have gotten similar results. Patricia Hausman reports:

"Dr. Thomas Lyon and his colleagues reported that recurrence of heart attack and death was four times as common in patients who admitted they were not adhering to the very lowfat diet prescribed by the doctors . . .

"Dr. A. Koranyi reported a study of 125 patients asked to follow a diet very low in fat. The death rate in the lowfat group was 9%, compared to 19% among patients not asked to restrict their fat intake."[82]

Such studies raise the interesting moral dilemma of whether, with our present state of knowledge, it is even ethical for doctors **not** to ask heart patients to restrict their fat consumption.

Remarkably, diet-style changes have sometimes produced spectacular results in even the most advanced cases. Writing in *Lancet*, and the *American Heart Journal*, two British doctors reported treating cases of severe angina pectoris with a pure vegetarian diet. All the patients had suffered severe chest pain due to a restriction of blood supply to the heart, were unable to exercise, and were considered most likely candidates for fatal heart attacks. After six months on a pure vegetarian diet, they were all free of angina pain, and "able to engage in strenuous activities." Five years later, the patients were all still alive, still adhering to the pure vegetarian diet, and still free of angina symptoms.[83]

THE FIGHT GETS ROUGH
Though these industries have not been successful in their attempts to impede the growing medical understanding regarding diet and heart disease, they have been remarkably successful in maintaining control

of our nation's food policies. In 1982, the Department of Agriculture was about to publish an article in its magazine *Food/2* which was mildly critical of diets high in saturated fat and cholesterol. The meat, dairy and egg lobbies, however, got wind of this, and brought the matter to the attention of Deputy Secretary of Agriculture Richard Lyng. A former president of the American Meat Institute, Lyng dutifully vowed the article would be "published over my dead body."[84]

The article was deleted,[85] and Mr. Lyng is not only still with us, but has now become the Secretary of Agriculture, placing him in an even better position to oversee what the government tells the public, and what it does not.

The political power of the saturated fat industries is remarkable. In 1961, when the American Heart Association first publicly and officially urged Americans to substitute polyunsaturated fat for some of the saturated fat in their diets, the dairy industry did not find this turn of events to their liking, and quickly got the FDA to prohibit margarine and vegetable oil companies from calling attention to the fact that their products were polyunsaturated. So successful was the immense pressure exerted by the dairy industry that the word "polyunsaturated" was virtually made taboo. By law, no product could be labeled polyunsaturated, even if it were 100% polyunsaturated.[86]

For many years, the American Heart Association and many other public health groups have asked that foods containing saturated fat be so labeled. But the saturated fat lobby has thwarted every effort in that direction, thereby keeping the vast majority of Americans unaware which of their food choices expose them to this danger.

The lengths to which the saturated fat industries are willing to go to defend their profits speaks of how shaky they know the ground to be on which they stand. When the American Heart Association publicly announced its massively documented position condemning saturated fat and cholesterol as agents of heart disease, the dairy industry countered by threatening them with multi-million dollar lawsuits, unless they stopped giving "misleading" advice to the public. Though not particularly delighted by the prospect of a drawn out and costly court battle, the American Heart Association bravely stood its ground and would not retract its position.

The dairy industry then went to work on the various state chapters of the Heart Association, seeking to undermine its foundations. In Wisconsin, the state known as "America's Dairyland," dairy farmers exerted tremendous pressure on the local chapter, threatening they would never raise another cent if the state chapter went along with the diet recommendations of the national Heart Association. When the state chapter protested that it was not in their legal power to differ from the national guidelines and set their own course, the dairy interests were less than sympathetic. They promised a multi-million dollar lawsuit, unless the state chapter repudiated the national policy.

Frightened by the prospect of a costly legal battle that would break them financially, intimidated by the prospect of dwindling donations, and aware that the dairymen had the money to carry out their threats, the Wisconsin chapter of the American Heart Association capitulated.[87] They formed a "Task Force on Nutrition and Cardiovascular Disease" to review the matter and make recommendations. Membership on the Task Force included such legendary champions of science in the public interest as the executive director of the Dairy Council of Wisconsin.[88]

The Task Force recommended a policy that came as no surprise to anyone who knew its membership. It recommended that the Wisconsin chapter of the American Heart Association repudiate the official position of the national organization.

The dairy industry was ecstatic, and the Dairy Council's national office sent a letter of congratulations. The Wisconsin Dairy Council passed a formal resolution commending the Wisconsin chapter of the American Heart Association for it's "wisdom" in recognizing that:

". . . diets to lower blood cholesterol . . . are not warranted by the general public." [89]

The American Heart Association was appalled. But there was little they could do, because by now the Wisconsin chapter had been virtually taken over by the dairy interests. The public health messages of the Wisconsin Heart Association, instead of drawing attention to the role of saturated fat and cholesterol in producing heart disease, acted as if there were no connection. In fact, if people requested this information, what they received was a copy of the Task Force's statement, written under the watchful eye of the executive director of the Dairy Council. In case that wasn't enough to discredit the saturated fat and cholesterol "theory," they also received a statement from the Dairy Council, reassuring the inquirers they could put their full faith in dairy products.[90]

You might wonder how on earth the Wisconsin chapter of the American Heart Association could justify not informing the public that diets high in saturated fat and cholesterol lead to heart disease. One high-ranking official of the state chapter explained:

> *"We don't aggressively promote it (the message that saturated fat and cholesterol promote heart disease) any more than a tobacco state would promote the tobacco (link with cancer) message."*[91]

But on closer inspection, that statement is telling, for every day, the meat, dairy and egg industries are finding themselves more and more in a posture as medically untenable as that held by the tobacco industry. Every year the research incriminating these foods becomes more incontrovertible.

THE CLINCHER
In 1984, the United States Federal Government announced the results of the broadest and most expensive research project in medical history.[92] It took over ten years of systematic research, and cost over $150,000,000. The project director of the study, Basil Rifkind, concluded that the mammoth undertaking:

> *". . . strongly indicates that the more you lower cholesterol and fat in your diet, the more you reduce your risk of heart disease."*[93]

George Lundberg, editor of the *Journal of the American Medical Association*, which first published the results of this gargantuan study, said that 25 years from now this study would be looked upon as the one:

> *". . . that secured the cholesterol theory in heart disease."*[94]

The study not only demonstrated that our blood cholesterol levels directly determine our risk of heart disease, it also proved that even very small changes in our blood cholesterol levels produce considerable changes in heart disease rates.[95]

Dr. Charles Glueck, director of the University of Cincinnati Lipid Research Center, one of the twelve major centers participating in the project, noted:

> *"For every one percent reduction in total cholesterol level, there is a two percent reduction of heart disease risk."* [96]

Columbia University Cardiologist Robert Levy, who directed the entire project, agreed:

> *"If we can get everyone to lower his cholesterol by ten to fifteen percent by cutting down on fat and cholesterol in the diet, heart attack deaths in this country will decrease by twenty to thirty percent."* [97]

Even that small reduction would save more lives in a year than are lost to motor vehicle accidents in a decade!

FINALLY
The meat, dairy and egg industries to this day maintain that we "shouldn't jump to any conclusions," because "all the facts aren't in." When asked what kind of study would be adequate, their demands have been so prohibitive as to be utterly absurd, in one case demanding a study involving at least 50,000 people, lasting a minimum of 30 years, and costing over a billion dollars.[98]

As time has gone along, however, and study after study after study has pointed an ever more accusatory finger at saturated fat and cholesterol, some industry spokespeople have finally been forced to admit that their products promote atherosclerosis. Even then, however, they declare:

> *"Consumers have an inalienable right to clog up their arteries if they want to."* [99]

But in the last thirty years scientists have learned for the first time how we can **stop** clogging up our arteries. And we are now certain that of all the factors involved in heart disease—including obesity, lack of exercise, sugar consumption, total fat consumption, caffeine consumption, smoking, high blood pressure, lack of fiber in the diet, and chlorinated drinking and cooking water[100]—there is one culprit that towers mightily above the rest. We now know that culprit is saturated fat and cholesterol.

NOW

We know today how to prevent heart attacks and strokes. We know how to prevent the killers that account for more than half of the deaths in the United States every year. But most of us, thanks to the dedicated endeavors of the meat, dairy and egg industries, have not gotten the good news. We still think we must eat animal products in order to be healthy. We still think heart attacks and strokes are a regrettable but more or less inevitable byproduct that comes with living well and growing old. The heart attack has become so much a part of American life as to virtually be an institution. We take it for granted.

Few of us know that our passive attitude is perpetuated by the deliberate efforts of those who profit from our staying hooked on the foods that cause heart disease.

As long as we remain passive we cannot make the real choices that empower us. Although there are people who do not want us to make such choices and are willing to do almost anything to confuse us, we now have for the first time in history, sufficient knowledge to take control over our bodies and our lives. Now we can make food choices which we know will dramatically improve the health of our cardiovascular system, prevent heart disease and strokes, and at the same time reduce the suffering in the world.

A well-known publication editorialized:

"A vegetarian diet can prevent 97% of our coronary occlusions."[101]

This publication was not the *Vegetarian Times*, nor was it the *New Age Journal*. It was *The Journal of the American Medical Association*.

LOSING A WAR WE COULD PREVENT

> *"When Health is absent*
> *Wisdom cannot reveal itself,*
> *Art cannot become manifest,*
> *Strength cannot be exerted,*
> *Wealth is useless and*
> *Reason is powerless."*

-HEROPHILIES, 300 B.C.

I N 1971, PRESIDENT Nixon signed the Conquest of Cancer Act, thereby officially inaugurating what has become known as the "War on Cancer." Today, the war continues. Every day the National Cancer Institute spends over three million dollars. They are joined in the fray by organizations such as the American Cancer Society, which spend another million dollars a day.[1]

You might think that with so much money being spent, we'd be making progress. But the war on cancer isn't going very well. We aren't massacring the enemy; it's massacring us.

"Everyone should know the war on cancer is largely a fraud."[2]

(DR. LINUS PAULING, TWO-TIME NOBEL PRIZE WINNER)

The most common cancers—cancers of the lung, colon, breast, prostate, pancreas and ovary—together account for most cancer deaths. The death rate from these cancers has either stayed the same, or increased, during the past 50 years.[3] And the statistics for the less common cancers are equally bleak.

The three cancer treatments most fashionable today are surgery, radiation and chemotherapy. Each is invasive; each has devastating side effects; each treats only symptoms. And their rate of success is thoroughly underwhelming.

HALFWAY WHERE?

Organizations like the National Cancer Institute and the American Cancer Society appeal for funds by pleading: "Don't Quit on Us Now, We're Halfway There." But they have had a hard time documenting their "progress."

One man who knows to what lengths these organizations are sometimes forced to go in their effort to retain public confidence is John Bailar, former editor of the *Journal of the National Cancer Institute*. Bailar, who worked for the Institute for 25 years, told the 1985 annual meeting of the American Association for the Advancement of Science that today more people with benign or mild diseases are being included in the statistics, in order to make it seem like more cancer victims are being cured.[4]

Another tactic, which makes it appear things are getting better than they are, is to define a cancer patient as "cured" if he or she has survived for five years after being diagnosed, and is free of obvious symptoms. With early enough detection, many cancer victims will indeed fit this criteria of "cured." However, in many cases, this early detection does not change the date of death, but only the length of time the person is aware he or she has cancer.[5] One prominent physician who has seen more than enough of modern cancer treatment has grown very cynical:

> *"The real beneficiaries of early detection are the providers of health care, who now have a longer time in which to treat the victims before they die. This means they can charge more for doctor's visits, more procedures, more tests, and longer hospital stays. The American Cancer Society . . . has put hope up for sale. Unfortunately to date, it has been selling mostly false hope."*[6]

Today, treating cancer is a huge business. Every 30 seconds another American is diagnosed as having the disease. Typical cancer patients spend over $25,000.00 to try to treat their condition, often exhausting savings that took a lifetime to accumulate. Sadly, they don't get very much today for their money. Every 55 seconds, another American dies of cancer.

TWO SEARCHES

There is a tragedy here. Billions upon billions of dollars are being poured into the search for the "magic bullet" that will cure cancer, a search that has thus far been utterly unsuccessful. And yet, at the same time, another search has been underway which has borne great fruit. Unbeknownst to the public, we have been learning more and more about how to prevent the disease in the first place.

The tragedy is that the American people have been continually cajoled into putting their trust and their money into the thus-far-futile search for a cure, and have not been told what has been learned about prevention. Without this information, Americans every day unknowingly choose to eat foods that contribute heavily to their risk of cancer.

In 1976, the United States Senate Select Committee on Nutrition and Human Needs, under the chairmanship of Senator George McGovern, convened public hearings on the health effects of the modern American diet. After listening to the testimony of the nation's leading cancer experts, McGovern was not particularly delighted with the war on cancer, calling it a "multi-billion dollar medical failure."[7]

At one point in the proceedings, McGovern pointedly asked National Cancer Institute director Arthur Upton how many cancers are caused by diet. The head of the largest cancer organization in the world replied "up to 50 percent."[8]

McGovern was dumbfounded. "How can you assert the vital relationship between diet and cancer," he demanded, "and then submit a preliminary budget that only allocates a little more than one percent (of National Cancer Institute funds) to this problem?"

Dr. Upton responded sheepishly: "That question is one which I am indeed concerned about myself."

The problem is that diet is not a "magic bullet." It is a way of preventing cancer, but only in rare cases a way of cure. Organizations like the National Cancer Institute are not encouraged to focus much attention on prevention because there is vastly more money to be made in treatment, and far more glamour in the possibility, however remote, of a cure. Attention is further drawn away from prevention by food industries whose products are known to be involved. They apply immense pressure on government and public health organizations to keep them from informing the public as to what is known about dietary prevention. The result is that you and I are continually being told to put our faith and our money into cancer treatment, and into the hope for an eventual cure. We are not told how to keep cancer from happening in the first place.

The tragic result is that we are losing a war we could prevent.

PREVENTION

Meanwhile, with 1,400 Americans dying of cancer every day, cancer researchers have investigated just which lifestyle factors produce high rates of cancer.[9] In the prestigious *Advances in Cancer Research*, they conclude:

> *"At present, we have overwhelming evidence . . . (that) none of the risk factors for cancer is . . . more significant than diet and nutrition."* [10]

Conducting hearings on the health effects of the modern American diet, the Senate Select Committee wanted an expert opinion on what medical science now understands about diet and cancer. They summoned Dr. Gio B. Gori, the Deputy Director of the National Cancer Institute's Division of Cancer Cause and Prevention. Dr. Gori's credentials are indeed impressive: he is also the director of the National Cancer Institute's Diet, Nutrition and Cancer Program. He testified:

> *"Nutritional science is coming of age . . . No other field of research seems to hold better promise for the prevention and control of cancer and other illnesses, and for securing and maintaining human health."* [11]

Of course, the Senate wanted to know just what the dietary influences are that promote cancer. Most of us think of chemical additives, such as preservatives, artificial colors and flavors. But bad as these are, it turns out they are not the chief culprits. Dr. Gori told Congress:

> *"Until recently, many eyebrows would have been raised by suggesting that an imbalance of normal dietary components could lead to cancer and cardiovascular disease . . . Today, the accumulation of . . . evidence . . . makes this notion not only possible but certain . . . (The) dietary factors responsible (are) principally* **meat and fat intake**." [12]

You will recall that the meat, dairy and egg industries didn't open their arms wide to welcome the news that saturated fat and cholesterol cause heart disease. Nor have they been all that pleased about what has been learned about the causes of cancer, for once again, meat and fat intake have been increasingly implicated.[13]

The Federal Trade Commission wanted an impartial expert witness to assist their efforts in determining whether the same diets that cause heart disease could also cause cancer. They called in a nutritional scientist from Harvard University, Dr. Mark Hegstead. He testified:

> *"I think it is clear that the American diet is indicted as a cause of coronary heart disease. And it is pertinent, I think, to point out the same diet is now found (guilty) in terms of many forms of cancer: breast cancer, cancer of the colon, and others . . ."* [14]

In light of this, the meat, dairy and egg industries have done the only thing they could. They have joined hands with the tobacco industry to do whatever they can to confuse the issue and make the public think "anything can cause cancer." The more people feel anything can cause cancer, the less they will focus attention on those specific things which, in fact, are known to cause cancer. The more confused and powerless people feel, the less likely they are to make the choices which would actually decrease their risk of cancer. It's not that these industries want people to get cancer; it's just that they want us to continue buying their products. The fact that their products do, in fact, cause cancer, is to their minds, a deeply unfortunate public relations issue.

COLON CANCER

Most of the medical researchers who have done the work investigating dietary causes of cancer are people who were, along with the rest of us, unknowingly schooled in the National Dairy Council brand of nutritional "education." Accordingly, most of them became members in good standing of the Great American Steak Religion. But then, in the 1970's, a number of studies were published in the *Journal of the National Cancer Institute* which reported what was then startling news. Researchers were finding that the incidence of colon cancer was high in precisely those regions where meat consumption was high, and low where meat consumption was low.[15]

It was found, in fact, that **there is not a single population in the world with a high meat intake which does not have a high rate of colon cancer**.

The meat industry, true to form, did what it could to deny the emerging truths, but the more studies were done, the clearer the correlation became. With each succeeding year, it became harder for even the meat industry's paid scientific consultants to avoid the conclusion that meat-eating is involved in the production of a killer that affects over 20% of the families in the United States. Even the conservative journal of the Association for the Advancement of Science concluded:

> *"Populations on a high-meat, high-fat diet are more likely to develop colon cancer than individuals on vegetarian or similar low-meat diets."* [16]

The meat industry countered by saying that genetic factors were responsible. They couldn't deny that those populations who eat the most meat get the most cancer; the evidence was too strong. But they said it was only a coincidence, and the real reason was that such populations were hereditarily disposed towards the disease.

Dr. John Berg and his associates at the National Cancer Institute decided to find out. It was known that the Japanese had lower rates of colon cancer than Americans, and that they ate less meat. Dr. Berg and his co-workers undertook a major study to see what happened to Japanese who immigrated to the United States and adopted the standard

American diet-style. If the industry point of view were correct, these people would maintain their lower colon cancer rates, even though they now ate more meat.

One more sacred cow toppled with the results of this rigorous study. The colon cancer rates of the Japanese immigrants had in fact risen to match the colon cancer rates of their American neighbors.[17]

The meat industry now found itself decidedly on the defensive, but countered by protesting that it could be anything in the American diet-style that was responsible. To single out meat as the culprit, they avowed, was unscientific.

In an effort to isolate precisely which dietary factors were responsible, Dr. Berg and his colleagues at the National Cancer Institute now undertook a major study that correlated colon cancer rates with intake patterns for no less than 119 specific foods. Dr. Berg then reported the results in the *Journal of the National Cancer Institute*. Meat didn't fare very well. In fact, of all foods studied, it was by far the most strongly associated with colon cancer. Wrote Dr. Berg:

> *"Risks of beef, pork and chicken all rose with frequency of use, and the composite picture suggests an underlying dose-response relationship."* [18]

Faced with rigorous data which told us what we could do to prevent colon cancer, spokesmen for the meat industry now parried by saying more studies needed to be done. They were confident, they said, that meat would be vindicated.

As more research was indeed done over the following years, things didn't work out the way the industry hoped. Further research discovered that another dietary factor involved in colon cancer is fat consumption. It became increasingly apparent that the more fat people consume, the greater their risk of colon cancer.[19]

Then another factor was isolated—fiber consumption. Researchers discovered that the less fiber in a person's diet, the more likely he or she is to get colon cancer.[20] These were not the results the meat industry had hoped for either, because meats, like eggs and most dairy products, are high in fat, and provide absolutely no fiber whatsoever.

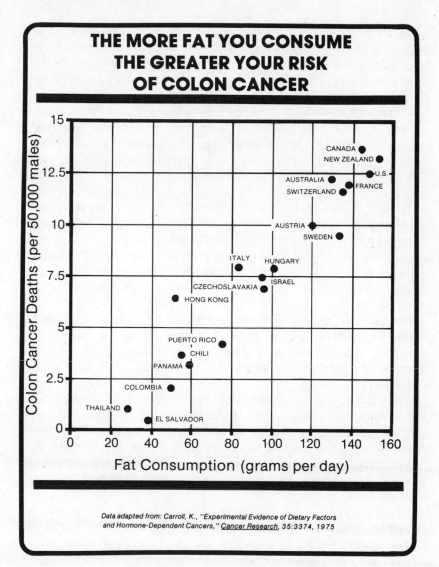

THE MORE FAT YOU CONSUME THE GREATER YOUR RISK OF COLON CANCER

Data adapted from: Carroll, K., "Experimental Evidence of Dietary Factors and Hormone-Dependent Cancers," *Cancer Research*, 35:3374, 1975

Until very recently of course, most of us didn't know that a lack of fiber in our diets was a problem. In fact, most of us didn't even know what fiber was, and for years National Dairy Council nutritional "education" materials ignored fiber altogether. But medical research is increasingly finding fiber to be a most important dietary component.

Fiber acts like a broom in your intestines, sweeping things along. Without it, waste gets blocked up, and the length of time your food takes to pass through your colon is greatly increased. This is particularly true if your diet contains animal fat, because animal fats are solid at body temperature. They clog up your intestines just as grease clogs up drains.

One of the functions of the bowel walls is to absorb moisture from the bowel contents. If, for some reason such as bacterial or amoebic contamination, the body discharges the bowel contents in a rush, without allowing time for the bowel walls to absorb moisture, what comes out will be watery. Victims of dysentery often become extremely dehydrated, and can, in extreme cases, die from the dehydration that results from diarrhea.

But without enough fiber the problem is the opposite. The waste material remains in the colon longer, and more moisture is absorbed by the colon walls. The longer it takes for the contents of the colon to complete their transit, the drier and harder will be the stools that finally emerge.

Researchers have found that the stools of people whose diets are low in fiber tend to be harder, drier, and smaller than the stools of people whose diets are higher in fiber. On a low-fiber diet, people typically have to strain to evacuate. People whose diets are high in natural fiber, in contrast, have been found to produce large, soft, moist and plentiful stools—and these are the same people who show low rates of colon cancer.

There seem to be a number of reasons why high-fiber diets protect against colon cancer, and fiber-deficient diets promote the disease. The longer transit times produced by low-fiber diets provide more opportunity for the bowel walls to reabsorb the toxins the body is trying to eliminate. In other words, the material hangs around longer, the toxicity of the colon increases, and the colon walls absorb more toxins. In addition, fiber helps to dilute, bind, and deactivate many carcinogens.[21]

FIBER CONTENT
OF COMMON FOODS

FOOD ITEM	FIBER (g/kg)	FOOD ITEM	FIBER (g/kg)
Blueberries	15.2	Ground Beef	0
Brussels Sprouts	13.5	Sirloin Steak	0
Oat Flakes	13.5	Lamb Chops	0
Pumpkin	12.0	Pork Chops	0
Cooked Carrot	9.6	Chicken	0
Brown Rice	8.1	Ocean Perch	0
Swiss Chard	6.8	Salmon	0
Lettuce	6.3	Cheddar Cheese	0
Cucumber	5.7	Whole Milk	0
Applesauce	5.3	Eggs	0

Source: *Nutritional Almanac* (Revised), Nutritional Research, Inc.,
John D. Kirshman, McGraw Hill Book Co., New York, 1979

With the growing awareness of the importance of dietary fiber, many meat-eaters are beginning to add bran or other fibers to their diets. This, in fact, is now the belated recommendation of the National Dairy Council which manages to get in a plug for dairy products as it recommends:

> *". . . bran flakes with milk, or cream, if you are concerned with fiber."*

Adding fiber to your diet will speed up transit time, which is good. And the extra fiber will help to absorb some of the toxins in the colon, which is also good. But just adding fiber to a meat-based diet may not help all that much in reducing the risk of colon cancer.

You see, the digestion of meat itself produces strong carcinogenic substances in the colon and meat-eaters must produce extensive bile acids in their intestines to deal with the meat they eat, particularly deoxycholic acid. This is extremely significant, because deoxycholic acid is converted by clostridia bacteria in our intestines into powerful carcinogens. The fact that meat-eaters invariably have far more deoxycholic acid in their intestines than do vegetarians is one of the reasons they have so much higher rates of colon cancer.[22]

Researchers who analyze and test human feces can distinguish the feces of meat-eaters from those of vegetarians by their smell.[23] They report that the eliminations of meat-eaters smell far stronger and more noxious than those of non-meat-eater. There is a serious reason. Putrefying animal products are far more toxic than rotting plant products, and meat-eater's colons are continually subjected to these toxins.

The human intestine has a very hard time handling the putrefying bacteria, high levels of fat, and lack of fiber that characterize meat, dairy products and eggs. There are other animals, though, whose intestines seem designed for the task.

The human intestine is anatomically very different from that of the natural carnivores, such as dogs and cats. Because of the design of their intestines, these animals are virtually guaranteed short transit times.

Our bowel walls are deeply puckered; theirs are smooth. Ours are full of pouches; theirs have none. Our colons are long, complex path-

THE BOWELS OF HUMANS AND CARNIVORES ARE STRIKINGLY DIFFERENT

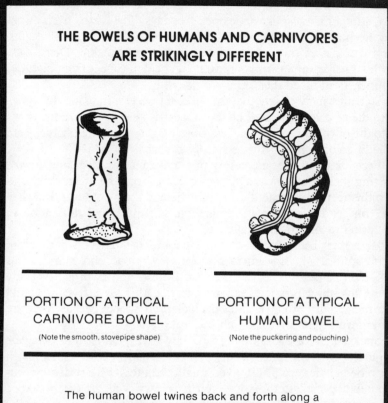

PORTION OF A TYPICAL CARNIVORE BOWEL

(Note the smooth, stovepipe shape)

PORTION OF A TYPICAL HUMAN BOWEL

(Note the puckering and pouching)

The human bowel twines back and forth along a convoluted pathway, with many twists and hairpin turns. Carnivores bowels, in contrast, take a relatively direct and straightforward route. As a result, their transition times are much shorter than ours. They can handle cholesterol and fat, and have much less need for fiber to move things along.

ways, like a winding mountain road full of hairpin turns; theirs are
short, straight chutes, like wide open freeways. The toxins from putrefying flesh are not the problem for them that they are for us because
everything passes through them so much more quickly. Dogs, cats,
and the other natural carnivores do not get colon cancer from high-fat,
low-fiber, flesh-based diets. But we do.

Statistics show clearly that the more fat we eat, the more likely we
are to die of colon cancer. The more meat we eat, the more likely we
are to die of colon cancer. The less fiber we eat, the more likely we are
to die of colon cancer.[24] It's as simple as that.

Faced with an ever-increasing preponderance of medical evidence
indicting their products as agents of colon cancer, the meat, dairy and
egg industries have found it difficult to defend their products. But they
have time and again shown remarkable ingenuity and dedication in
attempting to rise to the challenge.

With their backs to the wall, these industries have made much of
several studies which seem to associate low blood cholesterol levels
with colon cancer.[25] They have claimed these studies prove that low
blood cholesterol promotes colon cancer. If this were true, it would
make meat, dairy products and eggs look pretty good, because they are
well known for raising blood cholesterol levels.

Spokesmen for the saturated fat lobby have even tried to persuade
the public, governmental agencies, and even cancer researchers that if
your blood cholesterol is high you might tend to get heart disease, but
if your blood cholesterol is low you may very well get colon cancer.
The more likely you are to get one, the less likely you are to get the
other. So it balances out in the long run, and there's no point worrying.

But as the figure on page 261 shows, the mortality pattern for
these two diseases is far indeed from opposite. In fact, they often run
quite parallel, and both correlate explicitly with meat consumption.

The real reason why some people with low blood cholesterol levels
have higher rates of colon cancer is actually quite simple. While most
people carry diet-derived cholesterol in their blood, and deposit it in
their arteries, thus causing heart disease, there are some people who
instead send the excess cholesterol to their bowels. Accordingly, these
people show low levels of blood cholesterol, even if their diets are high

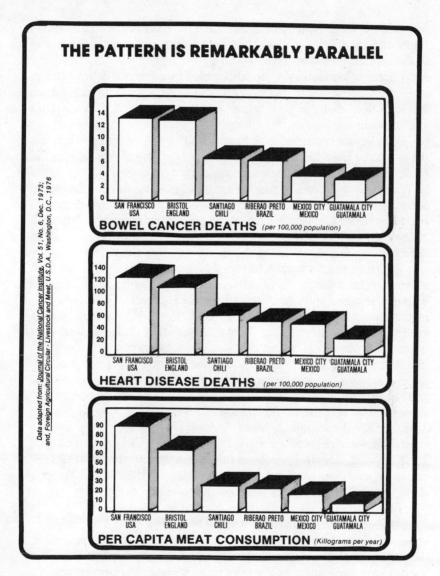

in saturated fat and cholesterol. But they have very high levels of cholesterol in their stools and in their intestines—and very high rates of
colon cancer.[26]

On the other hand, people whose blood cholesterol is low because
their intake of saturated fats and cholesterol is low do not show high
levels of cholesterol in their stools and intestines, and their rates for
colon cancer are, in fact, very low.

But the saturated fat lobby has a point in all this, even if it is not
the one they wish to make. When it was first found that high blood
cholesterol causes heart disease, there was a rush to find ways to lower
it. When it was discovered that the intake of polyunsaturated fats could
accomplish this purpose to some extent, many felt an answer was to
replace saturated fats in the diet with polyunsaturated fats. It wasn't
known, yet, that polyunsaturated fats lower the levels of cholesterol in
the blood by driving it out of the blood and into the colon.[27]

The answer isn't simply to replace saturated fats in the diet with
polyunsaturated fats, as was once thought. The answer is to lower the
intake of fats, per se, in order to be protected across the board. Replac-
ing saturated fats with polyunsaturated fats will help some, because
saturated fats are far and away the worst offenders, guilty of producing
heart disease, strokes, cancer, and just about every other degenerative
disease known to man. But too much fat of any kind is not good.

Vegetarians need to be aware that not only meat, eggs and dairy
fats are harmful to health. Vegetable fats such as salad oils and marga-
rines need to be used in moderation. And much the same is true for
nuts, seeds, olives and avocados.

We know today with remarkable accuracy which diet-styles promote colon cancer. But you wouldn't know it from the statements of
the meat, dairy and egg industries. On May 7, 1976, John Morgan,
president of Riverside Meat Packers, announced:

*"We shouldn't jump to any conclusions and do something foolish
just because some study seems to say something that we know from
common sense isn't true. Beef is the backbone of the American diet
and it always has been. To think that meat of all things causes
cancer is ridiculous."* [28]

On March 13, 1982, John Morgan died of cancer of the colon.[29]

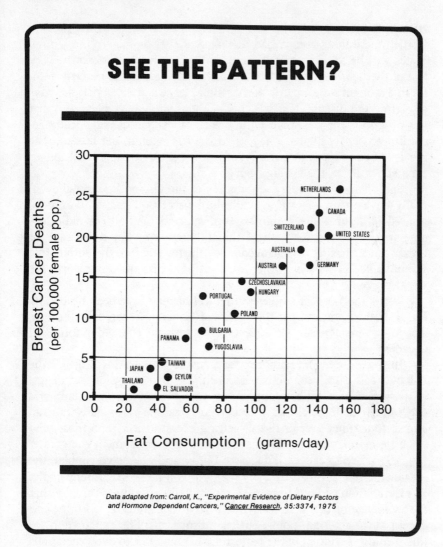

SEE THE PATTERN?

Breast Cancer Deaths (per 100,000 female pop.)

NETHERLANDS
CANADA
SWITZERLAND
UNITED STATES
AUSTRALIA
AUSTRIA
GERMANY
CZECHOSLAVAKIA
PORTUGAL
HUNGARY
POLAND
BULGARIA
PANAMA
YUGOSLAVIA
TAIWAN
JAPAN
THAILAND
CEYLON
EL SALVADOR

Fat Consumption (grams/day)

Data adapted from: Carroll, K., "Experimental Evidence of Dietary Factors
and Hormone Dependent Cancers," *Cancer Research*, 35:3374, 1975

BREAST CANCER

In the time it takes you to read this chapter, 100 women in the United States will be told by their doctors that they have breast cancer. Very few of them will ever have been told that the higher the percentage of fat in a woman's diet, particularly animal fat, the greater risk she runs of getting the disease. Nor will any of them likely have been told that the prognosis for a woman with breast cancer varies statistically according to her fat intake. The less fat she has eaten in her lifetime, the greater hope she has, statistically, of beating the disease, and the longer time she will, on the average, survive.[30]

Sadly, one out of every ten women in the United States will eventually develop breast cancer, while billions of dollars continue to be poured into surgical techniques, sophisticated methods of radiotherapy, and the widespread use of chemotherapy. Yet the death rate for breast cancer has hardly changed since the days before the automobile was invented. It is a classic and truly tragic case of losing a war we could prevent.

The largest cancer studies in medical history have been headed by Dr. Takeshi Hirayama, at the National Cancer Research Institute in Tokyo, where as many as 122,000 people have been monitored for decades.

In one study, Dr. Hirayama and his co-workers investigated the risk of breast cancer for women according to their intake of meat, eggs, butter and cheese.[31] The findings were not easy for the meat, dairy and egg industries to swallow. Those who consume meat daily face an almost four times greater risk of getting breast cancer than those who eat little or no meat. Similarly, the more eggs consumed, the greater the risk of breast cancer. The more butter and cheese consumed, the greater the risk of breast cancer. (See figure on page 265) Interestingly, an examination of Dr. Hirayama's report makes it appear initially that the incidence of breast cancer rises with a rising intake of butter and cheese up to a certain point, but then drops off. The explanation for this seeming deviation in the pattern is that many lacto-ovo vegetarians consume butter and cheese daily, and yet, because they do not eat meat, their breast cancer rates are lower than those for meat-eating women who eat less cheese and butter.

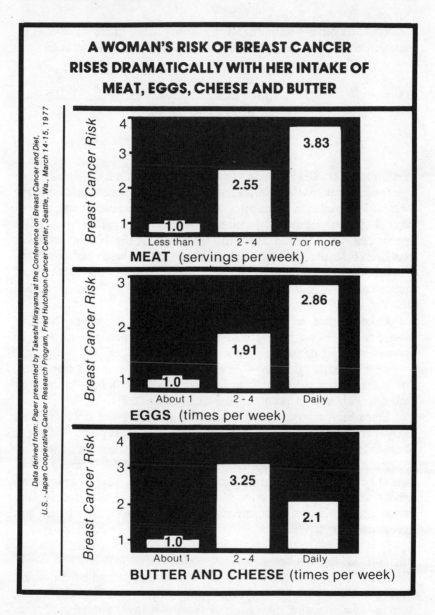

Data derived from: Paper presented by Takeshi Hirayama at the Conference on Breast Cancer and Diet,
U.S. - Japan Cooperative Cancer Research Program, Fred Hutchison Cancer Center, Seattle, Wa., March 14-15, 1977

**A WOMAN'S RISK OF BREAST CANCER
RISES DRAMATICALLY WITH HER INTAKE OF
MEAT, EGGS, CHEESE AND BUTTER**

Breast Cancer Risk

1.0 — Less than 1
2.55 — 2 - 4
3.83 — 7 or more

MEAT (servings per week)

Breast Cancer Risk

1.0 — About 1
1.91 — 2 - 4
2.86 — Daily

EGGS (times per week)

Breast Cancer Risk

1.0 — About 1
3.25 — 2 - 4
2.1 — Daily

BUTTER AND CHEESE (times per week)

This and other studies reveal the same pattern for breast cancer as has been found true for heart disease, strokes, and colon cancer:

Breast Cancer Mortality
(Highest Incidence ranked first)
1. *Meat-eating women*
2. *Lacto-ovo vegetarians*
3. *Pure vegetarians*

A number of studies have found that vegetarian girls have later menarche (onset of menses) than meat-eating girls. In Japan, as diets have become less traditional and more Western, with increasing amounts of animal fat, one result for Japanese girls has been earlier and earlier menarches. Dr. Hirayama and his colleagues at the National Cancer Research Institute have found that women who have an earlier menarche (under thirteen years of age) have over four times the incidence of breast cancer as women who have a later menarche (over seventeen years of age).[32]

Other studies, from other parts of the world, corroborate the Japanese findings. The more fat in a young girl's diet, the earlier her menses will begin, and the higher will be her risk of breast cancer.[33]

Studies have also shown that as animal fat consumption rises, menstrual periods become heavier, further apart, longer, and more painful, with greater premenstrual difficulties.

Diets high in meats, dairy products and eggs not only force an early menarche, they also delay menopause.[34] A report published in the *British Medical Journal* found that women whose diets are high in fat and protein reach menopause at an average age of 50. They stand in marked contrast to women whose diets are low or void of animal fat, who reach menopause at an average age of 46. Sadly for meat-eating women, there is a distinct correlation between later menopause and breast cancer.[35]

CERVICAL CANCER
Cervical cancer, is frequently linked to injuries sustained by the cervix during childbirth; however, like breast cancer, it is highest among women who consume diets high in fat, particularly animal fat.[36]

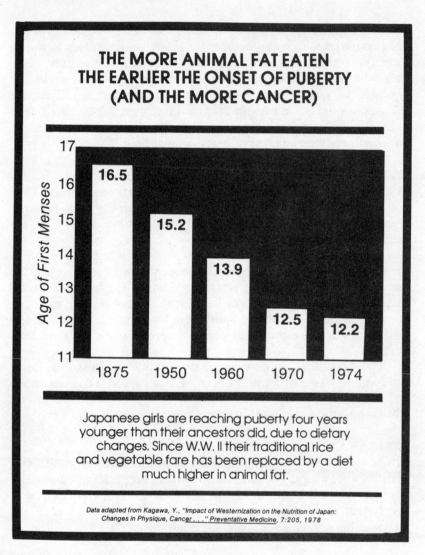

THE MORE ANIMAL FAT EATEN THE EARLIER THE ONSET OF PUBERTY (AND THE MORE CANCER)

Japanese girls are reaching puberty four years younger than their ancestors did, due to dietary changes. Since W.W. II their traditional rice and vegetable fare has been replaced by a diet much higher in animal fat.

Data adapted from Kagawa, Y., "Impact of Westernization on the Nutrition of Japan: Changes in Physique, Cancer . . ." Preventative Medicine, 7:205, 1978

Studies show the incidence of cervical cancer in women in developed countries who began intercourse before age seventeen is two to three times higher than for those who began later. Poignantly, those girls who have the earliest sexual encounters in these countries are typically the same ones who have the earliest menarches. They are thus more susceptible to both breast and cervical cancer. Both their difficulties have repeatedly been correlated to diets high in protein and fat, most notably animal protein and animal fat.[37]

CANCER OF THE ENDOMETRIUM (UTERUS)

Many women today take estrogen pills to prevent osteoporosis. They don't know they could accomplish the same purpose by simply not eating concentrated animal proteins.[38] Nor do they know they are greatly increasing their risk of developing uterine cancer.[39]

The relationship between fat consumption and uterine cancer is the same as it is for the other female cancers: the more fat eaten, the more cancers. In fact, almost every single one of the factors currently acknowledged as a risk indicator for uterine cancer—obesity, early puberty, late menopause, estrogen pills, high blood pressure, and diabetic tendencies—occur disproportionately in women whose diets are high in fat.

Those countries, with the lowest consumption of fat such as Japan and Nigeria, have the lowest rates of uterine cancer. Those countries with the highest consumption of fat, such as the United States and other meat-eating countries, have the highest rates of uterine cancer.[40]

OVARIAN CANCER

The July 19, 1985 issue of the *Journal of the American Medical Association* contained a report by Dr. John Snowden, an epidemiologist at the University of Minnesota's School of Public Health, summarizing a twenty-year study of diet and ovarian cancer. The results were a tremendous blow to an already-reeling egg industry:

"Women who ate eggs . . . three or more days each week had a three times greater risk of fatal ovarian cancer than did women who ate eggs less than one day per week."

WHICH ARE REALLY
THE HIGH FAT FOODS?
(Percentage of Calories As Fat)

VIRTUALLY ALL FAT (80-100%)

Butter	100%	Coconut	85%	Avocado	82%
Salad Oils	100%	Pork Sausage	83%	Bologna	81%
Cream, Light	92%	Sirloin Steak	83%	Frankfurters	80%

VERY HIGH FAT (60-79%)

Half and Half	79%	Sunflower Seeds	71%	Eggs	65%
Brick Cheese	72%	Peanuts	69%	Ground Beef (Lean)	64%
Cheddar Cheese	71%	Swiss Cheese	66%	Tuna (Oil packed)	63%

HIGH FAT (40-59%)

Chicken (Dark w/skin Roasted)	56%	Salmon, Sockeye	49%	Ice Cream	48%
Mozzarella (part skim)	55%	Yogurt	49%	Sirloin Steak (Lean)	47%
Bass, Black Sea	53%	Milk	49%	Chicken (Light w/skin Roasted)	44%

MEDIUM FAT (20-39%)

Soybeans	37%	Low Fat Milk	31%	Non-Fat	
Cottage Cheese	35%	Low Fat Yogurt	31%	Cottage Cheese	22%

LOW FAT (0-19%)

Oatmeal	16%	Macaroni	5%	Apricot	4%
Garbanzo Beans	11%	Whole Wheat	5%	Artichoke	3%
Cabbage	7%	Spaghetti	5%	Peach	2%
Green Beans	6%	Brown Rice	5%	Potatoes	1%

Source: "Nutritive Value of American Foods in Common Units," U.S.D.A. Handbook No. 456

As with the other female cancers, the incidence of ovarian cancer rises not only with egg consumption, but with the consumption of any form of animal fat. Dr. Ronald Phillips concluded a report in *Cancer Research* by saying the evidence is now overwhelming: vegetarian diets strongly reduce the incidence of breast, uterine, ovarian, colon, and many other cancers.[41]

PROSTATE CANCER

Prostate cancer is one of the most virulent forms of a virulent disease. It has usually spread before it is detected, and is usually fatal.

Prostate cancer is highly correlated to fat consumption.[42] The figure on page 271 shows why the meat, dairy and egg industries do not particularly want to publicize the world-wide pattern. Nor are they encouraged by studies such as the one done at California's Loma Linda University. This twenty-year undertaking involved over 6,500 men, and found that those who consumed large amounts of meat, cheese, eggs and milk had 3.6 times the incidence of prostate cancer as men who ate those foods sparingly, or not at all.

Even for men who do not come down with prostate cancer, the effects of different diet-styles on the health of their prostates can be considerable. By the age of 60, 40 percent of U.S. males have enlarged prostates. While most of these are not malignant, they can be forerunners of cancer, and are often quite uncomfortable.

Worldwide, autopsies reveal that wherever the diet-style is similar to the American fare—with high animal fat consumption—close to 25 percent of all men develop latent cancer of the prostate by their old age.[43]

The hormonal changes that high-fat diets cause in men are not as easily observable as those produced in women, because men do not have such obvious milestones in their sexual evolution as menarche and menopause. But there are strong indications that high-fat (and particularly high animal fat) diet-styles stimulate the early development of sexuality in boys as much as they do in girls. And just as girls with early menarche run into the most trouble later on with breast cancer, boys with early onset of puberty later find themselves the most susceptible to prostate enlargement and prostate cancer—particularly if they continue this diet-style throughout their lives, as they usually do.

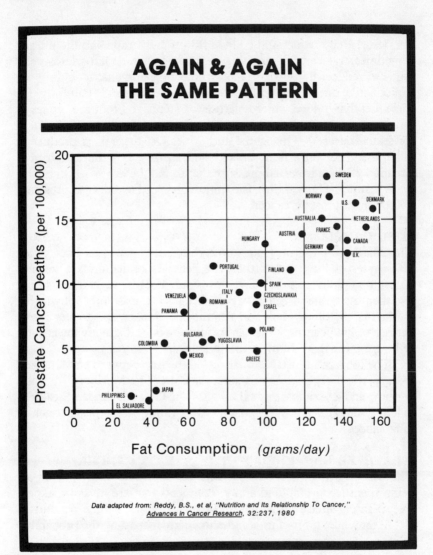

AGAIN & AGAIN
THE SAME PATTERN

Data adapted from: Reddy, B.S., et al, "Nutrition and Its Relationship To Cancer,"
Advances in Cancer Research, 32:237, 1980

Diets high in saturated fat and cholesterol tend to clog up our arteries, thereby reducing the blood flow to our hearts and brains, and sometimes, tragically, obstructing them altogether. Atherosclerosis also tends to reduce the flow of blood to our other organs, including our reproductive ones, thus producing impotence in men.[44] Painfully, the same diet that induces atherosclerosis also tends to produce high levels of androgens, the male sex hormones, which may lead to a greater need for sexual release.[45] Thus some authorities feel these diets produce in older men, not only heart attacks and strokes, but the unfortunate situation of chronic sexual pressure that cannot be expressed in a satisfying manner. The resulting frustration may lead to enlarged prostates, and often to prostate cancer.

LUNG CANCER
The Marlboro Man may not know this, but vegetarians have much lower rates of lung cancer than the general population.[46] The meat industry would like us to believe this is only because vegetarians smoke less than meat-eaters. But many studies have consistently shown that the higher the blood cholesterol count of a smoker, the greater his or her risk of lung cancer.[47] Vegetarian smokers have distinctly lower rates of lung cancer than do meat-eating smokers.[48]

The tobacco industry capitalizes on the link between smoking and meat, particularly in their ads aimed at men. The Marlboro Man is a cowboy, and a veritable embodiment of the Great American Steak Religion. I sometimes wonder which will get him first, a heart attack or lung cancer.

WHATEVER HAPPENED TO THE WAR ON CANCER?
The war on cancer is a tragedy. Billions upon billions of dollars are being spent to develop and apply treatments that are invasive, expensive, painful, often mutilating, and in many cases of little benefit.

Meanwhile, most of us are unknowingly increasing the probability of cancer with our every meal.

The more I've learned about diet and cancer, the more stunned I've been at our ignorance of their close relationship. We do not have to quake helplessly in the face of cancer, "hoping" to escape its clutches.

We do not have to sit by passively, watching our loved ones succumb to this disease. We do not have to spend our life savings, undergoing painful and devastating treatments that do little or no good. We are blessed now with the knowledge which enables us to make clear, life-giving choices. We need only make them in time.

AN OUNCE OF PREVENTION

> *"Loyalty to a petrified opinion never yet broke a chain or freed a human soul."*
>
> (MARK TWAIN)

OVER THE LAST twenty-five years, there have been unprecedented breakthroughs in our understanding of food choices and health. However, there is an enormous gap between what has been discovered and what the public has learned of it. As a result, tens of millions of American men, women and children are suffering needlessly.

We have been given an extraordinary opportunity. We now hold an infinitely precious gift in our hands—our health, the health of our children, the possibility of a truly healthy world. These are no longer mere dreams; they could be our destiny.

The time is at hand when heart disease, atherosclerosis, strokes and cancer could be things of the past. And I can see a future when people would hardly be able to believe the ancient legends, that once, before they knew better, human beings sickened themselves by eating the corpses of animals whose lives had been hell.

With a diet-style that is compassionate and healthy, we can become something far healthier and greater than we have yet been. Compared to what is possible, our present physical bodies are like light bulbs without current, waiting to be lit.

The more I've learned about the diet-health connection, the more amazed I've been by how much is already known. Not only heart disease and cancer, but many other diseases have been traced directly to today's dietary blindness. Scientific studies have shown not only that these diseases, and the immense suffering they entail, can often be prevented by intelligent food choices; in many cases they can be treated by diet-style changes with direct, consistent, and powerful benefits.

DIABETES

Diabetes is a good example. Millions of Americans suffering enormously from this disease do not know their agony could be greatly relieved by different food choices.

One of the reasons diabetes is the 8th leading cause of death in the United States is that diabetics are extremely vulnerable to atherosclerosis.[1] Highly prone to heart attacks and strokes, their life expectancies are much shorter than normal.[2] But it is not just that their lives are shortened; the damage atherosclerosis does to their cardiovascular system has profound consequences to the quality of their lives. Degeneration in the arteries bringing blood to their eyes is so severe that 80% of diabetics suffer serious eye damage, and diabetes is the leading cause of new cases of blindness in the country. The blood supply to their kidneys is often compromised and as a result diabetics have 18 times the average rate of serious kidney failure. Many spend the last years of their lives tied to the ordeal of a kidney machine. Circulation to their extremities is cut down to such an extent that an infection in a toe which for most of us would be minor can, for a diabetic, easily lead to gangrene, may require amputation of a foot or a leg, and can even be life-threatening. As if this weren't enough, since atherosclerosis decreases circulation to the reproductive organs, diabetic males have a much higher rate of impotence than the general population.[3]

Yet, with all the terrible damage atherosclerosis does to diabetics, most of them do not know which diets promote atherosclerosis and which diets reduce it. Most eat the standard American diet. As a result, within 17 years of the onset of their illness, most diabetics today suffer a major health catastrophe, such as heart attack, kidney failure, stroke or blindness.[4]

This is especially tragic because it is so needless. Different diet-styles produce very different results.

In *Lancet*, Dr. Inder Singh reported a remarkable study in which 80 diabetic patients were restricted to very lowfat diets—20 to 30 grams a day—and forbidden any sugar consumption.[5] Within six weeks, over 60% of the patients no longer required insulin. In the weeks that followed, the figure rose to over 70%, and those who still needed insulin therapy needed only a small fraction of what they had required before the diet change. All 80 cases were monitored for periods ranging from 6 months to 5 years, and the success of the dietary changes was confirmed over time.

There's a reason why the lowfat diet helped so much. The pancreas operates according to a kind of thermostat. Just as a heater governed by a thermostat will switch on and off as the temperature changes in the room, the pancreas secretes insulin in response to sugar in the blood in order to keep blood sugar levels within a certain range. Many diabetics need to give themselves insulin shots, but this is not, as commonly thought, because the pancreas is not secreting enough insulin. In fact, many diabetics produce more insulin than a normal person, yet still need these injections.[6] The reason is that their insulin is not able to do its job, and their blood sugar levels skyrocket out of control unless medication is given.

It turns out that a common cause for the malfunction of the diabetic's own insulin is the high level of fat in their blood.[7] Thus the reduction of dietary fat, particularly saturated fat, can be of greatest significance to diabetics, for it lowers the concentration of fat in the blood, and thus allows their own insulin to do its job.

The *American Journal of Clinical Nutrition* reported a study in which 20 diabetics, all of whom needed insulin, were put on a high-fiber very lowfat diet. After only 16 days, 45% of these patients were able to discontinue the insulin injections.[8]

Other studies have produced similar results.[9] Approximately 75% of diabetics who have needed insulin therapy, and 90% of diabetics who have needed diabetic pills (sulphonylureas), can be freed from their need for medication in a matter of weeks on a lowfat high-fiber diet.

For a diabetic to be freed from his or her need for medication is a great blessing, for compared to the pancreas, medications are a vastly inferior means of controlling blood sugar levels. Furthermore, they have serious side effects. The pills more than double the risk of heart attack, and sometimes cause jaundice, skin rashes and anemia.[10] Overdoses of medication are common because the body's needs change all the time, and are impossible for patients to monitor with anything remotely resembling the accuracy of the pancreas. Insufficient food intake can easily precipitate disorienting bouts of hypoglycemia (low blood sugar). The insulin pump is a recent, sophisticated improvement, but it is expensive, must be worn at all times, produces infections at the injection site a third of the time, and markedly worsens the eye diseases so common to diabetics.[11] Additionally, the pumps are machines; machines can malfunction; and a malfunctioning insulin pump can be fatal.

Lowfat diets, particularly those without any saturated fat, have demonstrated a remarkable success rate in allowing diabetics to dispense with their pills, shots and pumps.[12] Happily, these are the very same diets which protect against the ravages of atherosclerosis to which diabetics are otherwise so terribly prone.

There is a rare and very serious form of diabetes called childhood-onset diabetes which is in many ways a different disease. It is not the result of the body's own insulin being rendered ineffective, but is rather a situation in which the pancreas has been seriously injured, and either cannot secrete insulin at all, or does not secrete enough. Even for victims of this singularly destructive form of diabetes, however, wise food choices are of enormous value. Those who omit meat and other high-fat low-fiber foods need 30% less insulin, have more stable blood sugar levels, are (in medical terms) less "brittle," and are significantly protected from the complications of atherosclerosis that otherwise would cause them such immense suffering.[13]

The scientific breakthroughs of the past 25 years have found that the same diet-styles which can do so very much to help diabetics are the very ones that prevent the disease in the first place. Worldwide, the disease is rare or nonexistent among peoples whose diets are primarily grains, vegetables and fruits. If these same people switch to rich meat-based diets, however, their incidence of diabetes balloons.[14]

In Micronesia there is a small island called Nauru, near the equator, just west of the Gilbert Islands. Before World War II, the native Polynesians lived here in isolation, and were such a healthy and happy people that the island used to be known as Pleasant Island. On this island there are enormous deposits of bird dung that have accumulated over the centuries. After the war, the phosphates from this bird dung were coveted by the industrialized nations. As a result, the Nauruans became very wealthy, and began to emulate the West—gorging themselves on rich foods, canned and frozen meats, fish, oils, white rice, soft drinks. Their consumption of fiber plummeted and their consumption of fat skyrocketed. Now the island is not so pleasant. Tragically, over one-third of these people have developed diabetes.[15]

An enormous scientific project, which studied more than 25,000 people for 21 years, found that vegetarians have a much lower risk of diabetes than meat-eaters. One of the authors of the study, University of Minnesota epidemiologist Dr. David Snowden, summarized the findings:

> *"We suspect it is the absence of meat that may explain our findings. In this study we looked at various levels of meat consumption, and as those levels got lower and lower, the risk of diabetes also decreased."* [16]

In a more personal vein, Dr. Snowden confided:

> *"My meat consumption has dropped significantly . . . since completing the diabetes study."* [17]

HYPOGLYCEMIA

The disorientation caused by mild cases of hypoglycemia is so common in the United States today that most people think it's "normal." They do not realize the sense of weakness, dizziness or confusion they sometimes experience is the result of a drop in their blood sugar level. And they also do not realize this is a product of their food choices. Hypoglycemia is found wherever people consume significant amounts of meats, sugar and fats.[18]

In its mildest form, hypoglycemia causes feelings of confusion, uncertainty and a lack of confidence in oneself. In more difficult cases, victims may temporarily not know who or where they are. The result in extreme cases can be coma and death.

You may assume that moderating your sugar consumption is the chief factor in preventing hypoglycemia; but fat consumption is also greatly involved.

Dr. S. Sweeney fed young healthy medical students a very high fat diet for two days. Then he gave them a glucose tolerance test. All of the subjects showed signs that their blood sugar metabolism had been driven completely out of whack by the excess fat. On another occasion, Dr. Sweeney fed the same students a diet consisting of sugar, candy, pastry, white bread, baked potatoes, syrup, bananas, rice and oatmeal. After two days of this high sugar, high starch fare, he administered another glucose tolerance test. The blood sugar metabolism of the subjects was not nearly as off balance as it had been from the high fat diet.[19]

If you want to get hypoglycemia, or if you already have it and want to make it worse, eat lots of fat, sugar, animal protein, dairy products and processed foods. Stay away from fresh vegetables and whole grains. Don't believe all that stuff you hear about smoking and meat being dangerous to your health. And don't worry about getting your vitamins and minerals from your food—you can always a pop a vitamin pill any time you want. There is no need for regular meals, as long as you really load up when you have the chance. Remember that coffee is the key to mental alertness, and alcohol is the path to relaxation and freedom from your fears. And, God forbid, don't exercise. Such a regime is guaranteed to make your pancreas forget it ever knew health, and alter your consciousness in a decidedly unpleasant direction.[20]

MULTIPLE SCLEROSIS

Today's doctors have been taught in medical school that nothing can be done to prevent Multiple Sclerosis, and nothing can be done to treat it. They tell their patients that this terrible disease is incurable. This represents one of the most profound examples of needless suffering perpetuated by an ignorance of what has been learned about diet and health. If you know anyone who suffers from Multiple Sclerosis, please share this information with him or her.

The onset of M.S. usually occurs in the mid-thirties. Women have a slightly higher incidence than men. It is the most common disease of the central nervous system in Americans aged 20 to 50 years of age. Over 250,000 Americans are afflicted with this devastating disease, and the numbers are rising daily.

Multiple Sclerosis is a disease that attacks the brain, spinal cord, and nervous system over a period of years. According to conventional medical doctrine, the attacks just keep coming, and the patient can only look forward to getting ever worse. There is no way to predict when the next attack might occur, or what might set it off. Today's doctors tell their M.S. patients nothing can be done to prevent the attacks from seriously injuring their nervous system, causing weakness, dizziness, numbness, and/or blindness. Modern orthodox medical opinion says that within ten years of most M.S. victim's first attack they will be permanently and seriously disabled.

The pessimism of conventional medicine is indeed warranted—for M.S. victims who consume the standard American diet. For those on a different diet, however, another outcome is possible.

During World War II, when the diets of people in occupied western European countries were dramatically reduced in animal fat consumption, researchers noticed that M.S. victims in these areas suddenly had fewer attacks, less frequent hospitalizations, and fewer deaths. This observation gave rise to studies which revealed that there is a great variation in the worldwide incidence of the disease. It is most common where consumption of animal fats is high, and least common where such consumption is low or nonexistent. Per capita fat intake in the nine nations with the greatest prevalence of M.S. ranges from 105 to 151 grams per day; per capital fat intake in the nine nations with the least incidence of M.S. ranges from 24 to 60 grams per day.

Investigators also did brain tissue analysis of persons with M.S. and found a higher saturated fat content than in people without the disease.[21]

The next piece of the puzzle came into place when it was discovered that children who are fed cow's milk formulas grow up into adults with a higher susceptibility to M.S. than children who are breast fed.[22] Cow's milk contains only one-fifth the linoleic acid of human milk, and skim cow's milk is utterly void of this important nutrient.[23] Linoleic acid is an essential nutrient for human nervous systems, which is just where M.S. strikes. Researchers suspect that the nervous system of children raised on a diet that derived its fat from animal sources such as cow's milk might be deprived of sufficient linoleic acid at a critical juncture in the development of their nervous systems, and so become more susceptible to M.S. in later life.

Ironically, one of the arguments put forth by the meat, dairy and egg industries to justify consumption of saturated fats is that "fats contain essential nutrients." In fact, the only nutrient we must get from fat is linoleic acid, and animal fats are very poor sources. One tablespoon of safflower oil, for example, provides as much linoleic acid as a cup-and-a-half of butter, and more than two whole cups of beef fat.

The standard American diet—beginning with the substitution of cow's milk for breast milk, and continuing on with high levels of animal fat—is thus a breeding ground for Multiple Sclerosis. Different diet-styles, however, not only serve to prevent M.S., but have actually been shown to be of great benefit in treating it. In fact, most people would be astounded if they became familiar with the nutritional research on this supposedly "incurable" disease.

Dr. Roy Swank, head of the Department of Neurology at the University of Oregon, began treating "incurable" M.S. patients with a very lowfat diet.[24] In one instance he put 146 M.S. patients on a diet that was very low in fat (30-40 grams a day), low in protein, and supplemented with moderate doses of Vitamins A, C, D, and B-complex. Then he carefully monitored their progress over a period of twenty years.

The results Dr. Swank obtained in this and many other studies border on the miraculous.

About 90% of the M.S. patients who began the lowfat diet during the early stages of the disease not only arrested the disease process, but actually improved over the next twenty years. Of those M.S. victims who began the diet when their disease had already reached an intermediate stage, over 65% were able to prevent further damage, and even after seven years on the diet had suffered no further deterioration. Perhaps most amazing were the results for those M.S. victims who entered Dr. Swank's care and began the lowfat diet when their disease had already progressed to an advanced stage of severe disability. Over 30% were able to arrest the inexorable devastation of the disease, and showed no further decline.

In this and many other studies, a very lowfat diet for Multiple Sclerosis produced a profound reduction in the frequency of attacks, the severity of attacks, the damage done by the attacks, and the death rate.[25]

Dr. Swank has now treated several thousand M.S. patients with a lowfat diet over a period of 35 years. His results have met every challenge presented by the medical community, and are enormously superior to those achieved by any other known form of treatment to this otherwise crippling and usually fatal disease.[26]

Dr. Swank has found that if M.S. is caught early enough, then M.S. victims stand a 95% chance of arresting the disease and not getting any worse. For many, there is the very real possibility of a cure.[27]

Other physicians have followed up on Dr. Swank's work, and achieved results comparable to his. One clinic found that a pure vegetarian diet, very low in fat, has been of significant benefit even to the most advanced cases of Multiple Sclerosis.[28]

ULCERS
Peptic (digestive) ulcers occur as a result of the mucus membranes of the stomach and/or duodenum being literally eaten away by gastric secretions. This happens when the gastric secretions become extremely acidic.

With stomach ulcers as common and as painful as they have become today, a great deal of work has naturally been done to determine the effect of different diet-styles on ulcers.[29] But the public, by and large, has not learned the results of these studies. There are powerful economic interests who'd prefer we not know that ulcers occur most frequently, and most seriously, in people whose diets are acid-forming, low in fiber, and high in fat. Meats, fish and eggs are the most acid-forming of all foods. Meats, fish, dairy products and eggs contain no fiber. With few exceptions, these foods are all high in fat.

Orthodox western medicine traditionally prescribed dairy products and antacids to treat digestive ulcers—a treatment approach called
the "Sippy diet." This treatment originated when doctors noticed that
ulcer patients obtained immediate pain relief by drinking milk and
taking antacids. However, investigators who sought to find out
whether this treatment actually does any good, beyond the temporary
relief of pain, found that dairy products produce no improvement in
ulcer disease, and in fact often make things worse. Milk does contain
calcium, which tends to neutralize stomach acids, providing temporary
relief. But they found that milk actually increases natural acid production, which further erodes the linings of the duodenum and stomach.[30]

Researchers also found another excellent reason for staying away
from milk. Ulcer disease patients treated with dairy products were
found to have two to six times the number of heart attacks as ulcer
patients treated without dairy products.[31]

Fortunately for ulcer sufferers, there are foods which tend to neutralize excess stomach acids which do not stimulate the body to produce more of them, and do not increase the risk of heart attacks. Members of the cabbage family—cabbage, broccoli, cauliflower, and even
more potently, mustard greens, turnip greens, kale and collards—
contain a substance so effective in treating ulcers it has sometimes been
called "Vitamin U."[32] This substance is not stored in the body, however, so ulcer patients would be advised to eat these foods regularly.

Chewing one's food well is also quite important in the treatment
and prevention of ulcers because human saliva is highly alkaline. It
acts as a buffering agent in the duodenum and stomach, protecting the
linings of the digestive organs from becoming too acidic. People who
don't chew their food well, who "wolf" it down, are unknowingly
courting ulcers.

Wolves and other natural carnivores, by the way, can "wolf" down
their food without getting ulcers because their digestive systems (unlike ours) are anatomically designed to be highly acidic environments.
Their saliva is highly acidic, while ours is highly alkaline. Their digestive secretions are far more highly acidic than ours, so highly acidic, in
fact, that they can dissolve the bones of their prey. The natural carnivores are designed to "wolf" down their food. Their teeth are long and

pointed, suited for seizing prey and ripping off chunks of flesh. Our teeth, in contrast, are designed for the grinding of grains, vegetables and fruits. Without the aid of steak knives and cooking, we'd be hard-pressed indeed to handle flesh.

That we tend to get ulcers if we "wolf" down our food is an example of how eating habits which are anatomically unnatural to our species create disease. Heart attacks and strokes are other examples, because, as we have seen, the natural carnivores can tolerate any amount of cholesterol without their arteries suffering. Fortunately, the suffering caused by ulcers, like that caused by atherosclerosis, is entirely preventable, and in many cases can be cured by a natural vegetarian lowfat diet.

CONSTIPATION AND OTHER INTESTINAL PROBLEMS

"A good reliable set of bowels is worth more to a man than any quantity of brains."

(HENRY WHEELER SHAW)

"We aren't what we eat. We are what we don't shit."

(HUGH ROMNEY)

With diets that are low in fiber, there is little in the intestines to form a stool, except bacteria. It is not uncommon for the feces that ensue from low-fiber, meat-based diets to be as high as 75% bacteria.[33] On the average American diet, the "average American turd" is actually half bacteria!

This creates problems. With little roughage to stimulate peristaltic action, the material takes a long time to transit through the colon. The longer it takes, the drier it gets, and old dry feces do not gently plop from the body, but have to be pushed out by force.

Laxatives are often employed to move the bowels when the stools have become stuck, but in the long run these only make things worse because they irritate the bowel walls. The real answer is a diet low in fat and high in fiber. People who choose foods such as sprouts, whole grains, vegetables and fruits tend to have large, soft, moist well-formed stools that glide along easily through the intestines.[34]

Hemorrhoids, commonly known as piles, also result from diets that are low in fiber and high in fat. South African whites consume one of the highest fat and lowest fiber diets in the world, and have one of the highest hemorrhoid rates in the world. The diet of South African blacks, in contrast, is much lower in fat and higher in fiber, and these people suffer virtually no hemorrhoids.[35]

Researchers once thought that this striking contrast might be due to heredity. But those blacks in South Africa who do eat meat have higher hemorrhoid rates than the other blacks; and American blacks have the same incidence of hemorrhoids as American Caucasians.

In the United States, millions of people buy over-the-counter preparations which they are told will shrink their hemorrhoids. Sadly, these people are rarely told the real causes of their suffering and the road to its healing. Straining to eliminate hard, dry stools increases the pressure of blood in the veins of the rectum and legs. Over a period of time this leads to the formation of hemorrhoids, which are actually varicose veins of the rectum.[36] Varicose veins of the legs also commonly result from the same mechanism.

Diets high in fiber and low in fat yield soft, moist, plentiful stools, eliminate the need for straining, and are of great help in preventing and treating not only constipation, but hemorrhoids and varicose veins.[37]

There are additional problems that arise from straining to push hard, compact stools out of the colon. Such effort forces the stomach up against the diaphragm. Eventually, this repeated pressure enlarges the diaphragm opening, and part of the stomach may be pushed through the opening. This is called a hiatal hernia, and results in chest pains, indigestion and belching. This discomfort can be extremely intense, and is entirely preventable with lowfat high-fiber diets.[38]

A very high percentage of elderly people in the United States experience intractable constipation, bleeding and abdominal pain. What has happened is that the continual presence of old, dry material in their intestines has pushed the colon out of shape, forcing the formation of little pockets called diverculi.

Though this condition, called diverticulosis, is very rare in countries where fiber intake is high and fat intake is low, it is so common as to be considered almost inevitable in countries where the consumption of meats, dairy products, and other high fat foods are the norm.[39] In the United States, over 75% of those over the age of 75 suffer from diverticulosis.

These people experience repeated attacks, during which the intestines become inflamed and bleeding increases. Not knowing what's really going on, many turn to laxatives which unfortunately further irritate the intestinal linings. Eventually, in many cases, relief can only be obtained by undergoing major surgery in which segments of the colon are removed.

The good news is that none of this is necessary. Not only can diverticulosis be prevented by a diet that is high in fiber and low in fat, but it can often be successfully treated with such a diet as well.[40]

A report in the *American Journal of Digestive Disorders* tells of 62 diverticulosis patients who were put on a high-fiber diet. Fully 85% of the patients reported complete disappearance of their symptoms.[41]

In another study, 70 diverticulosis patients were put on a high-fiber diet. In this case, 88% of their symptoms were relieved or eliminated. And the number of patients requiring laxatives was reduced from 49 to 7.[42]

If you wish to add fiber to your diet in a supplementary form, psyllium husks are a better choice than wheat bran. They are milder, smoother, and less abrasive in their intestinal action. Take them with plenty of water, an hour or more before a meal. However, a health-supporting high-fiber diet is not achieved by merely adding fiber to a low-fiber diet. Studies in which such shortcuts have been employed have not been nearly as successful as when fiber-deficient and high-fat foods are eliminated, particularly those high in saturated fat.

The most common gastrointestinal disease seen by physicians in general practice in the United States today is known as "irritable colon syndrome," or "spastic colon." The chief symptoms are usually pain in the lower abdomen, alternating constipation and diarrhea, and mucus appearing in small-caliber stools. Today's doctors have been taught that this condition is caused by emotional disturbances, but doctors who have switched their patients to a high-fiber lowfat diet have consistently seen this "psychological" problem cured.[43]

Appendectomies are the most frequent emergency operation in the United States today. They are needed when the opening of the appendix becomes blocked. In such an occurrence the appendix cannot drain properly, bacteria multiply, and the appendix swells painfully. The appendicitis victim experiences acute pain, usually in the right lower quadrant of the abdomen.

The culprit that blocks the appendix and creates all these problems is very often a small piece of hard dry feces. The underlying reason behind most appendicitis is a diet-style that produces slow-moving, fiber-deficient stools. This results in the small, dry concretions of fecal matter, called fecaliths, which lodge in and block the opening to the appendix.[44]

The incidence of constipation, hemorrhoids, hiatal hernias, diverticulosis, spastic colons and appendicitis corresponds very closely to the amount of fiber and fat in people's food choices. Unfortunately, many people who do not understand the enormous impact our food choices have on the health of our intestines end up requiring surgery and undergoing constant pain. This is particularly sad because it is so unnecessary. It is hard to exaggerate the amount of suffering from these diseases that could be prevented by high-fiber, lowfat diets.

OBESITY

Yankee Stadium was originally built in the 1920's to accommodate the great crowds who wanted to see Babe Ruth play baseball. When it was renovated in the 1970's, the seating capacity had to be reduced by 9,000 seats. The seating reduction was necessary because, in the 50 years since the Babe swung his bat, the average American fanny had increased in width by four inches. And so the ballpark seats had to be widened from 15 to 19 inches.[45]

Television ads tell us "why beef is great if you're watching your weight." In other ads, we are shown feasts of beef fit for the bulging banquet tables of a king. The decorations are lavish, the music elegant, the furnishings posh, the people gorgeous, and the costumes speak of great wealth. "All of this," we are told, "for only 300 calories."

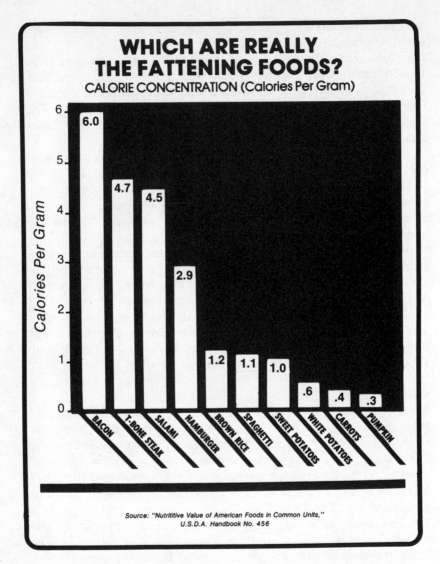

WHICH ARE REALLY THE FATTENING FOODS?

CALORIE CONCENTRATION (Calories Per Gram)

Source: "Nutrititive Value of American Foods in Common Units,"
U.S.D.A. Handbook No. 456

We are never told it is actually an undersized, surgically defatted sliver of beef that has "only 300 calories."

The meat and dairy industries have spent many millions of dollars to promote the belief that carbohydrates, such as potatoes, bread and pasta are the real culprits that cause excess weight gain. But literally thousands of impartial studies have shown this to have no basis in fact. Due to their high fat content, meats are far indeed from "calorie conscious."

The renowned Harvard nutritionist, Dr. Jean Mayer, explained the matter this way:

> *"In becoming a vegetarian, you will eat a greater percentage of your calories from cereal grains, dried beans and peas, potatoes and pasta—the very foods most dieters avoid with zeal. And you will lose weight."* [46]

Because people eating the standard American diet eat such a very high percentage of their calories as fat, most of them fight a never-ending "battle of the bulge." But obesity is not merely an aesthetic issue. It has been found to be a significant co-factor in all the degenerative diseases that kill and cripple modern man. The obese, and to a lesser but still significant extent the overweight, have higher rates of heart disease, diabetes, liver disorders, gallbladder disease, cancer, arthritis, and virtually every other degenerative disease. [47] Infant mortality rates are far higher for babies born to obese mothers. Obese teenagers have a life expectancy that is 15 years shorter than normal.

Clinically, the term "obesity" refers to excessive levels of body-fat. It is, quite literally, a case of "being fat."

From a clinical standpoint, the body weight most of us think of as "normal" is anything but healthy. As one authority wrote:

> *"A teenager who remains 20% under the normal weight enjoys a 15 year increase over and above normal life expectancy. Lower than normal weight is also associated with marked reductions in the incidence of cancer, cardiovascular diseases, diabetes, and other degenerative diseases. In a very real sense, then, U.S. and European*

weight standards are excessive, and the overwhelming majority of Americans and Europeans are detrimentally overweight . . .

   "The U.S. Public Health Service estimates 60 million Americans are overweight. In reality, the number of Americans who are above optimal weight may be three times the government estimate." [48]

When we realize that so-called "normal" weights are actually too high for optimum health, and a very high percentage of Americans are above even these weights, a picture emerges that is neither flattering nor healthy. What is considered "normal" in our culture is actually a moderate form of obesity.

Major studies published in the *Journal of Clinical Nutrition*, the *New England Journal of Medicine* and elsewhere have found that vegetarians suffer far less from being overweight than do meat eaters.[49] And pure vegetarians tip the scales in an even healthier fashion.

Most everyone has observed that the more body fat people have, the less they are likely to exercise. We all know people whose only exercise seems to be moving the food from their plate to their palate. Usually, we tend to think their weight problem is caused by a lack of exercise. But research is showing that it works the other way around, too.

The higher a person's percentage of body fat, the less he or she typically **wants** to exercise. Obese individuals tend to spend more time in bed, and remain otherwise sluggish. Studies of people playing tennis showed that the higher their percentage of body fat, the less calories they burned per minute, even though with their additional weight to move around they burned more calories per movement.[50] Their movements were less frequent, smaller and slower.

Thus the overweight person tends to be caught in a classical dilemma, where lack of exercise increases the weight problem, which in turn lowers the willingness to exercise—an unfortunate vicious circle, which can't help but contribute significantly to a speeding up of the system's degeneration.

ARTHRITIS
Many of the elderly in the United States—and quite a few of the not-so-elderly—experience terrible pain in their joints. Their fingers may

become twisted and swollen, and they may be unable even to button a coat without large doses of anti-inflammatory drugs such as aspirin. Many come to feel crippled and useless.

By the age of 35, 35% of Americans have diagnosable arthritis in their knees. At least 85% of those over the age of 70 have it, and many have it severely. There are 180,000 people in the country today who are bedridden or confined to a wheelchair because of this disease.[51]

The official position of the Arthritis Foundation is that diet and arthritis are not related. But, astoundingly, there has been very little research done to justify this assertion.[52] Up until now, virtually all arthritis research money has gone to test drugs.

At Wayne State University Medical School, however, there were a few medical researchers willing to investigate the heresy that diet might have something to do with arthritis. They put six rheumatoid arthritis patients on a fat-free diet. The results were startling. In seven weeks, all of the subjects showed total disappearance of their symptoms. When fats were reintroduced into their diets, it took only three days for the symptoms to reappear.[53]

In 1981, the *British Medical Journal* reported another instance that suggests the Arthritis Foundation's conclusions might be premature.[54] It involved a 38-year-old woman, who for 11 years had been suffering from steadily worsening rheumatoid arthritis. Three weeks after doctors removed all dairy products from her diet she showed signs of improvement. In four months, her arthritic symptoms had completely disappeared. She remained free of symptoms until, in the interests of scientific curiosity, she once again ate some cheese and milk. The next day her joints were swollen, stiff and painful. Fortunately, her symptoms again disappeared as she resumed her abstinence from dairy products.

In parts of the world where the diets are low in fats and cholesterol, and moderate in protein, and where the consumption of processed and junk foods is minimal, even old people who have done hard physical work their whole lives are essentially free of arthritis.[55] This presents quite a contrast to the United States, where so many are crippled by the disease that it is rare to find an older person who is not affected.

One study found not a single case of rheumatoid arthritis in a rural black South African community of over 800 people who ate no meats or dairy products.[56] Another study found that black South Africans who ate significant amounts of meat and other high-fat foods had almost four times the incidence of arthritis as those whose diet was very low in meat and fat.[57]

Arthritis patients characteristically suffer severely from atherosclerosis, and their blood cholesterol levels tend to be higher than normal. There is evidence that the fat and cholesterol which accumulates on the linings of the blood vessels in atherosclerosis prevent the normal transfer of oxygen to the joint tissues. Joint tissues which are thus deprived of oxygen become inflamed, and arthritic. As well, nodes or knots made up primarily of cholesterol are frequently found near arthritic joints. And arthritis patients often have severe atherosclerosis in the body's main artery, the aorta.[58]

Gouty arthritis is acknowledged even by the Arthritis Foundation as being diet-related. In fact, gout is one of the most easily controlled of all diseases when proper dietary quidelines are followed.[59]

Gout occurs when uric acid in the body forms needle-like crystals which become deposited in a joint. When that happens, there is severe pain and swelling in a joint, often the big toe.

Avoiding foods that are high in either purines or protein has been shown to be of enormous benefit to gouty arthritis sufferers.[60] Shellfish, fish, poultry, beef, pork and legumes are all high in purines.

Some people, particularly Filipinos, are especially susceptible to gout.[61] But on a low-purine, low-protein diet, gout is almost nonexistent, even among those people most genetically disposed toward it. During World War II, when gout sufferers in occupied European countries were suddenly forced to consume less meats and dairy products, the incidence of gouty arthritis plummeted.

There are many kinds of arthritis, including osteoarthritis, rheumatoid arthritis, gout, lupus erythematosus and ankylosing spondylitis. The connection with diet and gout is crystal clear, but far more work needs to be done for the other forms of arthritis. The evidence strongly suggests that diets very low in saturated fat, low in protein, high in fiber, and without any cholesterol would be best for the prevention of arthritis, and as an important element in treatment.

KIDNEY STONES

Kidney stones cause indescribable pain, and have been referred to as one of the most painful ordeals known to medicine. The severe pain they cause is completely unnecessary and preventable. Over 99% of all kidney stones can be prevented by low-protein, high-fiber, lowfat diets that contain no cholesterol, saturated fat or empty calories.[62]

Kidney stones vary according to their chemical composition. Some are made up chiefly of calcium oxalate, others of calcium phosphate, and others of uric acid. The formation of all of these types of kidney stones is directly attributable to diets high in animal protein. The more animal protein we eat, the more calcium our kidneys have to excrete. When our urine is high in calcium, it tends to precipitate out little crystals of calcium in the urinary system. It is around these crystals that kidney stones grow. So sensitive are our urine calcium levels to protein intake that the concentrations of calcium in our urine can be lowered in a matter of hours by decreased protein consumption.

Vegetarians in the United States have fewer than half the kidney stones of the general population.[63] Pure vegetarians have almost none.

GALLSTONES

The main ingredient in almost all gallstones is cholesterol. The more cholesterol in the diet, the more will be present in the gallbladder fluids, and the more readily gallstones will form.[64]

Dietary fiber also influences gallstone incidence, but in the other direction. Fiber tends to bind cholesterol and carry it out in the stool. Diets high in fiber produce lower rates of cholesterol gallstones. Worldwide, the greatest incidence of gallbladder disease, gallstones, and gallbladder cancer is found in people whose food choices are low in fiber, high in cholesterol and high in fat, such as the average American.[65]

Gallstone sufferers usually turn to surgery to relieve the intense pain. But lowfat, high-fiber diets not only prevent gallstones; they have been clinically shown to often relieve the pain of gallstones so significantly as to make surgery unnecessary.[66]

HYPERTENSION (HIGH BLOOD PRESSURE)

Each year Americans make 275 million visits to their doctors. The most common of all reasons, accounting for one out of every eleven visits, is high blood pressure. Nine times out of ten they leave with a prescription for a drug. More prescriptions are written in this country for hypertension that for any other disease.[67] Hypertension is so common in America today that, like heart attacks, we tend to think of it as an inevitable price we must pay for growing old.

Doctors prescribe so many drugs for hypertension because they know how dangerous the disease can be. If your blood pressure is high, compared to a person your age whose blood pressure is normal, you have:

> ***Double the risk of dying in the next year*
> ***Triple the risk of dying from a heart attack*
> ***Quadruple the risk of heart failure*
> ***Seven times the risk of a stroke*[68]

Studies of people whose blood pressure remains low as they age, however, have revealed these people share certain characteristics.[69] Their diets are low in fats, cholesterol and salt, and high in fiber. They eat whole grains, fresh vegetables and fruits, and their intake of processed and refined foods is minimal. Their body fat levels are low, and they get plenty of exercise.

In countries where the intake of salt, fats and cholesterol is low, hypertension is unknown.[70] In many cases, people in their 80's have the same blood pressure as teenagers. These are the same countries where strokes and heart attacks are few and far between.

This is not because these people are genetically favored. When people from these lands move to other countries and take on diets high in saturated fat, cholesterol and salt, their blood pressure levels shoot right up alongside ours.

Salt increases blood pressure by drawing water into the blood, increasing the pressure on the arterial walls. But salt is not the only cause of high blood pressure. If you partially block the end of a hose with your thumb, thereby increasing the resistance against which the water flows, it will shoot out under greater pressure. This is akin to what happens in our blood streams if we suffer from atherosclerosis. The deposits clogging our arteries narrow the channels, thereby increasing the resistance against which our blood flows, raising our blood pressure.[71]

Hypertension is an announcement that the circulatory system is not well. When the blood pressure is very high, this announcement should be construed as a veritable fire alarm, calling for immediate attention to serious trouble in the cardiovascular system.

Sadly, the conventional medical response is all too often simply to prescribe drugs to silence the alarm, while doing nothing about the problem the alarm is trying to draw to our attention.[72] Lowering blood pressure without doing something to improve the health of the cardiovascular system is like turning off the fire alarm and going back to sleep, without fixing what set it off in the first place.

In addition, these drugs have disturbing side effects. The Beta Blockers (propanolol, metoprolol, nadolol, atenolol, etc.) often make patients feel fatigued and listless.[73] The diuretics (hydrochlorothiazide, other thiazides, chlorthalidone, furosemide, spironolactone, etc.) raise blood cholesterol levels, and double the risk of fatal heart attacks.[74] And the blood vessel dilators (apresoline, hydralizine, etc.) have a wide range of common and unpleasant side effects, most commonly producing impotence in males.[75] The blood vessels are expanded to the point that the blood supply simply cannot engorge the penis and produce an erection. Females experience a decrease or total loss of sexual interest with blood vessel dilators.

These drugs do have a part to play in hypertension treatment, since they do bring down the blood pressure, which can be life saving. But would it not be a far greater service to show patients that by changing their diets they can accomplish the same results without all the disturbing side effects? Then these drugs could be used with discretion in the transition period, as a temporary bridge to a healthier life.

And it's not hard to know what the proper diet should be, for the same food choices that raise blood cholesterol levels also raise blood pressure levels. In fact, high blood pressure is almost invariably accompanied by high blood cholesterol.[76]

You may recall that the dairy industry greeted the news that saturated fat and cholesterol promote heart disease with something less than humble respect for the truth. They have responded similarly with respect to high blood pressure, for the same reason: their products are deeply implicated, this time on two counts. Cheese is among the highest foods in salt content; and the dairy industry is American's second leading seller of saturated fat, tipping its hat only to the meat industry.

But as you know by now, the dairy industry has not felt shy about taking profound liberties with the truth in order to defend its products. True to this form, the National Dairy Council has issued reports saying drinking milk and eating cheese lower blood pressure, and that eating salt does not raise it.

Impartial scientists have been amazed at such audacity. The association between foods high in saturated fat and cholesterol, such as dairy products, and high blood pressure, has been established and documented in literally hundreds of rigorous studies.[77]

The Dairy Council claims that the increased calcium from dairy products will lower blood pressure, but the truth is that such a decrease is minimal at best, and if obtained via dairy products, any such temporary benefits are more than outweighed by the increased development of atherosclerosis.

Their claim that eating salt does not raise blood pressure testifies profoundly to a lack of respect both for the truth and for the health of the American public.

Hypertension patients can get almost immediate relief from some of the problems of high blood pressure when they cease to consume saturated fats and cholesterol. Saturated fats cause blood clotting elements in the blood, called "platelets," to stick together, forming clumps that slow down the flow of blood. These clumpings cause the blood pressure to rise sharply within hours of a meal rich in saturated fat, and account for the many heart attacks that occur within hours of rich meals.[78]

Many studies have compared the blood pressure levels of people who have different diet-styles.[79] Even when the data has been adjusted to eliminate salt as a variable, the following pattern is consistent:

Blood Pressure Levels
(Highest ranked first)
1. *Meat-eaters*
2. *Lacto-ovo vegetarians*
3. *Pure vegetarians*

One study, reported in the *American Journal of Epidemiology*, found the blood pressure levels of vegetarians to be "significantly less" than the levels found in meat eaters, even when the data had been adjusted to compensate for any conceivable advantage the vegetarians might have had from their generally lesser intake of salt, alcohol, tobacco, tea and coffee.[80] The study's author attributed the difference in blood pressure readings to: "intake of animal protein and animal fat."

This information is not having an easy time finding its way into the public awareness. The meat and dairy industries do not like what has been learned, and are up to their usual shenanigans to prevent people from knowing.

But it is not only the meat and dairy industries. The incentive for those who would educate the public is small. In a drug-oriented culture fond of instant results with a minimum of effort, it's an uphill battle all the way. If you come up with a drug that lowers blood pressure, you can make millions of dollars. But if you want to show people how to eat so their blood pressure won't become elevated in the first place, enthusiasm dwindles.

There are millions of Americans at this very moment suffering profoundly from the consequences of high blood pressure. This is especially tragic because it is so thoroughly needless.

ANEMIA

The belief that vegetarians tend to be anemic is common among people who have been unknowingly schooled according to the "basic four" nutritional propaganda. This is a classic example of how ignorance can cause needless suffering. Such people may very well sense that dropping meat is a good idea, yet still find themselves reluctant to do so because they have been so deeply conditioned to believe that they would become iron deficient.

It turns out, however, that hardly anything could be further from the truth. Impartial and rigorous studies have consistently shown that vegetarians suffer less anemia than do meat eaters.

The figure on page 298 shows the iron content of various foods, according to official U.S. government figures. Popeye wasn't far off the mark. Calorie per calorie, spinach has 14 times the iron of a typical

IRON CONTENT OF FOODS
Milligrams per 100 Calories

VEGETABLES

Spinach	11.3
Beet greens	11.2
Mustard greens	8.3
Turnip greens	6.5
Cucumber	6.0
Cauliflower	4.2
Kale	4.0
Chinese cabbage	4.0
Iceburg lettuce	3.8
Collards	3.4
Bell peppers	3.3
Broccoli	3.1
Mushrooms	3.0
Zucchini	2.7
Peas	2.7
Green beans	2.7
Tomatoes	2.4
Red cabbage	2.4
Celery	2.4
Green cabbage	2.4
Carrot	1.8
Beet	1.6
Onion	1.4
Sweet potatoes	0.6

DAIRY PRODUCTS

Cheddar cheese	< 0.1
Bleu cheese	< 0.1
Cottage cheese	< 0.1
Mozzarella cheese	< 0.1
Low fat (2%) milk	< 0.1
Ice milk	< 0.1
Low fat Yogurt	< 0.1
Whole milk	< 0.1
Ice cream	< 0.1
Whipping cream	0.0
Butter	0.0

FRUITS

Strawberries	2.7
Dried apricots	2.3
Lemons	2.0
Blueberries	1.7
Raspberries	1.6
Blackberries	1.5
Peaches	1.3
Cantaloupe	1.3
Grapefruit	1.1
Plums	1.0
Pineapple	1.0
Banana	0.8
Orange	0.8

MEATS AND FISH

Sirloin steak, lean only	1.9
Pot roast, lean only	1.2
Ground beef, lean only	1.1
Tuna, canned and drained	0.9
Ham roast	0.9
Pork chop	0.9
Salami	0.9
Sirloin steak	0.8
Chicken breast	0.8
Turkey, light meat	0.7
Ocean perch	0.6
Salmon	0.6
Bacon	0.6
Rib roast	0.6
Leg of lamb	0.6
Bologna	0.6
Frankfurter	0.5
Lamb chop	0.3

GRAINS, SEEDS, LEGUMES

Lima beans	2.3
Navy beans	2.3
Lentils	2.0
Pumpkin seeds	2.0
Sunflower seeds	1.4
Split peas	1.4
Oats	1.1
Rye	1.1
Wheat	1.0
Walnuts	0.9
Almonds	0.8

Source: "Nutrititive Value of Foods," Consumer and Food Economics Institute,
United States Department of Agriculture, U.S. Government Printing Office, 1977

sirloin steak. Although meat is a decent source of iron, vegetables are actually better. The only iron deficient foods are dairy products, sugar, fats and processed foods. So iron deficient are dairy products that you'd have to eat a hunk of butter as big as your refrigerator to get as much iron as you would get from a bowl of broccoli.

For years our schools have been provided "nutritional education" materials by the dairy council and meat industry which compare the iron levels of different foods according to their weight. Intentionally or not, this has served to make meat appear unfairly advantageous when compared to vegetables and fruits, because the latter are high in water content, and the weight of the water in the plant foods dilutes their figures when so calculated.

Iron absorption is greatly assisted by the presence of Vitamin C.[81] In fact, a lack of this vitamin can prevent the body from effectively using the iron it is given. Fresh vegetables, sprouts and fruits are the best sources of Vitamin C; whereas meats, dairy products, eggs, fats and sugar provide none.

At least 20% of all women of child-bearing age in the United States are iron deficient. This is primarily due to their monthly loss of iron in their menstrual flow, coupled with their intake of sugar, dairy products and fats, none of which provide any iron to replace that which is lost. And meat eaters consistently have a heavier buildup of tissue on the inside lining of the uterus. The bleeding from these thickened tissues is heavier and longer, so more iron is lost per period than would be the case with a lighter diet. Vegetarian women, as a rule, have less estrogen in their bodies, lighter, shorter and easier periods, and so less iron loss.

Vegetarian women who do become anemic have frequently been so cowed by National Dairy Council propaganda that they fear something dreadful will surely happen if they don't "get enough protein." Not wishing to eat meat, they overconsume dairy products "just to be sure." Because dairy products are woefully iron deficient, these well-meaning women may unknowingly be eating their way into anemia.

Young children sometimes become anemic due to significant iron loss from intestinal bleeding. This problem has been the subject of very thorough study. The results of exceedingly conscientious and painstaking studies show that over half the intestinal bleeding in children is a reaction to dairy products.[82]

The misguided belief that vegetarians tend to be anemic is sadly ironic in light of the many studies which have measured the hemoglobin levels (which reflect the amount of iron in the blood) of people with different diet-styles. Vegetarians consistently fare better in these tests than do meat-eaters. Long-term studies show no iron deficiencies arising from lacto-ovo or pure vegetarian diets. The only people who run into trouble are the ones who eat a lot of dairy products, fatty foods, sugar, and junk foods.

A deficiency of Vitamin B-12 can result in a serious disease called pernicious anemia. Since only animal products reliantly contain appreciable amounts of this vitamin, it is possible that abstaining from all eggs and dairy products, as well as meat, may produce this serious condition. Accordingly, I advise all strict vegetarians to take supplementary B-12. Such supplements are readily available from plant sources and are very inexpensive. The sublingual form is far better absorbed by the body than swallowing the tablet form.

It is especially important for nursing mothers on a pure vegetarian diet to take supplementary B-12. This is necessary because the Vitamin B-12 stored in the mother's body will not go into her breast milk, thus exposing the infant to possible danger, unless the mother takes B-12 through a supplement.

ASTHMA

Researchers at the University Hospital in Linkoping, Sweden, put bronchial asthma patients, whose condition was so severe that they required cortisone or other medication, onto a pure vegetarian diet, without any eggs or dairy products. The results were extremely promising.

After one year of the diet, **more than 90%** of the patients who completed the project reported a major improvement in the severity and frequency of asthma attacks. Also, levels of medication dosages dropped an average of 50 to 90 percent. A number of the patients were so improved that they were able to discontinue medication altogether with the pure vegetarian diet.[83]

SALMONELLOSIS

Salmonellosis is a bacterial infection derived from contaminated animal products. The disease is, at best, a miserable nuisance; people experience nausea, diarrhea, abdominal cramps, fever, and sometimes vomiting and chills. For the aged, the ill, and infants, however, and for those whose immune systems are compromised, it's another story: the disease can be fatal.

Over four million cases of salmonellosis poisoning are known to occur annually in the United States. Many more than that are taken to be bad cases of the flu. But salmonellosis is far more than a flu. The National Research Council of the National Academy of Sciences evaluated "the salmonellosis problem" and stated:

"Salmonellosis is one of the most important communicable disease problems in the United States today." [84]

You may assume the meat you buy has been inspected for salmonellosis. But detection for this disease is not required by U.S.D.A. meat inspection regulations, and the meat packing plants are hardly eager to provide this or any extra service when not required to by law. There is, in fact, not a single meat packing plant in the entire country today which inspects its products for salmonellosis.

Knowing this, the American Public Health Association (composed of federal, state, and local public health officials), feels the public is woefully misled by meat inspection seals which seem to imply safety and wholesomeness. So upset was the American Public Health Association by this flagrant deceit that they filed a suit demanding a court order requiring meat labels to read:

"Caution—Improper handling and inadequate cooking of this product may be hazardous to your health." [85]

A frowning meat industry responded that it would be "unfair" to "stigmatize" meat by "warning consumers of the hazards associated with flesh eating." One meat industry spokesman pointed out that life is full of risks, as if that somehow justified keeping the public in the dark. He declared:

"Sure, you can get food poisoning from contaminated meat, but you can get it from unclean vegetables, too." [86]

Ironically, the man had a point, though I'm not entirely sure it was the one he wanted to make. Utensils, cutting boards, and human hands that come into contact with salmonellosis-infected meat can spread the disease. In a kitchen where meat is prepared, it can easily spread to salad vegetables. Since these foods are not cooked, the salad eater may get salmonellosis. And even cooked foods are placed in bowls, on plates, and eaten with cutlery that has been touched by hands that may have touched the contaminated meat. Thus the disease is liable to be spread in any kitchen that it enters, be it in a home, a restaurant, or a public service institution.

Congress wanted to know just how commonly meat in the United States today is infected with salmonellosis. They summoned Dr. Richard Novick, of the Public Health Research Institute, and asked for his expert testimony. The authority didn't mince his words:

"The meat we buy is grossly contaminated with both coliform bacteria and salmonella." [87]

One of the reasons our meat supply is so heavily contaminated with these disease agents is the way the animals are handled today. To begin with, they are sick creatures, due to how they are kept, and thus susceptible to just about any disease that comes down the pike. Then they are fed contaminated byproducts from the slaughterhouse, and crowded into cages, feedlots, trucks and holding pens which are perfect environments for diseases to spread. And as if that weren't enough, the slaughterhouses themselves could hardly be better designed for the spread of disease.

It is not just food reformers and vegetarians who are concerned. The *Journal of the American Veterinary Association* surveyed a cattle slaughterhouse and found a very high percentage of the carcasses were contaminated with salmonellosis. [88] When *60 Minutes* asked the head of the USDA Inspection Service, Dr. Donald Houston, about salmonella contamination, he answered (in March, 1987) that if you go into a supermarket anywhere in the United States and buy a chicken, the odds are better than one in three that it will be contaminated. Alarmed, *60 Minutes* conducted its own test, and the results brought no peace of mind. Over half the birds they purchased were found to be contaminated with salmonellosis. Amazed, they interviewed a number of meat inspectors, who publically acknowledged on national television that the inspection system provides no protection to the consumer.

Even the industry acknowledges this is the case. *Poultry Science*, a journal of the poultry trade, reported that 90% of the dressed product from a poultry processing plant was contaminated with salmonellosis.[89] The National Research Council, evidently not believing things could be this bad, conducted its own survey, and found out things were worse. No less than 90% of the poultry from a federally-inspected plant they examined were contaminated with salmonellosis.[90]

GOODBYE ANTIBIOTICS

At the same time, salmonella poisoning is becoming harder and harder to treat. The continuous feeding of antibiotics to livestock could hardly have been better designed to breed strains of bacteria, including salmonella, that are resistant to the drugs. Antibiotic-resistant bacteria flourish inside the animals as organisms vulnerable to antibiotics are killed off. As a result, diseases (including salmonellosis) which used to be treatable with antibiotics, are becoming increasingly dangerous, and much more often fatal.

Tragically, salmonella bacteria are only one of many disease-producing organisms that are becoming increasingly resistant to antibiotics, due to the continuous feeding of these drugs to livestock. For example, only a few years ago, less than ten per cent of staphylococci bacteria (notorious for causing skin, bone and wound infections as well as pneumonia and food poisoning) were resistant to penicillin. But today over 90% of staphylococci are resistant to penicillin.

Ominously, a major 1987 study by the Federal Center for Disease Control reported in the *New England Journal of Medicine* that the extremely hardy salmonella bacteria thriving in today's factory farms are not only increasingly resistant to antibiotics, they are also not all killed by most forms of cooking.[91] As a result, scientists predict that we will be seeing more and more cases of salmonella poisoning in the days to come, and that the cases will be increasingly serious. The chronic use of antibiotics in factory farms has created the likelihood (some say inevitability) of an epidemic of untreatable salmonella food poisoning.

It is no exaggeration to say that the indiscriminate use of antibiotics in factory farms is systematically producing disease-causing agents that are invulnerable to the modern wonder drugs. To keep the animals alive under such horrid conditions, antibiotics are, as a matter of course, placed in their feed. This use of the substances which are responsible for so many medical miracles is creating an "anti-miracle." It is a situation which could hardly have been better designed to breed and develop bacteria which are resistant to the medicines that have saved countless millions of lives from the epidemic scourges of the past. Unless we restrict the habitual use of antibiotics in livestock feed, these lifesavers are well on their way to becoming utterly ineffective, and physicians will find themselves as helpless in the treatment of many infectious diseases as they were in the pre-antibiotic Middle Ages.

Already, many of us who have eaten the products of factory farms have resistant organisms residing as members of our intestinal flora. We remain reasonably healthy, however, because their numbers are held in check by the many kinds of normal bacteria residing in our intestines. But as Dr. Kenneth Stoller, vice-president and public health affairs director for the American Association for Science and Public Policy, has explained, if we should require antibiotic treatment for any reason, "all hell can break loose." The normal organisms, which have not developed immunity to the medicines, are killed, and the resistant bugs can now multiply unchecked.[92]

The consequences can be severe. A recent review in *Science* revealed that over four per cent of infections caused by strains of salmonella which have become resistant to antibiotics are now fatal. For other infectious diseases also, our wonder drugs are rapidly losing their wonder.

This is why, in the 1970's, Great Britain and the European Economic Community (EEC) forbade the chronic use of antibiotics in livestock feed. But the pharmaceutical and livestock industries have to this day demonstrated something less than the utmost commitment to public welfare by successfully defeating every single attempt to follow suit in the United States.

AND NOW
We live in a crazy time, when people who make food choices that are healthy and compassionate are often considered weird, while people are considered normal whose eating habits promote disease and are dependent on enormous suffering.

Yet we are also living in a time of great discoveries, when every day we learn more about the consequences of our food choices, and so gradually grow more able to make our choices wisely.

The more I've studied the findings of the last few decades of medical research, the more I've realized that it is now really in our hands. Something is possible now that's never been possible before. We are learning how to create a truly healthy world.

I believe that each of us, at heart, wants to use our brief time in these bodies and on this planet to contribute something of value. I believe that each of us, at heart, wants to help make the world a better, safer place, a more loving and beautiful place. The healthier we are, the more able we will be to make whatever contribution we can.

We all know our world needs healing. Each of us experiences the planetary anguish of our time in our own way, but all of us know that not only our own lives, but the very existence of life on earth is hanging in the balance.

I have discovered that our eating habits affect the world we share far more profoundly than I had ever dreamed. They have an impact that extends far beyond issues of our own health. I have found that there are repercussions to our eating habits that are so immense and far-reaching as to make the matters of human health, as profound as they are, seem relatively trivial.

In the next two chapters, we will turn to how our food choices affect, not only our health, but our children, the gene pool, and the very possibility of life continuing to exist on earth. And we will explore the recent developments that speak in one voice, saying that never before in the history of mankind has a new direction in diet-style been needed with such aching urgency.

PART

THREE

*"Humanity, let us say, is like people packed
in an automobile which is traveling downhill
without lights at a terrific speed and driven by
a four-year-old child. The signposts along the
way are all marked 'progress.'"*

(LORD DUNSANY)

AMERICA THE POISONED

> *"There are those who want to set fire to our world;*
> *We are in danger;*
> *There is only time to work slowly;*
> *There is no time not to love."*
>
> (DENNA METZGER)

THERE IS A major problem with the medical research we have been discussing. It takes time for degenerative diseases to develop, and so the medical research which has correlated cancer, heart disease, and virtually every other degenerative disease of our time with conventional diet-styles is actually out-of-date. The cases of these diseases which modern medical research has studied actually developed, for the most part, on the meats, dairy products and eggs of the early and middle part of this century.

But today's meats, dairy products and eggs are vastly different commodities from those of even 30 years ago.[1]

For one thing, they are no longer the products of traditional farming methods. They are instead the products of assembly-line, mass production factory farming. Factory farm animals are much higher in fat than pasture-raised animals, because they get little or no exercise, and their feeds are intentionally designed to fatten them as rapidly and cheaply as possible. Further, their fat is far more highly saturated than that of free range livestock.

The 1975 World Conference on Animal Production issued a report titled "A Re-Evaluation of the Nutrient Role in Animal Products" which revealed the remarkable fact that factory farmed animals have as much as 30 times more saturated fat than yesterday's pasture-raised creatures![2]

While touted as suppliers of protein for the American public, today's factory farms are actually suppliers of saturated fat.

But as startling as this increase in saturated fat is, it is actually small potatoes compared to far more ominous changes that have occurred in today's meats, dairy products and eggs. Today's factory farm livestock are subject to vast quantities of toxic chemicals and artificial hormones. Residues are then transmitted to the people who eat their flesh and partake of their milk. Hardly any of these chemicals even existed before World War II, and so we have yet to witness the longer-term health consequences of eating the products of factory farms, which invariably contain residues from pesticides, hormones, growth stimulants, insecticides, tranquilizers, radioactive isotopes, herbicides, antibiotics, appetite stimulants and larvicides.

We have some important knowledge, though, about the long-range consequences of ingesting these substances, and I am not exaggerating when I say they are profoundly terrifying.

THE SEXUAL NIGHTMARE
The author of *Modern Meat*, Orville Schell, interviewed Dr. Carmen A. Saenz:

> " 'For years I have been encountering periodic cases of precocious puberty,' Dr. Saenz tells me when she is finished seeing the last of that morning's young patients. 'But in 1980, when I started finding one or two children like this in my waiting room every day, I knew that something quite serious was wrong. From the symptoms they were exhibiting, I was sure that they are being contaminated with some kind of estrogen.'
>
> "I ask Dr. Saenz to describe the symptoms. Without replying, she picks up a handful of polaroid photos from the top of her desk and hands them to me. Each shows the small body of a naked young girl. As I slowly thumb through them, Dr. Saenz gives me a case-by-case commentary in a tone of voice that matches the

*expression on her face—a mixture of outrage, sadness, and
determination.*

*"In the first photo, a four-and-a-half-year-old girl with delicate
coffee-colored skin, doelike brown eyes and almost fully developed
breasts lies on an examining table. She smiles with a sweet
innocence at the camera, seemingly unaware of the dramatic changes
that have gone on in her body.*

" 'She had an ovarian cyst,' says Dr. Saenz tersely.

*"A twelve-year-old boy stands against a white wall looking
with blank bewilderment into the camera. He wears a silver crucifix
around his neck, which dangles down between two grossly swollen
breasts.*

*" 'We've had to schedule him for surgery,' says Dr. Saenz
matter-of-factly. 'The emotional stress on him is incredible.'*

*"A one-year-old girl, whose teeth have not even completely come
in, lies on the examining table with a ruler stretched across her
chest to measure the diameter of her enlarged breasts. She has a
pacifier in one of her hands. Dr. Saenz says nothing. She just
shakes her head.*

*"A five-year-old girl, looking wild-eyed into the camera as if a
weapon were being aimed at her, lies on the examining table. Her
breasts are as large and well-developed as a fourteen-year-old's. Her
mons veneris is covered with a scraggly tangle of pubic hair.*

*" 'This one had a well-developed uterus and had begun to have
some vaginal bleeding,' says Dr. Saenz. 'These are developments
that we would not usually expect until 8 or 9 years of age at the
very earliest . . . I have seen hundreds of children like this, and I
am certain that there are thousands more going undiagnosed because
this problem has become so widespread that even many doctors are
no longer getting alarmed about it."* [3]

Dr. Saenz explained the cause of this epidemic of premature sexual
development in the February, 1982, *Journal of the Puerto Rico Medical
Association.*

*"The detailed analysis of histories on all of our patients discards
their use of medications or creams containing estrogens (as a cause),*

and none had neurological or other adrenal disorders . . . It was
clearly observed in 97 percent of the cases that the appearance of
abnormal breast tissue was . . . related to local whole milk in the
infant group. At a later age (the culprit was) . . . consumption of
local whole milk, poultry and beef." [4]

When Dr. Saenz was asked how she could be sure the children were
contaminated with hormones from meat and milk rather than from
some other source, she replied simply:

"When we take our patients off meat and fresh milk, their
symptoms usually regress." [5]

Regulations regarding hormone use in livestock are not enforced as
well in Puerto Rico as they are in the United States, and this partially
explains the epidemic there of premature sexual development. But
U.S. regulations are often laughed at in the rough and tumble world of
the American "cowboy," who tends to figure if a little is good, more is
probably better. As a result, doctors in the U.S. are seeing earlier and
earlier puberties in both boys and girls, more and more frequent cases
of small children developing sexual characteristics, and an ever expanding assortment of sexual aberrations. Other countries are also experiencing the same trend. An English medical journal reported that
hormone traces in the meat of chemically fattened livestock are causing
British school girls to mature sexually at least three years earlier than
in the past. [6]

There is no telling how many such cases occur, because when
children display symptoms of endocrine imbalance, doctors will almost
always blame it on a dysfunction of the child's endocrine system, unless the child has been taking hormone shots or pills. Few would ever
consider the possibility that the disturbance might stem from the use
of hormones in livestock production.

Meanwhile, both adults and children in our society are experiencing a plethora of behavior disorders connected to uncertain and confused sexual identities. The evidence that these arise at least in part
from hormonal imbalances is mounting steadily. We are also seeing a

startling increase in sexual abuse of children, and other tragic indications that human hormonal systems are haywire.

When hormones were first introduced into livestock production, after World War II, the meat industry was virtually ecstatic. The manufacturer of diethylstilbestrol, known as DES, humbly hailed the event as the most important moment in the history of food production. Because it produced more fat and more weight on the animals, and thus more profit for the meat industry, DES came to be used on more than 90% of America's cattle. It was called a "miracle."

Meanwhile, farmers who accidentally absorbed, inhaled or ingested even minute amounts of this "miracle" were not always fully able to appreciate its wonders.

"They exhibited symptoms of impotence, infertility, gynecomastia (elevated and tender breasts), or changes in voice register." [7]

Both adults and children were affected. The breast enlargement of a number of young children was directly traced to their having accidentally absorbed DES.[8] Nevertheless, literally tons of this hormone continued to be administered routinely to animals whose flesh and milk were destined for human consumption.

Then it was discovered that DES causes cancer even in the smallest doses imaginable. Lab animals developed cancer from daily doses of the hormone as low as one-quarter of a hundred-millionth of an ounce.[9] FDA biochemist Jacqueline Verret reported:

"Researchers from the National Cancer Institute assured Congressmen that it might be possible for only one molecule of DES in the 340,000,000,000,000 present in a quarter pound of beef liver to trigger human cancer . . ." [10]

After a fiercely fought political battle, it was finally made illegal to administer DES to livestock. But the meat industry simply shrugged its shoulders and carried on as usual. Several years after the ban went into effect, the FDA discovered how much respect the industry had for the law of the land. No less than half-a-million cattle were found to have been illegally implanted with DES.[11]

Today, many factory farms in the country continue to use DES illegally. Others have simply switched to the other sex hormones on the market which have the same effects and contain many of the same substances as DES. These hormones, such as Steer-oid, Ralgro, Compudose and Synovex, are used in virtually every feedlot in the country.[12]

SILENT SPRING

The loose-handed use of hormones in today's factory farms is sufficiently disturbing. But there is actually a far more ominous kind of contamination that people eating today's meats, dairy products and eggs unknowingly consume.

In 1962, Rachel Carson issued an epic warning to humanity in her prophetic book, *Silent Spring*.[13] She showed how pesticides were killing off birds, fish, and other wildlife at an alarming rate, in some cases to the point of extinction after only a few years use. The book drew its title from the fact that DDT and other pesticides were drastically reducing the populations of many bird species. Carson cautioned that the day was fast arriving when spring would come, but no bird songs would be heard:

> *"Over increasingly large areas of the United States, spring now comes unheralded by the return of birds, and the early mornings are strangely silent where once they were filled with the beauty of bird song. This sudden silencing of the song of birds, this obliteration of the color and beauty and interest they lend to our world have come about swiftly, insidiously, and unnoticed by those whose communities are as yet unaffected."*[14]

This is not what most of us would wish for our planet. But we have not heeded her warning about these lethal poisons.

We produce pesticides today at a rate more than 13,000 times faster than we did only 35 years ago.[15] Our environment and food chains are being inundated by a virtual avalanche of pesticides. What three decades ago took us six years to produce, we now produce every couple of hours.

It is hard for us to imagine how destructive these substances are. Pesticides are extraordinarily concentrated and powerful chemicals which have been intentionally developed to kill living creatures. In fact, some of them were originally developed to kill human beings. Phosgene, used today to produce chemical herbicides and insecticides, was originally developed for use in chemical warfare, and was, in fact, the agent of almost all deaths due to poison gas in World War I.[16] Zykon-B, another modern pesticide, is the substance which the Nazis used to produce deadly hydrogen cyanide gas, used to kill millions upon millions at Auschwitz, Dachau, and other concentration camps.[17]

Many of today's most widely used pesticides—including malathion and parathion—are members of the nerve gas family. So lethal is parathion that a chemist who swallowed an infinitesimal dose, amounting to 0.00424 of an ounce, was instantaneously paralyzed and died before he could take an antidote he had prepared in advance and had at hand.[18]

Pesticides are not the kind of substances you'd want to have hanging around in your environment. But hang around many of them do. In fact, the chlorinated hydrocarbon pesticides—DDT, aldrin, kepone, dieldrin, chlordane, heptachlor, endrin, mirex, PCB's, toxaphene, lindane, etc.—are extremely stable compounds. Ominously, they do not break down for decades, and in some cases, centuries.

THE FOOD CHAIN
Rachel Carson titled her book *Silent Spring* in memory of the song birds who have begun to disappear from our world. The reason it is birds, of all animals, who are the first to go, is that many of them are predators at the top of long food chains, and thus receive extremely concentrated doses of these chemicals.

You see, pesticides don't just affect the creature who ingests them first. They accumulate in the tissues of animals, and then, as one organism is eaten by another, they build up in ever higher concentrations at each successively higher rung on the food chain.

A worm living in the soil will store in its tissues all the pesticides it ever accumulates both from what it eats and what it absorbs through its skin. A bird which eats worms will thus ingest all the pesticides ever eaten or contacted by all the tens of thousands of worms it eats. At each successive stage up the food chain, the concentration of toxic chemicals is greatly increased. Thus, fish will accumulate in its body the total amount of poisons accumulated by all the thousands of smaller fish it eats. And each of these smaller fish will have collected in their flesh the total amount of toxic chemicals ever ingested by all the thousands of still smaller fish they have eaten. It's an exponential progression. Predator birds who eat fish often ingest extremely high concentrations of these deadly substances.

By the same token, a cow or chicken or pig will retain in its flesh all the pesticides it has ever consumed or absorbed, and factory farm animals build up especially high concentrations of chemical toxins for several reasons. 1) They are fed great quantities of fish meal. 2) Their other feeds are often grown on land heavily sprayed with the most dangerous pesticides. 3) They are dipped in, sprayed with, and intentionally fed many toxic compounds never encountered by animals raised in a more natural way.

These poisons are retained in the fat of the animals. With each inevitable step up the food chain, animals become ever more concentrated carriers of the most deadly chemicals ever known. Man, of course, sits at the very top of the chain whenever he eats fish, meats, eggs or dairy products.

The *Pesticides Monitoring Journal*, published by the EPA, chronicles scientific studies and research findings regarding these toxins. The journal confirmed what numerous studies have discovered:

"Foods of animal origin (are) the major source of . . . pesticide residues in the diet." [19]

Recent studies indicate that of all the toxic chemical residues in the American diet, almost all, 95% to 99%, comes from meat, fish, dairy products and eggs.[20] If you want to include pesticides in your diet, these are the foods to eat. Fortunately, you can overwhelmingly reduce your intake of these poisons by eating lower on the food chain, and not choosing foods of animal origin.

WHAT'S GOOD FOR DOW CHEMICAL COMPANY
Because the chlorinated hydrocarbon pesticides have such an extremely poisonous and persistent nature, environmentally aware peo-

ple have urged and pleaded and demanded and begged that this entire chemical family be outlawed. But the very poisonous and persistent qualities of these toxic chemicals have made them big money-makers for the chemical companies who market them aggressively. These corporations have applied enormous political and economic pressure to keep their products in use. The tragic result is that millions of pounds of these lethal agents continue to be used every year.

In the 1970's, mounting public concern overrode pressures from the chemical companies, the forced the passage of the Toxic Substances Control Act. But this Act has not in practice turned out to be the boon to environmental health it was intended to be. More than three years after the Act became law, the agency responsible for its administration had not yet ordered testing for a single one of the more than 50,000 toxic chemicals on the market.[21]

The Reagan administration was particularly instrumental in preventing the Toxic Substances Control Act from being enforced. Evidently believing "what's good for Dow Chemical Company is good for America," the Reagan administration abolished or crippled many of the country's most important health and environmental laws, including those regulations designed to protect the public from the misuse of pesticides.[22]

The current philosophy of toxic chemical management is to let the chemical companies regulate themselves. The chemical companies think this is a grand idea, though they know they must remain ever watchful lest the public become too concerned and require toxic pesticides to be legitimately assessed for their environmental impact. To prevent such a potentially embarrassing occurrence, they have come up with an ingenious and effective strategy: they have promoted the idea that dangerous chemicals have all been banned, and the government can be trusted to protect us, so there's nothing to worry about.

By and large the public has bought their story. President Reagan did. In fact he publicly complained:

> *"The world is experiencing a resurgence of deadly diseases spread by insects because pesticides like DDT have been prematurely outlawed."* [23]

But Reagan couldn't be more wrong.

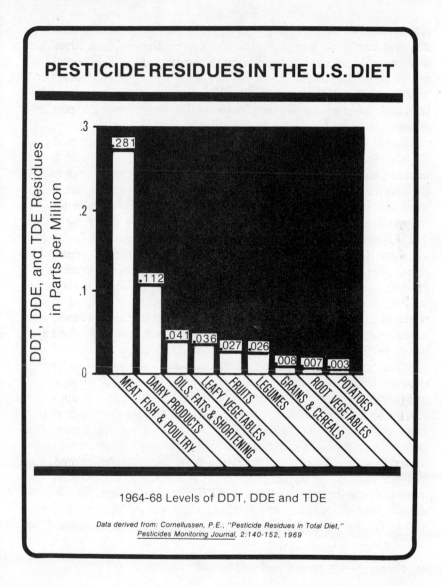

PESTICIDE RESIDUES IN THE U.S. DIET

1964-68 Levels of DDT, DDE and TDE

Data derived from: Cornellussen, P.E., "Pesticide Residues in Total Diet," Pesticides Monitoring Journal, 2:140-152, 1969

THE TRUTH

One reporter who uncovered the shocking truth regarding chemicals and our environment is the outstanding environmentalist Lewis Regenstein. In *How to Survive in America the Poisoned*, his superbly documented report on the use and effect of deadly chemicals, he writes that although the chemical industry wants us to believe that the really dangerous pesticides have been banned, this is not at all what has actually occurred:

> *"Despite the overwhelming evidence that pesticides cause cancer and are extremely dangerous to humans and the environment, almost none of these chemicals has ever been 'banned' by the government in the true sense of that word. In the very few cases where pesticides have been the subject of suspensions, cancellation proceedings, and/or court actions, the results have usually been restrictions or bans placed on some or most uses, while other applications have been allowed to continue."* [24]

Even in the few cases where the use of a pesticide has been restricted, the poison does not simply disappear from the environment. Quite the contrary, toxic chemicals like DDT take decades or even centuries to degrade. Even if by some miracle we stopped all pesticide use today, these chemicals would remain with us, contaminating our environment and our food chains for the foreseeable future.

DDT, one of the earliest pesticides, is one of a mere handful of these poisons that has actually been banned. Yet four years after the moratorium on DDT had been declared, the government tested soils in Arizona that had once been treated with DDT and found no measurable decrease in the amount in the soil. [25] Twelve years after the chemical was banned in the United States, researchers checked 27 bottle-nosed dolphins found dead off the coast of California. They found "extremely high" concentrations of DDT in every one. [26] So persistent is DDT in the environment that even now it continues to be found in the bodies of penguins and seals in Antarctica, seals in the Arctic ocean, and in frogs living at very high altitudes in remote regions of the Sierra Nevada mountains. [27]

THE TIP OF THE ICEBERG

While DDT has gotten most of the publicity, there are unfortunately many other toxic chemicals that are equally widespread in the environment, and actually more poisonous. The pesticide dieldrin, for example, is five times more poisonous than DDT when swallowed, and forty times more so when absorbed by the skin.[28] Yet, by the time dieldrin was finally banned in 1974, the FDA found it in 96% of all the meat, fish and poultry in the country, in 85% of all dairy products, and in the flesh of 99.5% of the American people![29] Sadly, dieldrin will remain with us for a long time; it is one of the most biologically stable of all pesticides, taking many decades to break down.

Dieldrin is also one of the most potent carcinogens ever known.[30] It causes cancer in lab animals at every dosage tested, down to the most infinitesimal concentrations measurable by modern, sophisticated equipment. In humans, low levels of exposure cause convulsions, severe liver damage, and rapid destruction of the central nervous system.[31] After a World Health Organization anti-malarial program used dieldrin, workers foamed at the mouth, went into convulsions, and died. Others, who had only the most minimal exposure to the substance, suffered convulsions for months afterwards.[32]

This doesn't sound like a substance you'd particularly want in your food. But for many years, dieldrin was applied to virtually all the acreage in the United States still used to grow corn, oats, barley, soybeans, and alfalfa for livestock feed.[33]

In March, 1974, the U.S.D.A. discovered that almost 10 million chickens in Mississippi were heavily contaminated with dieldrin, from feed grown on land to which the pesticide had been applied.[34] The chickens were destroyed, but the Agriculture Department admits it has no way of knowing how often this kind of incident occurs, and acknowledges that we are fortunate if we become aware of even the tiniest fraction of such occurrences. On June 26, 1980, the U.S.D.A revealed that turkey products from Banquet Foods Corporation contained intolerable levels of dieldrin. Eventually two million packages of frozen turkey dinners, turkey pies, and other turkey products were recalled.[35]

While dieldrin is no longer being applied to our soils as it once was, it remains in the soils to which it was once applied. These are the soils which grow the grains that are fed to the animals whose flesh, milk and eggs Americans consume. For the foreseeable future, dieldrin will continue to work its poisonous way up the food chain, collecting in the fatty tissues of the animals. The only bright side to this is that you can do a great deal to avoid consuming dieldrin by eating low on the food chain.

DIOXIN

During the Vietnam War, Agent Orange was sprayed by U.S. air forces over Vietnamese jungles and farmlands. The pilots who flew these missions were assured of the safety of the substance, and had a motto which expressed their flippant attitude towards their missions: "Only we can prevent forests." On some occasions they would engage in playful spray fights with Agent Orange, their cavalier attitude unfortunately exemplifying our national point of view towards toxic chemicals.[36]

Many Vietnam veterans no longer have a casual attitude towards these poisons. They have suffered grievously for their exposure to Agent Orange, and watched in dismay as their children were born with extremely high rates of birth defects.[37] One veteran, Michael Ryan of Long Island, testified before Congressional hearings on Agent Orange, and brought with him his daughter Kerrie, who was born with severe deformities, although neither of her parents had any family history of birth defects. A *Washington Post* reporter, Margot Hornblower, described the scene:

> *"During the emotion-laden hearing, Kerrie, a frail child with short brown hair, sat in her wheelchair gazing wide-eyed at the television cameras, the Congressmen high on the wood-paneled dais and the roomful of lobbyists and reporters.*
>
> *" 'She's a dynamite little kid,' said her mother to the committee.*
>
> *"Kerrie was born eight years ago with 18 birth defects: missing bones, twisted limbs, a hole in her heart, deformed intestines, a partial spine, shrunken fingers, no rectum. During surgery, a blood clot developed and she suffered brain damage. Doctors say she will never walk . . . "[38]*

It may seem to you and me that Agent Orange is a horrible weapon of war, and certainly not something to spray on land used to grow food. But its two active ingredients—2,4-D and 2,4,5-T—are in fact sprayed today on land used to grow food for livestock.[39] Millions of pounds continue to be used, even though 2,4,5,-T contains a particular substance which is so toxic it makes DDT look like a glass of champagne. 2,4,5,-T contains dioxin.

The head of the Toxic Effects Branch of the EPA's National Environmental Research Center, Dr. Diane Courtney, called dioxin:

". . . by far the most toxic chemical known to mankind." [40]

She also testified that dioxin is present in beef and dairy products from cattle that have grazed on land treated with 2,4,5-T.

The EPA has officially recognized the fact that cattle which graze on land sprayed with 2,4,5-T accumulate dioxin in their fat.[41] But Dow Chemical Company, which profits greatly from the sale of 2,4,5-T, would rather the public not be concerned. According to them:

". . . 2,4,5-T is about as toxic as aspirin." [42]

It would be a good thing if it were, because millions of pounds of this lethal chemical have been sprayed on land in the United States. And since dioxin is stored and concentrated as it moves up the food chain, cows, pigs and chickens contain in their flesh the dioxin residues from all the plants they have ever eaten. Pesticide authority Lewis Regenstein warns:

"Humans who eat beef . . . can get a concentrated dose of dioxin that has built up over several years." [43]

Dioxin causes cancer, birth defects, miscarriages and death in lab animals at the lowest levels possible to test—in some cases as low as 1 part per trillion. In fact, dioxin's toxicity makes it difficult to use in conducting cancer research; it tends to kill the test animals before they have a chance to produce tumors, even when given in the lowest possible doses, such as a few parts per trillion.[44]

A single drop of dioxin can kill 1,000 people. To kill a million people would take only an ounce.[45] Yet it could be in the meat, dairy products, and eggs sold in your supermarket.

HEPTACHLOR

When Rachel Carson first alerted the nation to the enormous dangers of the toxic chemicals we were flooding into the environment, and to the fact that these poisons tended to collect and concentrate in the food chain, the chemical companies were disturbed. Their response, however, did not demonstrate the most enlightened regard for the public welfare.

Before *Silent Spring* was published in book form, segments were serialized in the *New Yorker*. The Secretary and General Counsel of Velsicol Chemical Corporation, Louis A. McLean, responded by sending a threatening and intimidating letter to Carson's publisher, Houghton Mifflin, Inc., attempting to prevent the book from being published. The letter charged Carson had made "inaccurate and disparaging" statements about one of Velsicol's biggest money-makers, a pesticide named heptachlor.[46]

To their credit, Houghton Mifflin decided to print the book anyway, knowing the truth of Rachel Carson's dire warning that heptachlor accumulates in the food chain and has disastrous effects on living tissue. Velsicol Chemical did not give up its efforts to keep the substance in widespread use, however, and heptachlor continued to be sprayed on millions of acres of land used to grow corn for animal feed.[47] Finally, in October 1974, the Environmental Defense Fund (EDF) petitioned the EPA to ban heptachlor (and the associated compound chlordane), on the grounds that it posed "an imminent health hazard to man."[48] The EDF pointed out:

> *"The incidence of heptachlor in human food is currently very high in the United States, especially in meat, poultry, fish and dairy products . . . Heptachlor is carcinogenic at the lowest levels tested (one-half part per million) in laboratory experiments . . ."*[49]

In November, 1974, the EPA finally began hearings and appeals to determine if the chemical should be banned. But heptachlor was such a huge money-maker for Velsicol Chemical Corporation that the company spent literally tens of millions of dollars on legal maneuvers to fight a possible ban at every step of the way.[50] The company's tactics included withholding lab reports from the EPA which showed malignant tumors had been produced in animals exposed to heptachlor. When this "accidental oversight" was discovered, several company officials were indicted by a federal grand jury.[51]

In the meantime, Velsicol continued to manufacture and sell millions of pounds of heptachlor, and the poison is still used today for many applications. As a result, it will continue to accumulate in the food chain for years to come, slowly poisoning unknowing consumers of the foods highest on the food chain—meats, dairy products, and eggs.[52]

POISONED PORK

Several years after heptachlor was finally restricted, the Department of Agriculture discovered that, as part of its school lunch program, it had sent 40,000 pounds of heptachlor-contaminated ground pork to school systems in Louisiana and Arkansas. By the time they realized what had been done, over 14,000 pounds of poisoned pork had been consumed by the children.[53]

When we hear a phrase like "poisoned pork," most of us think of someone immediately getting sick, perhaps with stomach cramps, diarrhea, fever and so on, because these are the usual symptoms for bacterial poisonings which are carried in pork and other meats. But with pesticides, there is considerable "lag time" between the ingestion of these compounds, and the eventual manifestation of cancer, birth defects and other devastation. Of course, if the dosage is high enough there are immediate repercussions, including death. But for most of us, the problem is the gradual accumulation of these substances over a period of time. And it is a problem whose occurrence we have no way of recognizing until a deformed baby is born, a miscarriage or stillbirth happens, or a tumor appears. By that time we have virtually no way of tracing the mental and emotional disorders we experience to the toxic chemicals we have ingested.

In instances like the contaminated ground pork sent to the children in the South, we were very fortunate indeed to discover the high concentrations of heptachlor in these foods. But there is no way we can be aware of more than the tiniest percentage of such incidents. The tests to determine the existence of these chemicals in foods are expensive, time consuming, and require sophisticated equipment. As a result, they are rarely performed.

Heptachlor disasters will be with us for some time. In December 1986, Banquet Foods admitted that 200,000 chickens in Arkansas had to be destroyed because they were found to be contaminated with a variety of heptachlor known as chlordane. In April, 1986, milk contaminated with dangerously high levels of heptachlor had to be recalled in Arkansas, Texas, Louisiana, Kansas, Missouri and Oklahoma.[54] At the same time, beef supplied by the U.S.D.A. Donated Food Program to California elementary and high schools had to be recalled due to heptachlor contamination.[55]

Most frightening of all, Arkansas authorities found heptachlor contamination in the breast milk of 70% of nursing mothers.[56] Nevertheless, we are told not to be alarmed, even though a Hawaii study of 120 infants, whose supply of breast milk was discovered to be contaminated with heptachlor, found the development of the infants' brains to be significantly retarded.[57]

It is hard to avoid the feeling that we have seen only the barest glimmer of the top of the toxic chemical iceberg.

THERE GOES MICHIGAN

One of the saddest features of the pesticide story is that there are people who have been consistently successful in knowingly covering up the dangers. As a result, the public is still, for the most part, unaware of the gravity of what is happening.

It is not only the chemical companies who would like to keep us ignorant of the hazards of pesticides. Some government officials have also come to think we would be better off not knowing. A particularly dramatic instance of such a misguided attitude occurred in Michigan in 1973 and 1974, and involved one of the worst cases of pesticide poisoning yet to come to light.[58] Here, the poison involved was PBB's (polybrominated biphenyls). When the U.S. Congress finally investigated the fiasco six years later, they asked expert witnesses about PBB's. The answers were not reassuring. Impartial experts testified:

"PBB's are persistent and can be passed on for generations. PBB's are stored in the body fat, where they can remain indefinitely. During pregnancy, they can cross the placenta to the developing fetus . . . PBB is . . . capable of producing physical defects in offspring in utero." [59]

Not substances you'd particularly want in your hamburgers. Yet, in 1976 alone, several years after the PBB contamination occurred, Michigan residents ate over 5 million pounds of hamburger contaminated with PBB's. [60]

What had happened was that this toxic chemical had somehow gotten mixed into livestock feed which was dispersed throughout the state. When the PBB's were first discovered in virtually **all** of Michigan's meat and dairy products, state officials tried in every way to cover up the incident. Had the public been notified of the extreme urgency of the situation, a great deal of tragedy could have been avoided. But as it is, according to testimony before Michigan's Senate Commerce Subcommittee on March 29, 1977, nearly all of Michigan's residents now have unacceptable levels of PBB's in their bodies. [61] It is quite likely that every single person who consumed meats, dairy products or eggs in the state of Michigan during 1976 or 1977 now has significant amounts of these carcinogens in his or her organs. Tests in 1976 found that 96% of nursing mothers in Michigan had PBB's in their milk. [62]

It is very difficult for us to grasp the magnitude of today's toxic chemical pollution, and the degree to which our food choices can expose us to such dangers. And especially tragic is the fact that there are people who don't want the public to know, people who perceive it to be in their own interests to keep the public ignorant. There are industries who are profiting from our use of these chemicals, and from our continuing to make our food choices high on the food chain. They tell us all the bad pesticides have been banned, and the government is on top of things. They tell us there's nothing to worry about. But they lie!

Even in the few cases, such as DDT, where a pesticide has actually been banned, we are far indeed from off the hook. The Library of Congress estimates that over 2.2 million tons of DDT have been used worldwide, more than a pound for every human being on earth. [63] The

Environmental Defense Fund estimates that the American people today, have collectively, some 20 tons of DDT in their bodies—which
works out to one-and-a-half grams per person.[64]

In the face of such mind-boggling statistics there is a tremendous
temptation to go blank, to feel powerless and numb. We may want to
erect a wall of denial, to retreat back into ignorance. But one thing is
certain: in this case, ignorance is **not** bliss, though the companies that
profit from our ignorance would like us to believe it is. They see no
problem at all in the continuing use of these poisons, nor in you and
me unknowingly making food choices that daily expose us to residues
from the most toxic substances ever known to mankind.

OUR IMMUNE SYSTEMS AREN'T IMMUNE

We are presently seeing an enormous outbreak of immune system diseases that weren't a problem years ago—diseases like cancer, AIDS,
and herpes. Some immune system diseases, such as Chlamydia Trachomatis are so new that most people have never heard of them. Chlamydia Trachomatis struck close to 4 million Americans in 1985, and
the numbers are mounting rapidly.[65] In the early stages, women usually don't know they have Chlamydia. Untreated, however, it moves
into the uterus and fallopian tubes, causing pelvic inflammatory disease, chronic pain, fever, and in many cases, sterility.

In 1900, cancer was the tenth leading cause of death in the United
States, and was responsible for only three percent of all deaths. Today,
it ranks second, and causes about twenty percent of all deaths. More
Americans will die of cancer **this year** than died in World War II, the
Korean and the Vietnamese wars combined.[66]

Many scientists now feel that the presence of toxic chemicals in
our bodies is largely responsible for these epidemics. A case in point is
a substance that was once considered among the safest of germ-killing
compounds—hexachlorophene. Routinely used as an antiseptic in hospitals, clinics, and doctor's offices, hexachlorophene was never imagined to be a menace. Newborn infants were bathed in it, and to this
day hospital personnel sometimes wash their hands in it. The compound was widely used in baby creams, oil, and powders. It was routinely incorporated in many common household products, including

mouthwashes, anti-perspirant deodorants, shaving cream, first-aid kits, and over-the-counter medications for acne and psoriasis. In fact, hexachlorophene became practically a household word when Dial soap commercials brightly announced the good news that Dial soap now contained this wonderfully effective germ killer.

But it turns out that hexachlorophene is not the boon its manufacturers would like the public to believe.

In 1972, 35 healthy newborn infants in Paris, France, died after being dusted with talcum powder high in hexachlorophene.[67] In 1978, a Swedish study showed that nurses in Swedish hospitals who had regularly washed their hands in a hexachlorophene solution had given birth to an extraordinarily large number of deformed children.[68]

Hexachlorophene, it was discovered, contains trace amounts of dioxin.

The manufacturers of hexachlorophene still maintain the substance is safe. But there is growing evidence that the dioxin it contains severely damages the human immune system.

The April 18, 1986, issue of the *Journal of the American Medical Association* contained a major report by joint researchers from the Center for Disease Control in Atlanta, the Missouri State Health Department, and St. Louis Medical School.[69] To keep down dust in a Missouri mobile home park, sludge mixed with oil had once been sprayed on a dirt road. This is a fairly common occurrence, but in this case the sludge had come from a plant that made hexachlorophene. Researchers painstakingly studied the people who lived in the mobile home park over the years and compared them to a control group of men, women and children living in another mobile home park where the sludge had not been used. The text was exhaustively scrupulous. The two groups were virtually identical in race, employment, history of illness, use of pesticides, and use of tobacco and alcohol.

The results suggest why so many scientists today associate toxic chemicals with the current epidemic of immune system diseases. The researchers found:

> ". . . *significant damage to the immune systems of the exposed people.*"[70]

AIDS AND MORE

There is evidence that dioxin and other toxic chemicals damage the thymus gland, which plays a vital role in the body's immune system. Thus, people suffering from toxic chemical poisoning may be more susceptible to bacterial and viral infections of all kinds. They may experience the symptoms of common ailments, and have no way of tracking their impaired health to the pesticides they have slowly accumulated. And worst of all, with impaired immune systems, they may also become more susceptible to the frightening prospect of diseases such as AIDS and cancer.

Current estimates are that twenty-five to seventy-five percent of the people who are exposed to the AIDS virus (human T-cell lymphotropic Virus-III, also known as HTVL-III) are eventually stricken by this deadly disease of the immune system. There is much we don't know yet about AIDS. And while it is homosexuals and intravenous drug users who are especially at risk, the disease is unfortunately spreading rapidly into other segments of the populations. The presence of this disease, which could produce the most devastating epidemic in human history, makes the strength and health of your immune system particularly significant today.

We know that the accumulation of toxic chemicals in the body compromises the immune system. And we know that among people who are exposed to the AIDS virus it is those with weakened immune systems who are mostly likely to come down with the disease. Many scientists see the spreading of the AIDS epidemic as a consequence, therefore, at least in part, of the toxic chemical pollution of our environment, food chains, and bodies.

In today's world, anything we can do to strengthen our immune systems is especially important. In this light it is particularly sad how often people are ignorant of the role their food choices play. Not knowing the consequences of eating high on the food chain, they may expose themselves unnecessarily to the worst enemies our immune systems have ever known.

Given the immense quantity of these poisons we have spewed into the environment, you may wonder why there are not more glaring birth defects, and why there is not an even greater epidemic of cancers. Part of the answer lies in the "lag time" necessary before the most conspicuous problems arise.[71] A lab animal with a life span measured in months will develop cancer within months when exposed to these substances, whereas humans are on a much slower timetable, so it often takes decades for the damage to show up. It is only comparatively recently that the deluge of pesticides has occurred, though already the lamentable consequences are beginning to appear in our children. Forty years ago, cancer in children was a medical rarity. Today, more children die of cancer than from any other cause.

In lab tests, the offspring of animals exposed to pesticides can be killed and autopsied for evidence of internal birth defects. As a result of such tests, we know these substances cause birth defects in animals in even the most infinitesimal concentrations. It is not so easy, however, to determine the number of human children being born with birth defects, since most birth defects are not glaring external deformities of the kind suffered by thalidomide babies. Most are internal, and not immediately apparent at birth. Children with learning disabilities, hyperactivity, lowered I.Q.'s, lessened resistance to disease, weakened immune systems, damaged livers of kidneys, chronic ailments that resist diagnosis, and/or emotional problems are rarely studied to see if contamination by toxic chemicals in utero may have done the damage. I'm sure that if they were, the results would be very interesting.

There is no telling how many of us suffer from dullness of spirit, frazzled nervous systems, confusion, irritability, emotional instability, or some other form of unease due to toxic chemical pollution. And there is no way of measuring or tracing most of the damage that has been done. As a result, most people are unaware of the ominous dangers these poisons represent, and of the correspondingly crucial importance of our food choices.

This problem is particularly distressing because it is so needless and avoidable. A new direction for America's agriculture and diet-style might yet mean that our immune systems could be strengthened and our children grow up to live healthy lives and bear healthy children in a world increasingly safe from pollution.

PCB'S
Time and again I've been amazed to learn how widespread in the environment are the toxic chemicals that collect and concentrate in the

food chains. Probably the most widespread of all are the notorious PCB's. In the United States alone, nearly a **million tons** of PCB's have been produced—over five pounds for every man, woman and child.

Because of its biological longevity, almost all of this poison still persists in the environment. PCB's have been found in significant concentrations in wild polar bears and in fish from the deepest and most remote parts of the world's oceans. It is now likely that there is not a single human being anywhere on this planet who does not carry PCB's in his or her flesh.[72]

This does not bode particularly well for the health of our species or our world, for if there were a competition for the world's most toxic substance, PCB's would be right in there along with DDT, dieldrin, dioxin and the others. A few parts per billion can cause birth defects and cancer in lab animals.[73] Primates have developed fatal cancers and given birth to deformed children after ingesting doses as low as one part per million.[74]

Ominously, a recent government study found PCB's present in 100% of the human sperm samples tested.[75] They also found a correlation between high PCB levels and low sperm count.[76] PCB's are considered one of the chief reasons for the staggering fact that the average sperm count of the American male is today **only 70% of what it was only 30 years ago.**[77]

Tests done at several major universities have found that nearly 25% of today's college students are sterile.[78] This is a terrifying trend. Only thirty-five years ago, the sterility rate was less than one-half of one percent.[79]

Perhaps the leading researcher in the country in this field is Dr. Ralph Dougherty of Florida State University. He blames the drastic increase in sterility on the chlorinated hydrocarbons, such as PCB's, that have collected in the food chain.[80]

PCB's were first introduced by Monsanto, a company whose motto, "Without Chemicals, Life Itself Would Be Impossible," seems ludicrous in view of what PCB's are doing to human fertility. It wasn't long after Monsanto began producing PCB's that it became apparent that these chemicals posed major problems for human beings. Three years after production began, the faces and bodies of 23 out of 24 workers in the Monsanto plant had become disfigured.[81] But that didn't stop Monsanto. Since then, more than 750,000 tons of these deadly poisons have been produced. They can be found today in every river in America, in the snows of the Arctic and Antarctic, and probably in the tissues of every single fish in the waters of this planet.

SOMETHING SMELLS FISHY

Toxic chemical authorities agree that human contamination with PCB's comes mainly from eating fish from waters in which PCB levels are high.[82] Fish have a remarkable ability to absorb and concentrate toxic chemicals from their watery environments. For one thing, their food chains are extremely long, with phytoplankton being eaten by zooplankton, who are in turn eaten by tiny fish, who are then eaten by larger fish, and so on. More significantly, fish literally breathe the water they swim in, so they are also continually accumulating more and more contaminants in this manner. The net effect is almost as if they were underwater magnets for toxic chemicals. The EPA estimates fish can accumulate up to 9 million times the level of PCB's in the waters in which they live![83]

By the food chain effect, fish may thus become loaded with enormous concentrations of these toxic chemicals.

Shellfish that filter water, such as oysters, clams, mussels, scallops, and other mollusks, are especially vulnerable to pesticide saturation. An oyster will filter up to 10 gallons of water every hour. In only a month, an oyster will accumulate toxic chemicals at concentrations 70,000 times the amount in the water.[84]

While it is our lakes, rivers and other inland waterways that are the most polluted with toxic chemicals, the oceans, regrettably, have not been spared. Over 110 million pounds of DDT alone have ended up in the oceans of North America.[85] Tragically, there is substantial evidence that DDT levels in the oceans have damaged a major source of the world's oxygen supply—the microscopic phytoplankton.[86]

Livestock in today's factory farms are fed huge quantities of fish meal. Half of the world's fish catch is fed to livestock.[87] In fact, more fish are consumed by U.S. livestock than by the entire human populations of all the countries of Western Europe combined.[88] But don't bet too heavily on the meat or dairy industries voluntarily spending the amount of money it would require to test the fish meal they feed their animals for toxic chemicals.

When they do test, the results can be hard to stomach. Ritewood Farms in Idaho is one of the world's largest chicken factories. In 1979, the concentrations of PCB's in their chickens were found to be so high that one poultry sample could not even be measured.[89] Almost $3 million of egg and poultry products had to be destroyed. It remains anyone's guess how many Americans will never have children, or will give birth to deformed children, or will get cancer, as a result of eating products from the eggs and chickens that were not tracked down and destroyed. We have yet to see the impact of what has already been done. And the future is rapidly approaching.

Whenever cases like this are discovered, the chemical, meat and dairy industries often become extremely concerned about the public's response. One poultry executive justified his company's commitment to covering up the matter by saying:

"There's no point in scaring people. We have a duty to protect the public's peace of mind." [90]

These industries had a hard time doing their self-appointed "duty" in 1970, when 146,000 chickens in New York had to be destroyed because high levels of PCB's were found by the Campbell Soup Company.[91] And again in 1971, when 88,000 chickens and 123,000 pounds of egg products from North Carolina met a similar fate.[92] The chickens had eaten fish meal disastrously high in PCB's. In 1978, Ralston Purina had to recall 2,500,000 pounds of animal feed they had sold that was made from fish meal which they discovered, belatedly, to be heavily contaminated with PCB's.[93] Millions of eggs and almost half-a-million chickens were destroyed because the birds had already eaten the feed. It must have been hard for the companies involved to maintain the public's peace of mind when the FDA admitted it had no idea how many contaminated chickens and eggs were consumed.

Pesticide authority Lewis Regenstein writes of such occurrences:

"It can be assumed that such examples represent a tiny fraction of the number of actual incidents, and that most cases of PCB

contamination go undetected and/or unreported. Thus, most of the PCB's that contaminate our food end up being consumed by the public." [94]

KEEP IT DOWN . . . SOMEONE MIGHT BE LISTENING

It is remarkable how indifferent the companies that profit from these substances can be, not only to public health, but to the welfare of their own employees. In 1974, a Virginia plant began manufacturing the pesticide kepone. Within three weeks, workers became sick with tremors, dizziness and nervousness. When they sought medical help, what they received left a little bit to be desired. Many were given tranquilizers. One was referred to a psychiatrist. [95]

A year later, Virginia state officials found out that over 70 workers, plus 10 spouses and children, had been seriously poisoned by kepone. Many had become sterile. [96]

This did not stop Life Sciences, Inc., a subsidiary of Allied Chemical Corporation, from dumping great quantities of kepone into the James River in Virginia in the 1970's. [97] They did this despite knowing that this deadly chemical causes cancer, birth defects, and neurological disorders; and despite knowing that the James River is the seedbed for one-quarter of the country's oysters. [98] Predictably, the kepone spread into Chesapeake Bay, which produces 90% of America's softshell crabs, 40% of all commercial oysters, and 15% of all softshell clams, besides a significant percentage of the nation's commercial fishing catch.

Eventually the pollution was discovered, and traced to Allied Chemical. Their crimes discovered, Allied chemical stubbornly refused to repent.

According to Senator Patrick Leahy, who chaired a Senate committee investigating the matter:

> *"Allied Chemical took a position that makes Pontius Pilate look like Mother Theresa of Calcutta. That is giving them the benefit of the doubt."* [99]

As a result of the contamination, the entire area had to be closed to commercial fishing. Within a few years, however, pressures from the fishing industry caused the area to be reopened, even though kepone levels remained dangerously high.[100] Today, many of us eat fish from the James River and Chesapeake Bay, even though experts say these waters will remain seriously contaminated with kepone for another two centuries![101]

The least likely of all places in the world to find an uncontaminated fish is in the United States. We have the dubious distinction of being the world's largest producer of pesticides. We use 1.1 billion pounds of pesticides a year—about five pounds for every member of the population. This amounts to 30% of the entire world's use.[102] You may be wondering if any fish are safe. Unfortunately, even for research purposes, it is almost impossible now for scientists to find fish anywhere in U.S. waters which do not carry toxic chemicals in their flesh. Lewis Regenstein writes:

> *"From a health standpoint, the least dangerous fish to eat are smaller, deep-ocean fish that do not live or spawn near the coast, such as cod, halibut, and pollack, or freshwater fish from high-altitude streams that are not contaminated from industrial or agricultural runoffs or dumping. But even these fish will carry some pollutants. Unfortunately, uncontaminated fish and other animal products may simply no longer exist."* [103]

A major study reported in Tufts University's *Diet and Nutrition Letter* compared the offspring of 242 women who ate varying amounts of fish from Lake Michigan. The study found that the more fish the mothers had eaten, the more their babies showed abnormal reflexes, general weaknesses, slower response to stimuli, and various signs of depression. Even mothers eating the fish **only two or three times a month** produced babies weighing seven to nine ounces less at birth, with smaller heads.[104]

A 1986 follow-up study cast an even less favorable light on Lake Michigan fish. A definite correlation was found between the amount of fish the mothers had eaten, **even if it were only once a month**, and the children's subsequent brain development. The youngsters were given the "fixation to novelty" test, which is recognized as an accurate indicator of future verbal I.Q. Their scores were inversely proportional to the amount of fish their mothers had eaten. The more fish their mothers had eaten, the poorer they did.[105]

We are again and again told not to be alarmed. This is ridiculous because it is not too late to begin to reverse the damage. Our grandchildren might yet live in a healthy world, where people gather joyfully at night around crackling campfires, laughing about times in the distant past when human beings were so foolish as to spread such poisons into the environment. "It's a good thing," they might yet say happily, "that we learned better in time."

THE PHARMACEUTICAL FARM

We won't arrive at such a happy future eating the products of today's factory farms. These animals are not only fed huge quantites of often-contaminated fish, but they are subject to a distressing array of toxic chemicals. Cattle, pigs, sheep and other livestock are often routinely doused with a chemical called toxaphene to kill the parasites that breed in the crowded and grossly unsanitary conditions of modern factory farms.[106] This substance is a chlorinated hydrocarbon, a member of the deadly family that includes DDT, kepone, dieldrin, heptachlor and PCB's. Like other members of its chemical family, toxaphene is biologically stable, fat soluble, and a deadly poison. In the most microscopic doses it produces cancer, birth defects, and causes bones to dissolve in lab animals.[107] Even a few parts per trillion disturbs the reproduction of fish, and a few parts per billion turn their backbones to chalk.[108] Yet every day in the United States this chemical is routinely administered by untrained factory farm workers to the animals whose flesh and milk the public eats.

If there were a competition for the world's most deadly substance, toxaphene would definitely have its supporters, including, perhaps, Dr. Adrian Goss, the Chief Scientist for the EPA's Hazards Evaluation Division. A world renowned expert in toxic chemicals, he was formerly associate director of the FDA's scientific investigations office. His opinion of toxaphene is unequivocal:

> *"(It is) abundantly clear that toxaphene is an extremely potent carcinogen . . . I have never encountered an agent purposefully*

introduced into the environment . . . which had a carcinogenic
propensity as clearly marked and as pervasive." [109]

Yet each year in the United States over a million cattle are dipped in or
sprayed with several million gallons of toxaphene solution to kill parasites which thrive in factory farm environments.[110] This is done despite
the fact that toxaphene, like the other chlorinated hydrocarbons, can
be absorbed through the skin of animals and is retained in their flesh.

In December, 1978, veterinarians for the California Department of
Food and Agriculture were concerned about mange in the 850 head
herd of Chico, California farmer, George Neary. Neary pleaded with
them not to use toxaphene, but they assured him they knew what they
were doing, and insisted. Within a few weeks, nearly 100 cows had
died. Five hundred others either aborted their fetuses or gave birth to
calves that died soon after birth. A dog which ate some flesh from one
of the dead cows evidently did not find it to his liking. He dropped
dead seconds later.[111]

The administrators of the toxaphene program concluded they had
used too concentrated a solution. Sorry, George!

As if it's not enough, modern factory farms often swarm so thickly
with flies that farmhands have to turn on their windshield wipers in
order to be able to make it home from work. The flies can just about
drive the men crazy, and workers will go to great lengths to kill them.
Many of the sprays commonly used to kill flies around livestock (including Fly-Die, Duo-Kill, Vapona, and others) have as their primary
ingredient a substance that would also have some supporters in a competition for the world's worst poison—a chemical called dichlorvos.[112]

So toxic is dichlorvos that the World Health Organization has set
its acceptable daily intake at only 0.004 mg/kg, an amount exceeded by
someone who merely stays in the same room with a small No-Pest strip
containing the chemical for nine hours.[113]

But this doesn't prevent the decision makers in the meat industry
from giving the cows, chickens, pigs and steers in today's animal factories a continuing stream of dichlorvos products.

In their never-ending battle against flies, factory farm workers will
often mix toxic larvicides into the animal's feed. The poisons go in the

animals' mouths, through their stomachs and intestines, and out the other end—in so doing rendering the manure chemically toxic to the flies that would breed there.

One farmer told me these larvicides are a "nifty" idea. He laughed when I told him that the most popular of the larvicides, Rabon, has as its principal ingredient a substance that can cause extreme damage to the human nervous system and send people into convulsions, even in minute doses. He quickly pulled out an advertisement in which Rabon's manufacturer, Diamond Shamrock, says there is no need to worry about residues showing up in the meats and milk from animals fed Rabon. Indeed, they recommend feeding the poison to dairy cows while they are being milked, and to beef cattle right up to slaughter.

How trustworthy are the reassurances of such companies? When the manager of technical services and development at Diamond Shamrock was asked about problems with Rabon, he replied that the only problem was "getting the compound approved by the EPA."[114]

THE GOVERNMENT AS PROTECTOR

Twenty years ago, the amount of toxic substances used in animal farming was only a trickle compared to the torrent it has become today. Yet even then, when the U.S.D.A. tested 2600 poultry samples from every federally inspected plant in the nation, they could not find a single sample which was not contaminated with toxic pesticides.[115] In 1966, it was admitted in Congressional hearings that:

> *"No milk available on the market, today, in any part of the United States, is free of pesticide residues."* [116]

Unfortunately, the situation has grown steadily worse since then.

Most of us are deeply conditioned to believe that the government's meat inspection system takes good care of us, and would never allow unhealthy animals to reach the public. But in reality that is hardly the case. The animals often whiz by the inspectors faster than one per second, giving them only the briefest possible glimpse for the most glaring of problems. Detection of toxic chemicals requires complex laboratory equipment, and a great deal of time and expense.

In fact, the U.S.D.A. tests only **one out of every quarter-million** slaughtered animals for toxic chemical residues.[117] And even then, it tests for less than 10% of the toxic chemicals known to be present in the country's meat supply.[118] In 1976, less than 150 animals in the United States were condemned for drug residues, 57 for pesticidal residues, and 29 for miscellaneous residues. That's a grand total of less than 300 animals out of 119 million—not counting poultry.[119]

So low are our meat inspection standards that inspectors from the European Economic Community (EEC) in 1984 declared 11 of America's largest meat packers ineligible to export their products through the Common Market.[120]

The chemical companies would like us to believe that we are protected from harmful chemical residues, and that the problem is under control. But impartial scientists don't see it that way. Lewis Regenstein writes:

"A review of the government's policy in setting and enforcing tolerance levels for toxic pesticides leads to the inescapable conclusion that the program exists primarily to reassure the public that it is being protected from harmful chemical residues. In fact, the program, as currently administered, does little to minimize or even monitor the amount of poisons in our food, and serves the interests of the users and producers of pesticides rather than those of the public . . .

"The prime source of toxic pesticides and other chemicals for most Americans is in the consumption of food high in fat content, such as meat and dairy products. A vegetarian diet, or one that minimizes animal products, can substantially reduce one's exposure to most of these cancer-causing chemicals."[121]

The relationship between toxic chemicals and meat was ironically dramatized on April 5, 1973. On that day, the FDA finally banned the artificial coloring agent Violet No. 1 as a carcinogen. Up until then, the Department of Agriculture had been using the dye to stamp meats with the grades of "Choice," "Prime," and U.S. No.1 USDA." For over twenty years, the U.S.D.A. had been reassuring customers their meat was healthy by stamping the meat with a cancer-causing dye.[122]

THE GOOD NEWS

Fortunately, there are alternatives to pesticides. Agricultural techniques such as organic farming and Integrated Pest Management (IPM) are decidedly on the upswing today. These utilize natural insect controls, such as predatory insects, weather, crop rotation, pest-resistant varieties, soil tillage, insect traps, and other environmentally sound practices. IPM systems use chemicals when necessary, but recognize that tolerable quantities of pest insects may actually be desirable, because they provide food for beneficial insects.

Organic and IPM systems realize that "controlling" insects by poisoning them is not the best strategy. Even speaking strictly in terms of short term output and crop losses due to pests, pesticides are not the blessing the companies who sell them would like us to believe. Of the 25 most serious agricultural pests in 1970, 24 were either pesticide-aggravated or pesticide-induced pests.[123] Despite staggering increases in pesticide use, the percentage of U.S. crops lost to insects doubled between 1950 and 1974—mostly because the ecological balance has been so severely disturbed by the chemicals.

The chemical companies would like us to believe that the chemicals increase food production. But in their penetrating study of the causes of world hunger, *Food First*, Frances Moore Lappe and Joseph Collins found quite otherwise:

> *"In country after country, there is a regular progression of events. For the first few years (after pesticides are introduced) insects are controlled at reasonable cost and yields are higher than before. The growers, seeing the bugs literally drop from the plants, feel the pesticides give them power over forces that have always been beyond their control. Gradually, however, the pest species develop resistant strains through a survival-of-the-fittest selection.*
>
> *"It is not true that the only good bug is a dead bug. Some bugs are parasites or flesh-eating predators that live off the insect species doing the plant damage. Some eat only very specific parts of the crop plant. Studies show that the vast majority of insect species never cause sufficient damage to justify the cost of insecticide treatment. Their numbers are restricted below injury levels by the*

*action of these parasites and predators. But, when an insecticide
kills some of these parasites and predators, many ordinarily
insignificant pests are able to multiply faster."* [124]

A case in point is the spider mite:

*"Only 25 years ago, the spider mite was a minor pest. Repeated
use of pesticides supposedly aimed at other pests has decimated the
natural enemies and competitors of the mite. Today, the mite is the
pest most seriously threatening agriculture worldwide . . .*
   *"The irony . . . is that the more effective an insecticide is in
killing susceptible individuals of a pest population, the faster
resistant individuals evolve."* [125]

Fortunately, pesticides are not necessary. Organic and IPM techniques
not only work, but often work even in cases where the most powerful
pesticides won't. One of the worst pests corn growers face is the corn
rootworm, and chemicals have not been much help in this battle. The
worm has developed almost total resistance to the major pesticides.
Integrated Pest Management systems solved the problem by simply
rotating crops. The corn rootworm cannot eat the soybean plant. So,
when soybeans are planted alternately with corn, the rootworm has
nothing to eat, and cannot survive. The soybean plants have the added
benefit of supplying nitrogen to the soil, and so reducing the need for
fertilizer for the ensuing corn crop.[126]
   Unfortunately for pesticide-addicted agriculture, however, simply
switching to crop rotation after years of pesticide use can run into a few
difficulties. Some of the weedkillers used today on corn crops persist in
the soil and kill non-corn plants. Soybean plants die if planted in soil to
which these chemicals have been applied. Farmers who have been led
to rely on pesticides can find themselves in a vicious circle. They may
have created soil in which nothing will grow except corn. So they must
plant corn year after year, thereby virtually inviting insects, disease,
and weed problems.
   Earl Butz, Secretary of Agriculture under Nixon, used to say that
before the United States could consider organic farming, it would have
to decide which 50 or 60 million Americans were going to be allowed

to starve. His attitude exemplified the stance that government and agribusiness have taken in the past: that organic farming is a luxury we can ill-afford, and we need these chemicals to feed ourselves. The chemical companies, as you might imagine, have spent millions to reinforce this way of thinking.

But it could hardly be less true.

Up until World War II, American farmers grew huge harvests without relying on pesticides. And happily we could now do even better, thanks to our greatly increased understanding of IPM techniques. For example, it is now possible to rear large numbers of sterilized male insects, and then release them into an area in which this particular insect has become a problem. They mate with the females in the wild, and soon there is a drastic reduction in the population of the problem insect. It is also now possible to rear large numbers of beneficial insects, and release them to prey on the insect pests in an infested area.[127]

We could now do even better than ever without pesticides because our understanding of environmental systems is so much more sophisticated than it was before World War II, and because we can learn from the mistakes we have made. We know enough now to appreciate that while insects often become resistant to pesticides, no insect ever becomes resistant to a bird. And birds handle themselves pretty well around insects. A brown thrasher can eat 6,180 insects in a day. A swallow will devour 1,000 leafhoppers in 12 hours. A house wren will feed 500 spiders and caterpillars to its young during one summer afternoon. A pair of flickers considers 5,000 ants a mere snack. A Baltimore oriole eats 17 caterpillars a minute.[128]

In fact, government studies on the feasibility of organic types of farming have been extremely encouraging. A 1979 Agriculture Department Task Force of scientists and economists formed to study the matter came to:

". . . positive conclusions on the importance of organic farming and its potential contributions to agriculture and society." [129]

The U.S.D.A. Task Force found that some farmers actually experienced no reduction at all in yields when they gave up the use of chemicals. And those who did lose some production still made more money because they didn't have to pay for expensive chemicals.

Probably the most complete research project ever undertaken to assess the feasibility of organic agriculture was conducted by the Center for the Study of Biological systems at Washington University in St. Louis. This study matched a group of farms with similar soil conditions, crops and acreage, half of which used chemicals, while half did not. At the end of the study, the Center Director concluded:

> *"A five-year average shows that the organic farms yielded, in dollars per acre, exactly the same returns. In terms of yield, the organic farms were down about 10 percent. The reason why the economics came out is that the savings in chemicals made up for the difference."* [130]

You might think that a ten percent reduction in yield would mean food shortages. But it is important to realize that the vast majority of American agriculture does not grow food for people. It grows food for animals, whose flesh, milk and eggs we then consume. Most of it, actually, gets turned into manure, which cannot be recycled because it does not fall onto the land itself, but instead is concentrated in unbelievable quantities at feedlots and confinement sheds, and ends up in our already amply-polluted water.

If we were simply to grow food for people, we would need less than 30% of the yield we now require from our agricultural acreage. We could cut our yield in half, and still have far more than enough food to feed ourselves. And since the switch to IPM and other organic-type methods does not actually entail much loss of production, we could in fact feed the entire world if we grew food directly for people, instead of supplying what are really manure and saturated fat factories.

In doing so, we would also stop flooding the environment with lethal poisons. Our children might yet live in an increasingly safe and clean world.

REDUCING YOUR INTAKE OF PESTICIDES

The most effective way to reduce your intake of toxic chemicals is to minimize or eliminate your intake of meats, fish, dairy products and eggs. Choosing organic or unsprayed produce would be the next step. It also helps to reduce your intake of imported foods such as coffee, sugar, tea and bananas, because farmers in countries such as Ecuador, Mexico, Guatemala and Costa Rica use much greater concentrations of pesticides than even American agriculture is allowed to use. Pesticides, incidentally, which they often buy from U.S. chemical companies, and which are usually manufactured in this country.[131] It is likewise a good idea to beware of imported fruits and vegetables. You're safest if you stick with in-season, locally grown fruits and vegetables. U.S. regulations for pesticide use make many exceptions for Hawaii, with the result that fruit from Hawaii can be as heavily contaminated as that from Latin America. Among the worst of all foods are fast-food hamburgers, because they are often made from beef imported from Central America.

Some people feel that eating "organically raised" beef and poultry is a good way to limit their intake of pesticides. It is important to realize, though, that while meat products labeled "natural" or "organic" may be better than the typical factory farm commercial products, they still will include the concentrated toxins from all the foods the livestock ate. These lethal chemicals accumulate in the fatty tissues of animals in much greater concentrations than are found in fruits and vegetables. Pesticide authority Lewis Regenstein writes:

> *"Meat contains approximately 14 times more pesticides than do plant foods; dairy products 5 1/2 times more. Thus, by eating foods of animal origin, one ingests greatly concentrated amounts of hazardous chemicals. Analysis of various foods by the FDA shows that meat, poultry, fish, cheese and other dairy products contain levels of these pesticides more often and in greater amount than other foods."* [132]

In 1975, the Council on Environmental Quality concluded a lengthy analysis of the problem of pesticide residues in food by stating that dairy and meat products account for over 95% of the population's intake of DDT.[133] The same percentage holds true for the other pesticides. Sadly, people who have not been told this fact continue to eat high on the food chain, thus unknowingly exposing themselves day after day to large amounts of some of the most virulent poisons known to man. The bright side is that, knowing this, we can do something about it. A new direction for America's agriculture and diet-styles would mean that our children and their children might yet have healthy bodies and a healthy environment in which to live.

CONTAMINATED MOTHER'S MILK

You might think that any way toxic chemicals could possibly be eliminated from the human body would be a good thing. But, disturbingly, the most common way these stored-up poisons are released is in the breast milk of nursing mothers.

Just as dairy cows tend to excrete into their milk the stores of lethal chemicals they have absorbed, so, too, does human milk become contaminated from the stores of these poisons in the mother's body fat. The tragic results have been portrayed by the Ecology Action Center in a poster which shows a nude pregnant woman. On her effulgent breasts there is a label: "Caution—Keep Out of Reach of Children."[134]

Unfortunately, this poster is not intended as a joke. A nursing woman's body draws on its body fat reservoirs to make milk. Stored in her body fat reservoirs are virtually all the toxic chemicals she has ever ingested, inhaled, or absorbed through her skin. These poisons are thus incorporated into her milk. Breast-fed babies thereby may consume extraordinarily large amounts of the most toxic substances ever known to man.[135]

So high is most mother's milk in DDT, PCB's, dieldrin, heptachlor, dioxin, and so on that it would be subject to confiscation and destruction by the FDA were it to be sold across state lines.[136]

In 1976, the EPA found significant concentrations of DDT and PCB's in over 99% of mother's milk from every part of the country.[137] Other studies have confirmed these levels of saturation.[138] In 1975, the President's Council on Environmental Quality found DDT in 100% of the breast milk it sampled.[139] The other poisons which work their way up the food chain were similarly ubiquitous.

The EPA has concluded that the average American breast fed infant ingests nine times the permissible level of dieldrin, one of the most potent of all cancer-causing agents known to modern science.[140] As if that weren't enough, the EPA concludes that the average American breast fed infant also consumes ten times the FDA's maximum allowable daily intake level of PCB's.[141] In 1981, the breast milk of over a thousand Michigan mothers was tested for PCB's. Every single case showed residues of a chemical so toxic it causes birth defects and cancer in lab animals in doses as low as a few parts per billion.[142]

Some women are so alarmed by these terrifying facts that they decide not to breast feed their young. But this is not usually the best decision for a number of important reasons: 1) Human breast milk is nutritionally vastly superior for a human infant to any cow's milk formula. 2) The formulas are also likely to be contaminated with toxic chemicals. 3) Human breast milk contains antibodies which are crucial for the newborn. 4) Breast-feeding provides the bonding and emotional nurturance which are tremendously important to the well-being of both mother and baby.

Fortunately, there are ways a woman of childbearing age can minimize the risk to her young. Many studies have shown direct correlations between the amount of animal fat in a woman's diet, and the amount of residues in her milk. The less meat, butter, eggs, cheese, milk, poultry, and fish in a woman's diet, the less toxic chemicals will be found in the milk that flows from her breast to her young.[143]

In 1976, the EPA analyzed the breast milk of vegetarian women, and discovered the levels of pesticides in their milk to be far less than the average.[144] A study published in the *New England Journal of Medicine* made a similar comparison, and found:

> *"The highest levels of contamination in the breast milk of the vegetarians was lower than the lowest level of contamination . . . (in) non-vegetarian women . . . The mean vegetarian levels were only one or two percent as high as the average levels in the United States."* [145]

This is a tremendously important statistic. The breast milk of the average vegetarian nursing mother in the United States contains only **one or two percent** of the pesticide contamination as that experienced in the national average. If the national average for breast milk contamination were to be represented by the weight of a compact automobile (1600 pounds), the comparable vegetarian average would be equivalent to the weight of only a very small suitcase (16-32 pounds). No studies to my knowledge have been done on the breast milk of pure vegetarian women, but there is every indication their milk would be again many times safer.

Women, and even little girls, who think they may wish to have and breastfeed a baby in the future would do well to realize that the diet they eat today will greatly affect the health of their young. Any chemicals they ingest now will be stored in their tissues until released in their milk. And because mother's milk is often an infant's only source of food, the concentration of pesticides in its milk are crucial indeed. The Environmental Defense Fund has shown that the average American nursing infant receives 100 times more PCB's, on a body-weight basis, than the average adult.[146] Further, the effective dose is yet more toxic, since the infant's immature livers are completely incapable of detoxifying these chemicals. It is extremely important that young women know that by eating wisely today, they will be creating better breast milk for their babies tomorrow.

We know enough now to take the right path. The mothers of the future might yet nurse their babies, grateful in the knowledge that their milk is safe and pure. They might yet feed their young, with only a distant memory of the time when breast milk was a danger.

Men who think they may someday wish to father a child would do well to realize that the toxic chemicals they ingest today, including those especially damaging to sperm cells, tend to collect and concentrate in the male reproductive tract.[147] The result is that a very high number of birth defects stem from the male's absorption of these chemicals. This is why the offspring of Vietnam veterans who were involved with Agent Orange have such a high rate of birth defects; and why a University of Southern California Medical School study found distinct correlations between brain tumors in children, and their father's exposure to toxic chemicals.[148]

Even if a man does not father a child, he should be concerned. His sperm will still collect these chemicals. And, during intercourse, they will be transmitted to the female.[149] She will absorb them through her vaginal mucosa, and then store them in her womb, like the worst kind of biological time bomb, waiting to cause birth defects and cancer.

Fortunately, wise food choices today can do a great deal to protect the health of the as-yet unborn.

THE GENE POOL

It is almost impossible to exaggerate the profound threat toxic chemicals present to the human species. They can damage the very blueprint of life itself—the DNA molecule.[150] Hence the epidemic of the runaway cellular growth process we know as cancer; hence the epidemic of sterility; hence the epidemic of birth defects.

What is happening is that the human gene pool itself is in danger of being irreparably harmed. This gene pool is the culmination of at least three billion years of evolution, and is the primary resource of the human species. Defects in the DNA blueprint cause diseases which henceforth become hereditary. These tragedies will then persist for untold generations in the future. Scientists tell us:

> *"Changes in the chromosomes of sperm or our precursor cells may be transmitted to all future generations of humans. The heredity of man, his greatest treasure, is thereby at stake. Once irreversibly injured, the chromosomes cannot be repaired by any process known to man."* [151]

The mutagenic effect of these chemicals takes at least a generation to manifest. It is only in this generation that the biosphere and the food chains have been inundated with toxic chemicals which represent the highest summation of technological expertise at killing living creatures.

We have not yet seen the impact of what has already been done. But as Red Skelton used to say, "If we don't change the direction in which we are going, we will end up where we are headed."

NOW WHAT?

Facing this ominous future, I've been filled with many emotions. I've felt overwhelmed by the sheer quantity of these substances that have been produced; overwhelmed by such great damage which can be done by such infinitesimal amounts; and overwhelmed with rage at those who lie and profit from such abominations. It is not easy to see a man like Paul Oreffice, the president of Dow Chemical Company, appear on NBC's *Today* show, and tell us that "there's absolutely no evidence of dioxin doing any damage to humans." He said this despite knowing that the amount of dioxin sufficient to kill ten million people could fit in a space smaller than a human hand.

I don't think anyone could become aware of the immensity of what is involved and not feel pain for our world and our collective future. This pain goes beyond the personal, beyond any of our individual lives. It is the human journey itself that is now at stake.

Sometimes I've wished I could cover my eyes and it would all go away; I've wanted to believe that when the chips are down "they" would never allow our whole world to be poisoned. Other times, when my attempts to psychically numb myself have failed, and the reality of the situation has sunk in, I've felt other forms of grief. I've felt angry that we must see our lives and the lives of our children darkened by such avoidable tragedy. I've felt guilty, because as part of this society I can't help but feel implicated in this great misfortune. I've felt scared for what may yet lie in store. Mostly, though, there has been sorrow. Confronting what is happening can bring a sadness beyond the telling.

This sorrow belongs to us all, and I have learned it is not something to fear. For in the depths of our shared pain, we also experience our shared caring, our mutual prayers, and our common capacity to act. The pain we feel is the cracking of the shell that encloses our power to respond. Something precious can be born in times like these. In our shared pain we labor together to bring it to birth.

The pain we feel is not ours alone. It is rooted in caring, not just for ourselves and our children, but for all of humanity and all of life. Our distress is a statement of our interconnectedness with all beings. Something much larger than our individual selves and destinies is at work here. Our distress is an urgent statement from the depths of our being that this horrible pollution must not be allowed to continue. It is the awakening within our individual and collective conscience of the most profoundly transforming human responses. It is the source of the courage to redirect our lives.

Obviously the work of healing our world and ourselves is not a separate or passing chapter in our lives. The changes that are necessary won't come about simply because we stop eating meat, or simply because, on occasion, we meet or march or donate or lobby. It will take everything we are, and it will take all of us, and in forms we cannot yet even begin to imagine.

We will meet this challenge that asks so much because there is something inside us that is sacred, our conscience, that says this is what we are here to do.

I look out into the world and I see a deep night of unthinkable cruelty and blindness. Undaunted, however, I look within the human heart and find something of love there, something that cares and shines out into the dark universe like a bright beacon. And in the shining of that light within, I feel the dreams and prayers of all beings. In the shining of that beacon I feel all of our hopes for a better future. In the shining of the human heartlight there is the strength to do what must be done.

ALL THINGS ARE CONNECTED

"Destiny, or karma, depends upon what the soul has done about what it has become aware of."

(EDGAR CAYCE)

"Each of us is the last frontier."

(MERLE SHAIN)

THERE IS AN old story which tells of a man who lived a long and worthy life. When he died, the Lord said to him: "Come, I will show you hell." He was taken to a room where a group of people sat around a huge pot of stew. Each held a spoon that reached the pot, but had a handle so long it couldn't be used to reach their mouths. Everyone was famished and desperate; the suffering was terrible.

After awhile, the Lord said: "Come, now I will show you heaven." They came to another room. To the man's surprise, it was identical to the first room—a group of people sat around a huge pot of stew, and each held the same long-handled spoons. But here everyone was nourished and happy and the room was full of joy and laughter.

"I don't understand," said the man. "Everything is the same, yet they are so happy here, and they were so miserable in the other place. What's going on?"

The Lord smiled. "Ah, but don't you see—here they have learned to feed each other."

WASTING THE FOOD WE HAVE

The livestock population of the United States today consumes enough grain and soybeans to feed over five times the entire human population of the country.¹ We feed these animals over 80% of the corn we grow, and over 95% of the oats.²

It is hard to grasp how immensely wasteful is a meat-oriented diet-style. By cycling our grain through livestock, we end up with only 10% as many calories available to feed human mouths as would be available if we ate the grain directly.³

Less than half the harvested agricultural acreage in the United States is used to grow food for people. Most of it is used to grow livestock feed. This is a drastically inefficient use of our acreage. For every sixteen pounds of grain and soybeans fed to beef cattle, we get back only one pound as meat on our plates. The other fifteen are inaccessible to us. Most of it is turned into manure.

The developing nations are copying us. They associate meat-eating with the economic status of the developed nations, and strive to emulate it. The tiny minority who can afford meat in those countries eats it, even while many of their people go to bed hungry at night, and mothers watch their children starve.

"Love is feeding everybody."

(JOHN DENVER)

To understand the return on the food investment we get through cattle feeding, imagine you took a thousand dollars of your money and put it into a bank. A year later, you go to withdraw your money, expecting as well to collect the interest it has earned over the twelve months. But instead the bank teller hands you only a hundred dollars, and says that is all you get. All the rest is gone. Not only do you not get any interest on your investment, but you have lost 90 percent of it.

That is better than the protein efficiency of a meat-based diet. We lose over 90 percent of the protein we invest as feed in our livestock. Beef is the least efficient—we lose 94 percent of the protein we feed beef cattle. Dairy cattle are the most efficient—but here, too, we still lose 78 percent of our protein investment. With pigs and chickens our losses are in-between. We lose 88 percent of the protein we feed pigs, and 83 percent of our protein investment in poultry.⁴

"Forty thousand children starve to death on this planet every day."

(INSTITUTE FOR FOOD AND DEVELOPMENT POLICY)

To supply one person with a meat habit food for a year requires three-and-a-quarter acres. To supply one lacto-ovo vegetarian with food for a year requires one-half acre. To supply one pure vegetarian requires only one-sixth of an acre. In other words, a given acreage can feed twenty times as many people eating a pure vegetarian diet-style as it could people eating the standard American diet-style.[5]

Lester Brown of the Overseas Development Council has estimated that if Americans were to reduce their meat consumption by only 10 percent, it would free over 12 million tons of grain annually for human consumption. That, all by itself, would be enough to adequately feed every one of the 60 million human beings who will starve to death on the planet this year.[6]

"I've known what it is to be hungry, but I always went right to a restaurant."

(RING LARDNER)

By cycling our grain through livestock, we not only waste 90 percent of its protein; in addition, we sadly waste 96 percent of its calories, 100 percent of its fiber, and 100 percent of its carbohydrates.

Meanwhile, malnutrition is the principle cause of infant and child mortality in developing nations. In many of them, over 25 percent of the population die before reaching the age of four. In Guatemala, 75 percent of the children under five years of age are undernourished. Yet, every year Guatemala exports 40 million pounds of meat to the United States.[7] It borders on the criminal!

Many of us believe that hunger exists because there's not enough food to go around. But as Frances Moore Lappe and the anti-hunger organization Food First have shown, the real cause of hunger is a scarcity of justice, not a scarcity of food. Enough grain is squandered every day in raising American livestock for meat to provide every human being on earth with two loaves of bread.

Hunger is really a social disease caused by the unjust, inefficient and wasteful control of food. In Costa Rica, beef production quadrupled between 1960 and 1980. But almost all this beef is exported to the United States, and what does stay in the country is eaten by a tiny minority. Though more and more Costa Rican land is being turned over to meat production, the population is not eating more meat for the change. The average family in Costa Rica eats less meat than the average American housecat.

> *"The law, in its majestic equality, forbids the rich as well as the poor to sleep under bridges, to beg in the streets, and to steal bread."*

(ANATOLE FRANCE)

The world's cattle alone, not to mention pigs and chickens, consume a quantity of food equal to the caloric needs of 8.7 billion people—nearly double the entire human population of the planet.[8]

> *"He would daily throw out crumbs for the sparrows in the neighborhood. He noticed that one sparrow was injured, so that it had difficulty getting about. But he was interested to discover that the other sparrows, apparently by mutual agreement, would leave the crumbs which lay nearest their crippled comrade, so that he could get his share, undisturbed."*

(ALBERT SCHWEITZER)

According to Department of Agriculture statistics, one acre of land can grow 20,000 pounds of potatoes. That same acre of land, if used to grow cattlefeed, can produce less than 165 pounds of beef.[9]

In a world in which a child dies of starvation every two seconds, an agricultural system designed to feed our meat habit is a blasphemy. Yet it continues, because we continue to support it. Those who profit from this system do not need us to condone what they are doing. The only support they need from us is our money. As long as enough people continue to purchase their products they will have the resources to fight reforms, pump millions of dollars of "educational" propaganda into our schools, and defend themselves against medical and ethical truths.

A rapidly growing number of Americans are withdrawing support from this insane system by refusing to consume meat. For them, this new direction in diet-style is a way of joining hands with others and saying we will not support a system which wastes such vast amounts of food while people in this world do not have enough to eat.

"The day that hunger is eradicated from the earth there will be the greatest spiritual explosion the world has ever known. Humanity cannot imagine the joy that will burst into the world on the day of that great revolution."

(FREDERICO LORCA)

WAR IS HELL

Because the raising of livestock requires a much greater use of resources, it puts us in a situation where there is not enough to go around. In this kind of a dilemma there lurks a fear in us all that we will be the one who won't get enough. Thus, as long as there are people on this planet who are starving, we must all live in fear.

It is out of such fears that war arises. Conflicts stemming from territorial disputes become more frequent and more intense. Basic human needs become less important than property rights. We are set off against each other.

Fear is the real disease. The nuclear bombs are only symptoms. Is it not fear that makes us build and stockpile such terrible weapons? Whatever we can do to reduce fear reduces the possibility of war. We've already begun when we realize that our daily lives have a genuine impact on the level of fear in the world.

The understanding that meat-eating makes food scarce and puts us at odds with each other, so promoting war, is not new. The Bible is full of examples of conflicts arising from the competing needs of livestock raisers.[10] World history is full of battles that were fought because meat-eating societies needed more land to feed their stock.

In our century, we have had Gandhi urging us to "live simply so others might simply live." But his message was not new. Over 2,000 years ago, another wise man—Socrates—said much the same thing. In Plato's *Republic*, he extols the peace and happiness that come to people eating a vegetarian diet. Speaking to Glaucon, Socrates says:

> *"And with such a (vegetarian) diet they may be expected to live in peace and health to a good old age, and bequeath a similar life to their children after them."* [11]

But Glaucon is skeptical. He tells Socrates that he doesn't think people will be satisfied with so simple a life; they will want to eat "pig's flesh." Socrates answers that this would not be good, for people should avoid things "not required by any natural want." In fact, in describing the woes that will befall mankind if it eats animal flesh, Socrates seems uncannily prophetic—predicting both the medical consequences of meat-eating, which we are only now discovering, and the wars which throughout history it has brought in its wake:

> Socrates: *"And there will be animals of many other kinds, if people eat them?"*
>
> Glaucon: *"Certainly."*
>
> Socrates: *"And living in this way we shall have much greater need of physicians than before?"*
>
> Glaucon: *"Much greater."*
>
> Socrates: *"And the country which was enough to support the original inhabitants will be too small now, and not enough?"*
>
> Glaucon: *"Quite true."*
>
> Socrates: *"Then a slice of our neighbors' land will be wanted by us for pasture and tillage, and they will want a slice of ours, if, like ourselves, they exceed the limit of necessity, and give themselves up to the unlimited accumulation of wealth?"*
>
> Glaucon: *"That, Socrates, will be inevitable."*
>
> Socrates: *"And so we shall go to war, Glaucon, shall we not?"* [12]

Socrates spoke in a time when wars were ugly and vicious, but when the weapons of destruction were as nothing compared to today's nuclear stockpiles. Never before has it been so important as it is now to distinguish between basic human needs and excessive cravings. Never has it been more important to understand and defuse the fears that drive men to war. If any human being on the planet is starving, we all feel it.

Meat-eating contributes to the fear in the world by putting us in a position in which there is not enough to go around. But that's not all. Meat-eaters ingest residues of the animal's biochemical response to the horror of the slaughterhouse. Programmed by millions of years of evolution to fight or flee when in danger for their lives, the animals react to the slaughterhouse in sheer terror. Powerful biochemical agents are secreted that pump through their bloodstreams and into their flesh, energizing them to fight or flee for their lives. Like screaming air raid sirens, these chemical agents produce instinctual panic. Today's slaughterhouses virtually guarantee that the animals will die in terror.

Certain Indian tribes would not eat the flesh of an animal who died in fear, because they did not want to take into themselves the terror of such an animal. When we eat animals who have died violent deaths we literally eat their fear. We take in biochemical agents designed by nature to tell an animal that its life is in the gravest danger, and it must either fight or flee for its life. And then, in our wars and daily lives, we give expression to the panic in which the animals we have eaten died.

A new direction for America's diet-style would be a significant step towards a nonviolent world. It is a way of saying: "Let there be peace on earth, and let it begin with me." A nonviolent world has roots in a non-violent diet.

THE GROUND BENEATH OUR FEET

From dust we came and to dust we return. Archaeologists tell us that soil erosion played a determining role in the decline and demise of many great civilizations, including those of ancient Egypt, Greece and the Mayans. In *Topsoil and Civilization*, Vernon Carter and Tom Dale point out that wherever soil erosion has destroyed the fertility base on which civilizations have been built, these civilizations have perished.[13]

Topsoil is the dark, nutrient-rich soil that holds moisture and feeds us by feeding our plants. It is the most basic foundation of our sustenance upon this earth.

Two hundred years ago, most of America's croplands had at least 21 inches of topsoil. Today, most of it is down to around six inches of topsoil, and the rate of topsoil loss is accelerating.[14] We have already lost 75 percent of what may well be our most precious natural resource.[15] As a result, the U.S. Department of Agriculture says that the productivity of the nation's cropland is down 70 percent, with much of it on the brink of becoming barren wasteland.[16]

The U.S.D.A. admits this is an unparalleled disaster, but claims that:

> "... halting soil erosion and degradation would be prohibitively expensive."[17]

As long as we require our agriculture to feed our meat habit, this is no doubt true. But with a change in diet-style, we would need far less from our land. We would not have to force it artificially to supply the hyped-up demands we require to feed huge numbers of livestock. With a change in diet-style, halting soil erosion would cost us nothing. It would occur naturally, as part of sound soil management practices. Up until now we have resembled a sick man taking more and more pills to disguise his symptoms, even though the medications make him sicker. We have managed to mask the decline in our soil's fertility by saturating it with ever increasing amounts of chemical fertilizers and pesticides. American farmers now apply more than 20 million tons of chemical fertilizers to our farmlands every year, more than the combined weight of the entire human population of the country.

Although we have been virtually mainlining chemical fertilizers, our chemical "fixes" have done nothing to stop the erosion of our topsoil. In fact they have made it far worse.

It takes nature 500 years to build an inch of topsoil.[18] Currently, we lose an inch of topsoil every 16 years.[19] It takes nature a century to create 50 tons of topsoil on an acre of cropland. Today, thanks to the agricultural techniques we employ to produce massive amounts of livestock feed, one hard rainfall, or one strong wind, can erode that much topsoil from an acre of land in a couple of hours.[20]

"Food shortages will be to the 1990's what energy shortages have been to the 1970's and 1980's."

(ARMAND HAMMER, CHAIRMAN, OCCIDENTAL PETROLEUM)

The U.S. Soil Conservation Service reports that over 4 million acres of cropland are being lost to erosion in this country every year.[21] That's an area the size of Connecticut. Our annual topsoil loss amounts to 7,000,000,000 tons. That is 60,000 pounds for each member of the population.

Of this staggering topsoil loss, 85 percent is directly associated with livestock raising.[22]

"I never give them hell. I just tell the truth and they think it's hell."

(HARRY S TRUMAN)

Without a diet-style change, we are well on our way to losing what many scientists feel has always been the basis of our strength as a nation. If the present pace of soil erosion continues, it is just a matter of time until the people of the United States, the inheritors of the world's richest farmlands, will be forced to depend on foreign imports for food. That is, if there's any available.

Already, our agricultural practices are utterly dependent on foreign imports for the massive injections of chemical fertilizers on which our meat habit depends. We now import 85% of our potash, and significantly increasing amounts of nitrogen and phosphorous.[23]

A new direction for America's diet-style would reverse this pattern, making us far less dependent on foreign fertilizers, and thus less likely to be forced into intervening militarily in the affairs of other nations. It would allow us to feed ourselves, and help others, without destroying our land in the process. It would give us a chance to halt the erosion of our topsoil, and regain our footing in a sound and renewable agriculture.

> *"We don't inherit the land from our ancestors, we borrow it from our children."*

(PENNSYLVANIA DUTCH SAYING)

It is really quite astounding how much is to be gained from a shift in diet-style. Pure vegetarian food choices make less than 5% of the demand on the soil as meat-oriented choices.[24] By drastically reducing the demands on our soil, a new direction for America's diet-style would enable us to break our addiction to chemical fertilizers and pesticides. It would mean we could halt the horrendous overuse of nitrogenous fertilizers that are contributing to the destruction of the earth's ozone layer. It could mean we could stop raping the earth that sustains us. It would mean our children might yet have good rich soil in which to grow their food.

MOTHER EARTH

Over 100 years ago, the great Indian Chief, Seattle, was faced with the loss of his tribe's land. He responded out of his love and respect for the land, with utter honesty, and heartbreaking eloquence:

> *"We are part of the earth and it is part of us.*
> *The perfumed flowers are our sisters;*
> *the deer, the horse, the great eagle,*
> *these are our brothers.*
> *The rocky crests, the juices of the meadows,*
> *the body heat of the pony, and man---*
> *all belong to the same family.*
>
> *So, when the Great Chief in Washington sends word*
> *that he wishes to buy our land, he asks much of us . . .*
>
> *If we decide to accept, I will make one condition:*
> *The white man must treat the beasts of this land*
> *as his brothers.*
> *I am a savage and do not understand any other way.*

I have seen a thousand rotting buffalos on the prairie,
left by the white man who shot them from a passing train.
I am a savage and I do not understand how the smoking
iron horse can be more important than the buffalo
that we kill only to stay alive.

Where is man without the beasts?
If the beasts were gone, men would die
from a great loneliness of spirit.
For whatever happens to the beasts
soon happens to man.
All things are connected.
This we know.
The earth does not belong to man;
man belongs to the earth.
This we know.
All things are connected
like the blood which unites one family.
All things are connected.
Whatever befalls the earth befalls the sons of the earth.
Man did not weave the web of life,
he is merely a strand in it.
Whatever he does to the web,
he does to himself." [25]

TIMBER!

The current agricultural system, designed to supply America's meat habit, wastes almost all the food it grows by feeding it to livestock rather than people. This creates a constant pressure to get the highest possible immediate yields out of the land, at whatever ecological cost. As a result, we have lost hundreds of millions of acres to soil erosion.

In trying to replace it, we have spawned another major ecological catastrophe: we are destroying our forests. In fact, the United States has converted approximately 260 million acres of forest into land which is now needed to produce the wasteful diet-style most Americans take for granted. [26]

Since 1967, the rate of deforestation in this country has been one acre every five seconds.

"They took all the trees,
and put them in a tree museum.
Then they charged all the people
a dollar-and-a-half just to see them.
They paved paradise, and put up a parking lot . . ."

(FROM A SONG BY JONI MITCHELL)

Although Joni Mitchell rightly sensed the rapid deforestation of our land, she was wrong in attributing the destruction of our trees to urban development. For each acre of American forest that is cleared to make room for parking lots, roads, houses, shopping centers, etc., **seven acres** of forest are converted into land for grazing livestock and/or growing livestock feed.[27]

Deforestation is occurring to make land for meat production. In fact, researchers who have studied the uses to which deforested land are put concluded:

"More than three times as much meat is derived from
formerly-forested . . . land as is derived from range land. That
ratio is climbing each year as erosion and soil degradation claim
more and more of the nation's range land and ever more forest land
is converted to . . . land (for meat production)."[28]

It doesn't help matters that the Forest Service and the Bureau of Land Management do whatever they can to assist the meat industry. Enormous amounts of federal forest lands are leased each year to cattle ranchers at a tenth the price they would have to pay to graze their cattle on private land. And the cattlemen are allowed to clear-cut the forests on federal land to boot.

Forests, by the way, are one of the few places in the country where topsoil erosion isn't occurring. But after being cleared for use in livestock production, ex-forestland begins to lose topsoil rapidly.

Builders, and people wishing to buy firewood, have seen the price of wood skyrocket in the last few decades. But we have seen only the beginning if present trends continue. America's most important wood product is softwood lumber, yet our national resources of this essential natural resource fell 41 percent from 1952 to 1977. We have been importing more and more softwood from Canada, with the result that even Canada, with its seemingly limitless forests, is feeling the pinch. According to United Nations and Canadian Forest Service statistics, Canada's softwood reservoir could be exhausted in 40 years.[29]

The editor of *World Wood Review*, Herbert Lambert, tells us that we "will be unable to look northward beyond the year 2000" for our lumber.[30] The fact is that if present trends continue, we are fast approaching the time when there will be nowhere at all to look for lumber or any other wood products.

"I think that I shall never see
a poem lovely as a tree . . ."

(JOYCE KILMER)

At the present rate of deforestation in the United States, it won't be long before we never see a tree, period. I was stunned to learn that at the rate we are going, the United States will be stripped completely bare of **all** its forests in 50 years![31]

OUR OXYGEN PARTNERS
We need our forests. They are vital sources of oxygen. They moderate our climates, prevent floods, and are our best defense against soil erosion. Forests recycle and purify our water. They are homes for millions of plants and animals. They are a source of beauty, inspiration, and solace to millions of people.

The Bureau of Land Management and the Forest Service say there is nothing we can do to stem the tragic destruction of our forests. "People have to eat," said one agency official, shaking his head. And he's right—assuming the present meat habit, there is nothing we can do to save our forests. But diet-style changes could not only halt the process of deforestation, they could actually reverse it. Of the 260 million acres of American forest that have been converted into land now used to produce the standard American high-fat low-fiber diet-style, well over 200 million acres could be returned to forest if Americans were to stop raising food to feed livestock, and instead raise food directly for people.[32] Indeed, so direct is the relationship between meat production and deforestation that Cornell economist David Fields and his associate Robin Hur estimate that for every person who switches to a pure vegetarian diet, an acre of trees is spared every year.[33] A lacto-ovo vegetarian diet-style is also helpful, particularly if dairy and egg product consumption are low.

A new direction for Americans' diet-style would go a long way beyond just saving our forests, and rebuilding the ones we have destroyed. It would mean that our children could yet have wood with which to build and could yet live in a world rich with trees. It is probably the most potent single act most individuals can take at the present time in the effort to halt the destruction of our environment and preserve our precious natural resources.

HALF OF ALL SPECIES ON EARTH

It is not only American forests that are being cut down to support our meat habit. An ever-increasing amount of beef eaten in the United States is imported from Central and South America. To provide pasture for cattle, these countries have been clearing their priceless tropical rainforests.

It stretches the imagination to conceive how fast the timeless rainforests of Central America are being destroyed so Americans can have seemingly cheap hamburgers. In 1960, when the U.S. first began to import beef, Central America was blessed with 130,000 square miles of virgin rainforest. But now, only 25 years later, less than 80,000 square miles remain.[34] At this rate, the entire tropical rainforests of Central America will be gone in another forty years.

These tropical rainforests are among the world's most precious natural resources. Amounting to only 30 percent of the world's forests, the rainforests contain 80 percent of the earth's land vegetation, and account for a substantial percentage of the earth's oxygen supplies.

These forests are the oldest ecosystems on earth, and have developed extreme ecological richness. Half of all species on earth live in the moist tropical rainforests.

But these jewels of nature are being rapidly destroyed to provide land on which cattle can be grazed for the American fast-food market. According to the Meat Importers Council of America, we now import 10 percent of our beef consumption, and over 90 percent of that is from Central and Latin America.[35] In 1985, we imported over 100,000 tons of meat from Costa Rica, El Salvador, Guatemala, Honduras, Nicaragua and Panama. The Meat Importers Council reports that almost all of this meat ends up as fast-food restaurant hamburgers.

Interestingly, the rapidly growing trees and plants of the ageless Central and Latin American rainforests have consumed virtually all the minerals from the soil. Far more than in Northern forests, tropical rainforests store their nutrients in their trees and plants, and not in the soil. As a result, when these forests are cleared, the "grazing land" that is produced is not the same as, say, Texas grazing land. It is so poor in minerals that vegetation has a hard time growing back at all. Further, without a plant cover the heavy rains cause extremely rapid soil erosion. Immediately after clearing, two-and-a-half acres of ex-rainforest land can support a steer. But within a few years the land becomes so eroded that a single steer needs 12 acres. In ten years, so barren has the land become that a steer may now require 20 acres.

America's meat habit is turning the lush tropical rainforests into deserts useless even for cattle grazing.

Meanwhile, the native people suffer increasingly. As valuable farm land is used to grow food for cattle, the price and availability of native foods is pushed beyond the reach of many of the local people. The result is that many of them are starving to death. In addition, there is increased flooding and firewood scarcity. And, tragically, native rainforest tribes are being wiped out completely by the destruction of their environment.

What is left of the rainforests still contain much of the world's greatest treasures. Though a third of Costa Rica is today given over to cattle-raising, the remainder of this tiny country still houses more bird species than all of the United States combined.[36] But the continuing destruction of the rainforests jeopardizes the very existence of the animals, plants and peoples whose natural habitats are being rapidly hacked out of existence.

With the decimation of the Central American rainforests, many of our migratory birds are losing their winter homes. As a result, they are dying. This is tragic not merely because these birds provide so much beauty to our lives. They also play a major role in keeping down the populations of insect pests in the United States. The destruction of the rainforests in Central America is thus producing a substantial increase in pesticide use in this country.

This destruction is occurring just as Integrated Pest Management programs that entail selected breeding of adapted species of insects are showing great promise to supplant pesticides as a method of controlling insect pests. Ironically, many of the most promising biological control programs involve importing beneficial insects from the tropical rainforests.[37] At the present pace of our meat habit, however, many of the potentially beneficial insect species will be destroyed, along with their habitats, before we get a chance to use them to replace pesticides.

It is truly frightening to note that the current rate of species extinction in the world is 1,000 species a year, and most of that is due to the destruction of rainforests and related habitats in the tropics.[38] And as these environments continue to be destroyed, the rate of extinction is rising rapidly. If present trends continue, in the 1990's the figure will reach 10,000 a year (that's over one species every hour). In the next 30 years, over a million species will become extinct.

We still know very little about the natural treasures of the tropical rainforests, although it is clear that their preservation is essential to the ecology, not only of our hemisphere, but of the world. One-quarter of our medicines derive from raw materials found in these forests. Indeed, a child suffering from leukemia now has an 80% chance of survival instead of only a 20% chance, thanks to the alkaloidal drugs vincristine and vinblastine which are derived from a rainforest plant called the rosy periwinkle. Since less than one percent of the plant species of the tropical rainforests have been tested for medicinal benefits, researchers feel that here lie what could be the medicines of the future.

So damning is the evidence against U.S. hamburger chains in the destruction of the rainforests that the Rainforest Action Network has called for a national campaign to boycott Burger King. Calling the company "a driving force behind this environmental disaster," the Rainforest Action Network has purchased a series of ads in major newsmagazines to inform the public of the hidden price we pay for such meat:

> *"Before the rainforest was bulldozed and burned, it was home to thousands of rare and exotic species. After the cattle have come and gone, it's an eroded wasteland, practically empty of life . . .*
> *Activists in more than a dozen nations are fighting back—for the jaguars, orchids and howler monkeys. And for the millions of human beings who directly depend on the living rainforests for physical and cultural survival."*   .

A new direction for America's eating habits would go a long way towards saving the remaining tropical rainforests, and the countless species who will otherwise become extinct. The rainforests also produce extremely significant amounts of the world's oxygen supply. A new direction for America's diet-style would mean our children could yet have plentiful oxygen to breathe.

THE FOUNTAIN OF LIFE
Life on earth began in water, and has always depended for its very existence on water. With water, life can thrive and bloom; and deserts can be transformed into gardens, lush forests, or thriving metropolises like Tel Aviv or Los Angeles. Without water, we die.

Yet most of us are so used to having this precious resource at our fingertips that we have come to take it for granted. Sadly, we are fast approaching the time when we will be forced to learn the inestimable value of this natural treasure the hard way. Our supply of good water is disappearing at a terrifying rate.

The source of this ominous trend can be traced directly to our meat habit.

Over half the total amount of water consumed in the United States goes to irrigate land growing feed and fodder for livestock.[39] Enormous additional quantities of water must also be used to wash away the animals' excrement. It would be hard to design a less water-efficient diet-style than the one we have come to think of as normal.

To produce a single pound of meat takes an average of 2,500 gallons of water—as much as a typical family uses for all its combined household purposes in a month.[40]

To produce a day's food for one meat-eater takes over 4,000 gallons; for a lacto-ovo vegetarian, only 1,200 gallons; for a pure vegetarian, only 300 gallons. It takes less water to produce a **year's** food for a pure vegetarian than to produce a **month's** food for a meat-eater.[41]

The amount of water consumed by America's meat habit is staggering.

It takes up to a hundred times more water to produce a pound of meat as it does to produce a pound of wheat.[42] Rice takes more water than any other grain, but even rice requires only a tenth as much water per pound of production as meat.

It's not easy to conceive how huge are the quantities of water consumed in the production of meat. *Newsweek* magazine, with an eye to the picturesque phrase, portrayed the situation this way:

> "*The water that goes into a 1,000 pound steer would float a destroyer.*"[43]

Consumption of so much water has serious economic, as well as ecological, consequences. The economic costs are hidden from us, though, because our federal and state governments subsidize the meat industry's water consumption at every stage of the process. If these costs were not borne unknowingly by the taxpayer, but instead showed up at the supermarket cash register, the industry would long ago have gone bankrupt. If the cost of water needed to produce a pound of meat were not subsidized, the cheapest hamburger meat would cost more than $35 a pound!

Cornell economist David Fields and his associate Robin Hur have studied the fiscal consequences of water subsidies to the meat industry:

"Reports by the General Accounting Office, the Rand Corporation, and the Water Resources Council have made it clear that irrigation water subsidies to livestock producers are economically counterproduc tive. Every dollar that state governments dole out to livestock producers, in the form of irrigation subsidies, actually costs tax payers over seven dollars in lost wages, higher living costs, and reduced business income . . .

"The 17 Western states receive limited precipitation, yet their water supplies could support an economy and population twice the size of their present ones. But most of the water goes to produce livestock, either directly or indirectly. Thus, current water use practices now threaten to undermine the economies of every state in the region." [44]

When I first heard statements like these, I was flabbergasted. I could not understand how water subsidies to livestock producers could be "undermining the economies" of every Western state. I thought these economists must be exaggerating, to make a point. But the more I've learned, the more I've seen how severe indeed are the fiscal ramifications of pouring away such prodigious quantities of water to support our meat habit.

For example, in the Pacific Northwest (Oregon, Washington and Idaho), meat production accounts for over half the water consumed in the entire region. [45] And yet, even though the meat producers of the Pacific Northwest use such a disproportionate share of the area's water, they aren't all that productive. These states have to import most of their meat.

You may think the Pacific Northwest is amply supplied with rain and rivers. But the people of this area are paying an onerous price for spending so much water to produce so little meat, a price concealed in the region's soaring electrical costs. These states get over 80 percent of their electricity from hydropower plants, many of which are located along the Snake River in Idaho, and the Columbia River in Washington. [46] The water flowing in these rivers is the source of much of the state's electrical power. But the water used for livestock production in the Pacific Northwest also comes mainly from these same rivers, and it is taken from the rivers at points upstream from the power plants. The quantity of water taken from these rivers to grow livestock feed and otherwise produce meat is so huge that the amount of water left in the rivers to generate electricity is substantially reduced. Thus electricity becomes more expensive to produce, the price rises, and the government must look elsewhere for sources of electricity. Hence the need for nuclear power plants in the area.

Not only do livestock producers deplete the state's electrical power capacities through siphoning off water that would otherwise generate power, they also use enormous amounts of electricity to pump the water from the rivers to the point-of-use. All in all, economists calculate that the three-state area loses 17 billion kilowatt hours of electricity a year to the gluttonous water use of livestock production.[47] That's enough to light every house in the entire nation for a month-and-a-half.

The enormous loss of electrical power to the meat industry in the Pacific Northwest is one of the main reasons the region has had to continue the construction of the two nuclear power plants near Hanover, Washington, despite the fact that the cost overruns on these plants have been ludicrous, and hardly anyone is convinced they are safe.[48] Area residents have already had to pay $4,000 per household for the privilege of living in the shadow of these nuclear plants, and current estimates are that by the time the nuclear plants are in operation, each household will have to pay another $3,000. Those who cannot pay will have to go into debt. Many already have.

Due to their outrageous water consumption, the livestock industries of the Pacific Northwest account for more energy loss than will be gained by the nuclear plants.

Further south, we have the sunny state of California. California is known for its great grape vineyards, its lush fields of strawberries and artichokes, its vast acreages of lettuce and broccoli, its immense orange, lemon and avocado orchards. Yet, livestock producers are California's biggest water consumer.

You might think that all this water consumption would at least create jobs. But no other industry in the country even comes close to the meat industry when it comes to the paucity of jobs created per

gallon of water consumed. For every job created by livestock production in California, it uses 30 million gallons of water a year, far more
than any other industry.[49]

Economist Douglas McDonald estimates that if water subsidies
were withdrawn from California livestock producers, the income of the
state's other businesses and workers would rise over $10 billion annu-
ally.[50] Other economists have exposed the cost of water subsidies to the
meat industry that are hidden in the state's rising prices for water
rights, and thus, housing. Fields and Hur calculate the overall price of
subsidizing the California meat industry's water to be $24 billion.
That's a thousand dollars for every man, woman, and child in the
nation's most populous state—a state that imports most of its meat.

Though the economic consequences of water subsidies to livestock
producers are not always apparent to the uninformed public, they are
felt by every citizen in every part of the country. Economists Field and
Hur have concluded that while the meat industry likes to portray itself
as the backbone of the American economy, in truth it is more of a back-
breaking burden.

Half of the nation's grain-fed beef is produced in the High Plains
regions of Kansas, Nebraska, Oklahoma, Colorado, and New Mexico.
The enormous amount of water needed for what amounts to the lion's
share of the nation's meat production comes from a single source—the
Ogallala Aquifer.

Fifty years ago, the great Ogallala Aquifer remained virtually invi-
olate, hardly touched by the amount of water being pumped out of her
enormous reservoirs. But with the advent of factory farming and feedlot beef, the amount of water drawn from the Ogallala has risen dramatically. At the present time, over 13 trillion gallons of water are
being taken from this enormous aquifer every year, and the vast majority of that is used to produce meat. More water is withdrawn from the
Ogallala Aquifer every year than is used to grow all the fruits and
vegetables in the entire country.[51]

It took nature millions of years to form the great Ogallala Aquifer.
And she still contains as much water as any of the Great Lakes. But the
American meat habit is taking its toll on this priceless wonder of na-
ture. Water tables are dropping precipitously. Wells are going dry. And

water resource experts are estimating that at the current rate of water consumption, the Ogallala Aquifer may be exhausted in 35 years.[52] If this happens, the High Plains of the United States will be completely uninhabitable to human beings.

> *"The frog does not drink up*
> *the pond in which he lives."*

> (BUDDHIST PROVERB)

All over the country, the utterly disproportionate share of our water resources being used by the meat industry is creating shortages requiring deeper wells, which are more expensive to drill, and more expensive to pump. In many areas, people and industries are being forced to settle for water of poorer and poorer quality, at higher and higher costs.

Just in the last 20 years alone, Texas has used up one-quarter of its entire supply of ground water. Most of that water was used to grow sorghum to feed cattle. A new direction for America's diet-style would plug the drain through which our nation's water is being lost. It would enable us to conserve this most precious of natural resources. It would mean that our children could yet have ample water to drink.

QUITE A PILE

The standard American diet of today not only wastes prodigious amounts of water; it pollutes much of what is left.

Fifty years ago, most of the manure from livestock returned to enrich the soil. But today, with huge numbers of animals concentrated in feedlots, confinement buildings, and other factory farm locations, there is no economically feasible way to return their wastes to the soil. As a result there is a continuing decline in soil humus and soil fertility, an increasing dependence on chemical fertilizers and pesticides, and an accelerating loss of topsoil. It is far removed indeed from the natural ecological cycle, in which animal wastes return to the soil and provide the nutrients for next year's crops.

Sadly, instead of being returned to the soil, the wastes from today's animals often end up in our water. This is extremely significant, because the quantity of waste is so immense. It is a real challenge to our imaginations to conceive how much manure is produced by the animals in this country being raised for meats, dairy products and eggs. Every 24 hours, the animals destined for America's dinner tables produce 20 billion pounds of waste. That is 250,000 pounds of excrement a second.

The livestock of the United States produce **twenty times as much excrement as the entire human population of the country**![53] Over half this staggering production—over a billion tons a year—comes from confinement operations from which it cannot be recycled.

A typical egg factory, with 60,000 hens, produces 165,000 pounds of excrement every week.[54] But that's chicken feed, so to speak, compared to a relatively small pork operation, with, say, 2,000 pigs. Here an average day's production includes four tons of manure, and five tons of urine.[55]

When you start talking about cows, however, you really get into the big time.

> *"One cow produces as much waste as 16 humans. With 20,000 animals in our pens, we have a problem equal to a city of 320,000 people."*
>
> (HARRY J. WEBB, PRESIDENT, BLAIR CATTLE COMPANY,
> BLAIR, NEBRASKA)

The largest feedlots, with 100,000 cattle, "have a problem" equal to that of the most populous American cities. Unlike the residents of New York, Los Angeles, or Chicago, however, the residents of feedlots do not pay taxes out of which sewage systems can be constructed.

The result is that their waste tends to end up in our water.

Animal waste is high in nitrogen, which is one of the chief reasons it makes such good fertilizer if it's returned to the soil. But unreturned, much of the nitrogen converts to ammonia and nitrates. The dumping of livestock wastes into our water is one of the reasons more and more rural wells are encountering dangerously high nitrate levels. Even city water supplies are increasingly high in nitrates. This is an ominous trend, because levels of nitrates in water, which do no harm to adults, cause serious brain damage, and even death, to infants.

It may not seem to you or me that dumping vast amounts of live-stock wastes into our nation's streams, rivers and lakes makes ecological sense. But the U.S. Department of Agriculture used to encourage beef producers to locate their feedlots on hillsides near streams to make it easier to channel the wastes into the water.[56]

Feedlots are no longer encouraged simply to dump their wastes into our waterways, but a lot of it still ends up there. The result is algae overgrowth and oxygen depletion. As a consequence, many of our rivers, streams and lakes can now barely support fish or any other animal life.

When *Newsweek* asked Dr. Harold Bernard about the runoffs from U.S. feedlots, the E.P.A. agricultural expert did not mince words. He said feedlot wastes are:

> *". . . ten to several hundred times more concentrated than raw domestic sewage . . . When the highly concentrated wastes in a runoff flow into a stream or river, the results can be, and frequently are, catastrophic. The amount of dissolved oxygen in the waterway will be sharply reduced, while levels of ammonia, nitrates, phosphates and bacteria soar."* [57]

I must admit that I have had a hard time comprehending the overwhelming quantity of water pollution in the United States that ensues directly from livestock production. But animal wastes account for more than ten times as much water pollution as the total amount attributable to the entire human population![58] Astoundingly, the meat industry single-handedly accounts for more than three times as much harmful organic waste water pollution as the rest of the nation's industries combined![59]

A new direction for America's diet-style would do more to conserve and clean up our nation's water than any other single action. Indeed, each family who stops eating meat spares our waterways ever more pollution. A new direction for America's diet-style would mean that the water in our children's lives might yet be clean.

THE ENERGY CRISIS AND NUCLEAR POWER

When most of us think of the energy crisis, we think of lowering thermostats, weather-stripping doors and windows, and remembering to turn off the lights. We think of driving compact instead of luxury cars. We think of OPEC and the volatile price of oil. Some of us remember long gas lines, and the very real threat of oil shortages that could cripple the economy and devastate our lives. Some of us fear that our dependence on foreign oil may force us to become militarily involved in the Persian Gulf.

Very few of us realize how much our food choices have to do with all this.

Growing any kind of food, and getting it to our homes and restaurants, takes energy. But some foods take considerably more than others. Turning an amber field of wheat into Twinkies uses up a lot more energy than turning it into wholewheat bread. Refining and processing foods uses up more energy than consuming these foods in their more natural states. A regular size box of Wheaties costs $1.65 at my local market; yet it contains only $0.06 worth of wheat. The box itself costs more than that.

When it comes to resource and energy wastage, however, meat products are in a class by themselves.

Scientists compute the energy costs of foods by the value of the raw materials consumed in the production of that food. Frances Moore Lappe reports:

> *"A detailed 1978 study sponsored by the Departments of Interior and Commerce produced startling figures showing that the value of raw materials consumed to produce food from livestock is greater than the value of all oil, gas, and coal consumed in this country."* [60]

The same study revealed the equally startling fact that the production of meats, dairy products and eggs accounts for **one-third of the total amount of all raw materials used for all purposes in the United States.**

In contrast, growing grains, vegetables and fruits is a model of efficiency, using less than 5% the raw material consumption as does the production of meat.

A new direction for America's diet-style would mean a savings of over 30% of all the raw materials presently consumed in the country for all purposes.

Another way scientists compute the energy costs of various foods is to assess the amount of fossil fuel needed to produce them. An American scientist, David Pimental, calculates that if the whole world were to eat according to U.S. agricultural practices, the planet's entire petroleum reserves would be exhausted in 13 years.[61]

It is actually quite astounding how much energy is wasted by the standard American diet-style. Even driving many gas-guzzling luxury cars can conserve energy over walking—that is, when the calories you burn walking come from the standard American diet![62] This is because the energy needed to produce the food you would burn in walking a given distance is greater than the energy needed to fuel your car to travel the same distance, assuming that the car gets 24 miles per gallon or better. This remarkable fact does not arise because our cars deserve a gold medal for energy efficiency. They don't. They burn up enough energy to blow up a bridge every four miles.[63] But today's meat production systems are an energy conservationist's worst nightmare come true.

On a traditional farm, pigs and chickens kept warm in the winter by nestling in bedding. And in the summer they would cool off in shady, damp soil. In today's factory farms, however, there is no bedding, and no shady, damp soil. In order to maximize the animal's weight gain under these conditions, temperatures must be artificially controlled, and that takes energy.

Further heat is needed because the young animals are separated from the warmth of their mothers' bodies. Baby animals by nature are vulnerable to chills, and their situation is more precarious when they are taken from their mothers and put on cold concrete or drafty metal slat floors.

More energy is needed to bring feed to the animals. And more is needed to move their wastes away. In fact, the whole assembly line factory farming system is explicitly designed at every step to minimize human labor, and instead use machines that consume energy.

As a result, these factories provide hardly any jobs, considering the size of the operations. And they tend to use up our limited stores of fossil fuels as if there were no tomorrow. At the rate they're going, there won't be.

Agricultural engineers at Ohio State University compared the energy costs of producing poultry, pork and other meats with the energy costs of producing soybeans, corn, and other plant foods. They found that even the *least* efficient plant food is *nearly ten times* as efficient as the *most* energy efficient animal food:

> *"Even the best of the animal enterprises examined returns only 34.5% of the investment of fossil energy to us in food energy, whereas the poorest of five crop enterprises examined returns 328%."* [64]

Other studies show the same pattern. Corn or wheat provide 22 times more protein per calorie of fossil fuel expended than does feedlot beef. Soybeans are even better—**40** times more efficient than feedlot beef![65]

We can see why a feature article in *Scientific American* devoted to the energy crisis warned:

> *"The trends in meat consumption and energy consumption are on a collision course."* [66]

A new direction to America's diet-style would save an immense amount of energy. If we kicked the meat habit there would be no need for nuclear power plants. Our electric bills would be far lower than they are now. Our dependence on foreign oil would be greatly reduced. We would have the time and resources to develop solar and other environmentally sound energy sources. Our children might yet live in a world abundant with energy resources.

HARD-NOSED BUSINESSMEN
Over and over again, as I've envisioned the possibilities ensuing from a new direction for America's diet-style, I've been struck by what might be gained by such a move. I've seen how helpful it could be towards reducing world hunger, towards reducing the fear in the world that leads to wars, towards preserving our precious topsoil and forests, to-

wards saving thousands of species in the tropical rainforests from extinction, towards cleaning up and preserving our water. And I've been moved by how much animal suffering would be alleviated, how our health would improve, and how greatly we could diminish our use and intake of toxic chemicals that threaten so seriously the future of our species.

But there is yet another factor pointing in the same direction, one which might turn the heads of even the most hard-nosed American businessmen: it is actually quite astounding how good a new American diet would be for the economy.

Economists Fields and Hur report:

> *"A nationwide switch to a diet emphasizing whole grains, fresh fruits and vegetables—plus limits on export of nonessential fatty foods—would save enough money to cut our imported oil requirements by over 60 percent. And, the supply of renewable energy, such as wood and hydroelectric, would increase 120 to 150 percent."* [67]

Extrapolating from these energy savings, these economists have analysed the impact such a diet-style switch would have on the economy. The impact they see is formidable.

They see substantial increases in personal savings accruing from reduced expenditures for food, prescription drugs, medical care and insurance. And within a short time, they see even more personal savings accruing from savings on housing, energy, transportation and clothing. As a result, they say:

> *"A typical household of three could expect to save $4,000 a year in the short run. And, if they put aside 30% of those savings—and it is quite possible they could put aside up to half—the supply of lendable funds from personal savings would rise 50 percent."* [68]

Such a rise in lendable funds from personal savings would be extremely important to the economy. Personal savings are the economy's main source of funds for expansion. As the supply of such funds rose, the price of these funds—otherwise known as interest rates—would come down.

Interest rates would be brought down from another angle as well. Savings on energy imports would ease the pressure on the national debt. This, in turn, would substantially reduce government borrowing needs. Currently, to finance the ungodly growth of the national debt, the government has to siphon off half the reservoir of funds, mainly personal savings that are the fuel for the nation's economic growth. But the combination of increased personal savings, and lowered government borrowing, say economists Fields and Hur, would be a:

". . . double-barreled blast at high interest rates." [69]

As interest rates dropped, the snowball of economic benefits to the country would really get rolling. And meanwhile, a meatless diet-style would be saving enormous amounts of money presently spent on medical care, and person-hours lost to sickness. Say these economists:

"Savings on health care alone could be expected to reach $100 billion within five years." [70]

As the economy began to really hum with the decreased energy expenditures, savings would come from every direction, including reduced interest on the national debt as the government's borrowing needs continue to diminish. The savings on water subsidies to meat producers alone would be worth billions of dollars a year. Within five years, calculate Fields and Hur, total savings would reach $80 billion a year. In 20 years, according to their estimates, savings would reach $200 billion a year.

At present, the hideous growth of the federal deficit amounts to the mortgaging of our children's future. The legacy we are now leaving them is a debt so large many economists foresee no way they could ever hope to repay it. But if the economic scenario of Fields and Hur is correct, the savings deriving from a new direction in America's diet-style would enable the United States government to eliminate the federal deficit.

Perhaps our children might yet live in a sane and prosperous world.

THE UNFORGETTABLE DREAM

At the present time, when most of us sit down to eat, we aren't very aware of how our food choices affect the world. We don't realize that in every Big Mac there is a piece of the tropical rainforests, and with every billion burgers sold another hundred species become extinct. We don't realize that in the sizzle of our steaks there is the suffering of animals, the mining of our topsoil, the slashing of our forests, the harming of our economy, and the eroding of our health. We don't hear in the sizzle the cry of the hungry millions who might otherwise be fed. We don't see the toxic poisons accumulating in the food chains, poisoning our children and our earth for generations to come.

But once we become aware of the impact of our food choices, we can never really forget. Of course we can push it all to the back of our minds, and we may need to do this, at times, to endure the enormity of what is involved.

But the earth itself will remind us, as will our children, and the animals and the forests and the sky and the rivers, that we are part of this earth, and it is part of us. All things are deeply connected, and so the choices we make in our daily lives have enormous influence, not only on our own health and vitality, but also on the lives of other beings, and indeed on the destiny of life on earth.

Thankfully, we have cause to be grateful—what's best for us personally is also best for other forms of life, and for the life support systems on which we all depend.

The Indians who dwelt for countless centuries in what we now call the United States lived in harmony with the land and with nature. Their societies were each unique, yet all were founded on a reverence for life that conserved nature rather than destroying it, and which lived in balance with what we today call the ecosystem. To them, it was all the work of God. Every shining pine needle, every sandy shore, every mist in the dark woods, every humming insect was holy.

When the white man forced them to make the ultimate sacrifice and sell their land, the great Chief Seattle spoke for his people and asked one thing in return. He did not ask something for himself, nor for his tribe, nor even for the Indian people. There were, of course, many things of immense importance he must have wanted at such a time. He could have asked for more blankets, horses, or food. He could have asked that the ancestral burial grounds be respected. He could have asked many things for himself or for his people. But what stood above all else in importance had to do with the relationship between humans and other animals. His one request was as prophetic as it was plain:

> *"I will make one condition.*
> *The white man must treat the beasts of this land*
> *as his brothers.*
> *For whatever happens to the beasts*
> *soon happens to man.*
> *All things are connected."*

Chief Seattle spoke for a people whose bond with the natural world was unimaginably profound. Yet the white man called them savages, and utterly disregarded his plea. The factory farms that produce today's meats, dairy products and eggs are living testimony to how totally we have disdained the one condition he made.

The white man thought Chief Seattle an ignorant savage. But he was a prophet whose wisdom and eloquence arose from living contact with Creation. And his words are astoundingly similar to those of a book written long, long ago. The *Bible*, too, tells us the fates of humans and animals are intimately intertwined.

> *"For that which befalleth the sons of men befalleth the beasts.*
> *Even one thing befalleth them:*
> *as the one dieth, so dieth the other;*
> *yea, they have all one breath,*
> *so that a man hath no pre-eminence above a beast."*

(ECCLESIASTES 3:19)

Chief Seattle did not know that centuries before a book called the *Bible* had spoken in words almost identical to his own. But he spoke on behalf of life itself, and the wisdom of the ages poured through him. Today, when we have strayed so very far from an ethical relationship to other creatures and to the welfare of the world we share, his message remains with us as a light of immeasurable brilliance. Never before has the truth of his words been so apparent:

> *"One thing we know:*
> *Our God is the same.*
> *This earth is precious to Him . . .*
> *This we know:*
> *The earth does not belong to man:*
> *Man belongs to the earth.*
> *This we know:*
> *All things are connected*
> *Like the blood which unites one family.*
> *All things are connected.*
> *Whatever befalls the earth*
> *Befalls the sons of the earth.*
> *Man did not weave the web of life.*
> *He is merely a strand in it.*
> *Whatever he does to the web,*
> *He does to himself."*

RESOURCES

"This is the true joy in life: being used for a purpose recognized by yourself as a mighty one, and being a force of nature instead of a feverish, selfish little clod of ailments and grievances, complaining that the world will not devote itself to making you happy."

(GEORGE BERNARD SHAW)

"Liberty means responsibility. That is why most men dread it."

(GEORGE BERNARD SHAW)

RECOMMENDED COOKBOOKS

The New Laurel's Kitchen
Laurel Robertson, Carol Flinders and Brian Ruppenthal
Ten Speed Press
P.O. Box 7123
Berkeley, CA 94707

Ten Talents (no dairy or eggs)
Frank J. Hurd & Rosalie Hurd
Published by Frank J. Hurd
Chisholm, MN

The Farm Vegetarian Cookbook
(no dairy or eggs)
Edited by Louise Hagler
The Book Publishing Co.
Summertown, TN

Vegetarian Times Cookbook
Available from **Vegetarian Times** Bookshelf
P.O. Box 570
Oak Park, IL 60303

The McDougall Plan (very low-fat)
John McDougall
New Century
Piscataway, NJ

Complete Guide to Macrobiotic Cooking
Mushio Kushi
Warner Brothers
New York, NY

The Moosewood Cookbook
Mollie Katzen
Ten Speed Press
P.O. Box 7123N
Berkeley, CA 94707

Simple Food For The Good Life
Helen Nearing
P.O. Box 640
Stillpoint Publishing
Walpole, NH 03608

RECOMMENDED PERIODICALS

Vegetarian Times
141 S. Oak Park Ave.
P.O. Box 570
Oak Park, IL 60303

Animals Agenda
P.O. Box 5234
Westport, CT 06881

East-West Journal
17 Station Street
Box 1200
Brookline, MA 02147

Awaking in the Nuclear Age
P.O. Box 4742
Berkeley, CA 94704-4742

Environmental Action
1525 New Hampshire Ave., NW
Washington, D.C. 20036

Medical Self-Care
Box 717
Inverness, CA 94937
(415) 663-8462

Whole Life
89 Fifth Ave., Suite 600
New York, NY 10003

Mother Jones
1663 Mission St.
San Francisco, CA 94103

RECOMMENDED HUNGER ORGANIZATIONS

Food First
1885 Mission St.
San Francisco, CA 94103
(415) 864-8555

Oxfam America
115 Broadway
Boston, MA 02116
(617) 482-1211

Cultural Survival
11 Divinity Ave.
Cambridge, MA 02138

American Friends Service
    Committee
1501 Cherry St.
Philadelphia, PA 19102
(215) 241-7000

Grassroots International
P.O. Box 312
Cambridge, MA 02139
(617) 497-9180

Committee for Health Rights in
    Central America (CHRICA)
513 Valencia Street, Room #6
San Francisco, CA 94110
(415) 431-7760

Unitarian Universalist Service
    Committee
78 Beacon Street
Boston, MA 02108
(617) 742-2120

RECOMMENDED ENVIRONMENTAL ORGANIZATIONS

Greenpeace USA
1611 Connecticut Ave., NW
Washington, D.C. 20009
(202) 462-1177

Friends of the Earth
530 7th Street, SE
Washington, D.C. 20003
(202) 543-4312

National Coalition Against the
    Misuse of Pesticides
530 7th Street
Washington, D.C. 20003
(202) 543-5450

Sierra Club
P.O. Box 7603
San Francisco, CA 94120-9826
(415) 776-2211

International Wildlife Coalition
1807 H St., NW
Suite 301
Washington, D.C. 20006
(202) 347-0822

New Forests Fund
731 Eighth St.
Washington, D.C. 20003

Rainforest Action Network
300 Broadway
San Francisco, CA 94133

Citizens for a Better Environment
Suite 505
942 Market Street
San Francisco, CA 94102

The Cousteau Society
930 W. 21st Street
Norfolk, VA 23517

RECOMMENDED ANIMAL RIGHTS GROUPS

People for the Ethical Treatment of
  Animals (PETA)
P.O. Box 42516
Washington, D.C. 20015
(202) 726-0156

International Society for Animal
  Rights, Inc.
421 South State Street
Clarks Summit, PA 18411
(717) 586-2200

The Fund for Animals
200 W. 57th Street
New York, NY
212-246-2096

Friends of Animals, Inc.
11 West 60th Street
New York, NY 10023
(212) 247-8077

Friends of Animals, Inc.
1 Pine Street
Neptune, NJ 07753-9988
(201) 922-2600

Progressive Animal Welfare Society
  (PAWS)
P.O. Box 1037
Lynnwood, WA 98046
(206) 743-3845

Food Animals Concern Trust
P.O. Box 14599
Chicago, IL
(312) 525-4952

American Society for the
  Prevention of Cruelty to Animals
441 East 92nd St.
New York, NY 10128
(212) 876-7700

Animal Protection Institute of
  America
6130 Freeport Blvd.
P.O. Box 22505
Sacramento, CA 95822
(916) 422-1921

Farm Animals Reform Movement
P.O. Box 70123
Washington, D.C. 20088
(301) 530-1737

Humane Farming Association
1550 California Street, Suite 6
San Francisco, CA 94109
(415) 485-1495

In Defense of Animals
21 Tamal Vista Blvd.
Corte Madera, CA 94925
(415) 924-4454

National Anti-Vivisection Society
100 East Ohio Street
Chicago, IL 60611
(312) 787-4486

Animal Legal Defense Fund
333 Market St.
San Francisco, CA 94105
(415) 495-0885
  also
205 E. 42nd St.
New York, NY 10017
(212) 818-0130

Humane Society of the United
  States (HSUS)
2100 L St., NW
Washington, D.C. 20037
(202) 452-1100

The Culture and Animals
  Foundation
3509 Eden Croft Drive
Raleigh, NC 27612

Trans-Species Unlimited
P.O. Box 1553
Williamsport, PA 17703
(717) 322-3252

International Fund for Animal
  Welfare
P.O. Box 193
Yarmouth Port, MA 02675

Animal Rights International
Box 214
Planetarium Station
New York, NY 10024

Association of Veterinarians for
  Animal Rights
530 E. Putnam Ave.
Greenwich, CT 06830

Compassion in World Farming
20 Lavant Street
Petersfield, Hants,
ENGLAND

American Anti-Vivisection Society
801 Old York Road
Jenkintown, PA 19046
(215) 887-0816

HUMANE & HEALTHY DIET STYLE ORGANIZATIONS

North American Vegetarian Society
P.O. Box 72
Dolgeville, NY 13329

American Vegan Society
501 Old Harding Highway
Malaga, NJ 08328

San Francisco Vegetarian Society
1450 Broadway
San Francisco, CA 94109

East-West Foundation
P.O. Box 850
Brookline, MA 02147

Natural Hygiene Society
12816 Race Track Road
Tampa, FL 33625

American College of Health
  Science
6600-D Burleson Rd.
Austin, TX 78744

Canadian Natural Hygiene Society
P.O. Box 235
Station 'T'
Toronto, Ontario
M6B 4A1 Canada

OTHER GOOD PEOPLE TO KNOW ABOUT

SEVA Foundation
108 Spring Lake Drive
Chelsea, MI 48118

Interhelp
P.O. Box 331
Northampton, MA 01061

Interspecies Communication
273 Hidden Meadow Lane
Friday Harbor, WA 98250

Center for Science in the Public
  Interest/Americans for Safe Food
1501 16th St., N.W.
Washington, D.C. 20036
(202) 332-9110

FOOTNOTES

Chapter One—All God's Critters Have a Place in the Choir

1 --- Account adapted from Fox, M., *Returning to Eden*, Viking Press, 1980, pg 3; and Amory, C., *Animail*, Windmill Books, 1976, pgs 34-35; and elsewhere

2 --- Account adapted from Henkin, B., "Eight Unusual Dolphin Incidents," in Wallace, I., et al, *Book of Lists #2*, Bantam Books, 1980, pgs 107-108; and Amory, C., as per note 1, pgs 14-15; and elsewhere

3 --- Amory, C., as per note 1, pg 193

4 --- *Ogonyok*, cited in *The Extended Circle*, Wynne-Tyson, J. (ed), Centaur Press, 1985, pg 230; and Amory, C., as per note 1, pg 188

5 --- Kellert, Stephen R., and Felthous, Alan R., "Childhood Cruelty Toward Animals Among Criminals and Noncriminals," *Human Relations*, Volume 38, No. 12, pgs 1113-1120

6 --- Amberson, R., *Raising Your Cat*, Crown Publishers, 1969

7 --- Carson, G., *Men, Beasts and Gods - A History of Cruelty and Kindness to Animals*, Charles Scribner's Sons, New York, 1972, pg 65

Harwood, D., *Love for Animals - How It Developed in Great Britain*, New York, 1928, pgs 13-14 footnote

Morris, D., *The Human Zoo*, New York, 1969, pg 76

Pope Pius XII, quoted in Quinn, J., "A Proper Respect for Men and Animals," *U.S. Catholic*, June 1965.

Quinn, J., "A Proper Respect for Men and Animals," *U.S. Catholic*, June 1965

8 --- Schweitzer, A., letter to Japanese Animal Welfare Society, 1961

9 --- Schweitzer, A., quoted in *The Extended Circle*, as per note 4

10 --- Schweitzer, A., *The Animal World of Albert Schweitzer*, Beacon Press, 1951

11 --- Henkin, B., as per note 2

12 --- Ibid

13 --- Account adapted from Quaker Oats Co. Ken-L-Ration "Dog Hero of the Year Award," in Wallace, A., et al, *Book of Lists #3*, Bantam Books, 1983, pgs 124-128

14 --- Ibid

15 --- Amory, C., as per note 1, pg 18

16 --- Carson, G., *Men, Beasts and Gods - A History of Cruelty and Kindness to Animals*, Charles Scribner's Sons, New York, 1972, pg. 65

17 --- "Henry Bergh's Story," *Philadelphia Press*, Sept 22, 1884

ASPCA First Annual Report, New York, 1867, pgs 5-8

Coleman, *Humane Society Leaders*, pgs 42-43

18 --- As per note 17

19 --- Amory, C., as per note 1, pgs 31-32

20 --- Henkin, B., as per note 2

21 --- Ibid

22 --- Ibid

23 --- Fox, M., as per note 1, pg 4

24 --- Amory, C., as per note 1, pg 185

25 --- Dickson, L., *Wilderness Man*, First American Edition, Atheneum Press, New York, 1973

26 — Amory, C., *Man Kind? - Our Incredible War on Wildlife*, Harper and Row, New York, 1974
27 — Helfer, R., quoted in Amory, C., as per note 1, pgs 92-93
28 — Descartes, R., *Discourse on the Method of Rightly Conducting the Reason, and Seeking Truth in the Sciences*, trans. John Veitch, Chicago, 1920, pg iv.
29 — Ibid, pt. 5
30 — Sells, A., *Animal Poetry in French and English Literature and The Greek Tradition*, Bloomington, Indiana, 1955, pg xxv.
31 — Carson, G., as per note 16, pg 64
32 — Serjeant, R., *The Spectrum of Pain*, Hart-Davis, 1969, pg 72
33 — Amory, C., as per note 1, pgs 59-60
34 — Montagu, A., *Touching*, Columbia University Press, 1971
35 — Regenstein, Lewis, *The Politics of Extinction*, MacMillan Publishing Co., New York, 1975, pgs 52-59
36 — Ibid, pgs 163-185
37 — Rasmussen, R.K., in Wallace, I., as per note 2, pge 270
38 — Ibid
39 — Ibid
40 — Ibid
41 — Ibid, pg 271
42 — Ibid
43 — Ibid
44 — Fox, M., as per note 1, pgs 10-11
45 — Amory, C., as per note 1, pg 12
46 — Ibid
47 — Burnford, S., *The Incredible Journey*, Little and Brown, New York, 1961
48 — Fox, M., *Understanding Your Cat*, Coward, McCann & Geoghegan, New York, 1974, pg 78
49 — Amory, C., as per note 1, pgs 28-29
50 — Carter, K., quoted in Amory, C., as per note 1, pgs 190-192

Chapter Two—Brave New Chicken

1 — Smith, P., and Daniel, C., *The Chicken Book*, Little, Brown and Co., pgs 51-124
2 — Ibid
3 — Watson, E.L.G., *Animals in Splendour*, Horizon Press, 1967, pg 88
4 — As per note 3, pg 89
5 — Ibid
6 — Juvenal, cited in *The Chicken Book*, as per note 1, pg 160
7 — *Veg Times*, Jan. 1984, pg 64
8 — Singer, P., *Animal Liberation*, Avon Books, 1975, pg 102
9 — *Farmer and Stockbreeder*, Jan. 30, 1962
10 — Mason, J., and Singer, P., *Animal Factories*, Crown Publishers, 1980, pg 5
11 — *Wall Street Journal*, Aug. 9, 1967
12 — Morris, D., *The Clockwork Egg*, dist. by Food Animals Concern Trust (FACT, Inc.), Feb., 1983
13 — Duncan, I., "Can the Psychologist Measure Stress?" *New Scientist*, October 18, 1973
14 — "How Egg Industry Changed During the Last 20 Years," *Poultry Digest*, July, 1978, pg 232

15 — *Farming Express*, Feb. 1, 1962
16 — Singer, P., as per note 8, pg 99
17 — Ibid
18 — Angstrom, C.I., "Mechanical Failures Plague Cage-Layers," *Onondaga County Farm News*, Dec. 1970, pg 13
19 — Singer, P., as per note 8, pg 103
20 — Ibid, pg 97
21 — Reed, H., personal communication to author
22 — Mason, J., and Singer, P., as per note 10, pg 5
23 — Harrison, R., *Animal Machines*, Vincent Stuart Ltd., 1964, pg 147
24 — Singer, P., as per note 8, pg 112
25 — *Poultry Tribune*, March, 1974
26 — Bedicheck, R., *Adventures with a Texas Naturalist*, Univ of Texas Press, 1961
27 — *Upstate*, Aug. 5, 1973
28 — As per note 26
29 — *Poultry Tribune*, Feb., 1974
30 — Singer, P., as per note 8, pg 111
31 — As per note 27
32 — McWhirter, N., *Guiness Book of World Records*, Bantam Books, 1982, pg 377
33 — *National Geographic*, Feb., 1970
34 — North, J., "Catching Up on Smaller Profit Leaks," *Broiler Industry*, June 1976, pg 41
35 — Mason, J., and Singer, P., as per note 10, pg 42
36 — Gowe, R.S., Director of the Animal Research Institute, Agriculture Canada, at conference on "Livestock Intensive Methods of Production," Ottawa, Dec 6-7, 1978
37 — "Naked Chick Gets Serious Attention," *Broiler Industry*, Jan. 1979, pg 98
      ABC News Closeup, "Food: Green Grow the Profits," Dec. 21, 1973
38 — Dendy, M., "Broiler 'Flip-Over' Syndrome Still a Mystery," *Poultry Digest*, Sept. 1976, pg 380
39 — Wilson, W. "Poultry Production," *Scientific American*, July, 1976, pg 58
40 — Reed, H., personal communication to author
41 — Mason, J., and Singer, P., as per note 10, pgs 56-58
42 — Ibid
43 — Wall, R., "Cage Layer Fatigue," *Poultry Digest*, Jan 1976, pg 23
44 — Mason, J., and Singer, P., as per note 10, pg 29
45 — Ibid
46 — Singer, P., as per note 8, pg 110
47 — Shurter, D., and Walter, E., "The Meat You Eat," *The Plain Truth*, Oct-Nov. 1970
48 — *Poultry Tribune*, Jan. 1974
49 — Hightower, J., *Eat Your Heart Out*, Crown Publishers, 1975
50 — Stadelman, W., "Old-Time Flavor: New Injectables Possible," *Broiler Industry*, April 1975, pg 79
51 — Leonardos, G., "Brand Life May Depend on Unique Flavors," *Broiler Industry*, Oct. 1976, pg 33
52 — Babcock, M., "Shrinking Egg Market is Our Own Fault," *Egg Industry*, Jan 1976, pgs 29-30
53 — Mason, J., and Singer, P., as per note 10, pg 8
54 — Battaglia and Mayrose, *Handbook of Livestock Management Techniques*, Burgess Publishers, 1981
55 — Thompson, Bill, "In Search of the Natural Chicken," *East-West*, April 1986, pgs 38-45

Chapter Three—The Most Unjustly Maligned of All Animals

1 — Hudson, W. H., *The Book of a Naturalist*, George Duran Publishers, 1919, pgs 295-302
2 — Watson, E.L.G., *Animals in Splendor*, Horizon Press, 1967, pgs 43-47
3 — Hudson, W. H., as per note 1
4 — *The Animal World of Albert Schweitzer*, ed Joy, C., Beacon Press, 1950, pgs 114-115
5 — Ibid, pgs 116-117
6 — Schell, O., *Modern Meat*, Vintage Books, 1985, pg 59
7 — Ibid, pgs 61-62
8 — Brynes, J., "Raising Pigs by the Calendar at Maplewood Farm," *Hog Farm Management*, Sept. 1976, pg 30
9 — Hall, M., "Heating Systems for Swine Buildings," *Hog Farm Management*, Dec. 1975, pg 16
10 — Black, N. "Let's Give USDA to Do-Gooders, Gardeners," *National Hog Farmer*, Aug. 1976, pg 26
11 — *Farm Journal*, Aug. 1966, and elsewhere
12 — Ibid
13 — Ibid
14 — *Farm Journal*, Nov. 1968
15 — Ibid
16 — Mason, J., and Singer, P., *Animal Factories*, Crown Publishers, 1980, pg 30
17 — Singer, P., *Animal Liberation*, Avon Books, 1975, pg 117
18 — *Farm Journal*, May 1973
19 — *Farmer and Stockbreeder*, July 11, 1961
20 — Messersmith, J., personal communication to author
21 — Taylor, L., *National Hog Farmer*, March 1978, pg 27
22 — *Farm Journal*, April 1970
23 — Singer, P., as per note 17, pg 118
24 — cited in Singer, P., as per note 17, pg 118
25 — Ibid
26 — Mason, J., and Singer, P., as per note 16, pgs 30-31, 42
27 — Mason, J., and Singer, P., as per note 16, pg 42
28 — Ibid, pgs 43-44
29 — Schell, O., as per note 6, pg 186
30 — Ainsworth, E., "Revolution in Livestock Breeding on the Way," *Farm Journal*, Jan. 1976, pg 36
31 — Messersmith, J., personal communication to author
32 — Mason, J., and Singer, P., as per note 16, pg 45
33 — "Scientist Studies 'Test Tube Pig,'" *Hog Farm Management*, April 1975, pg 61
34 — "New Treatment Boosts Pigs Per Litter," *Farm Journal*, March 1976, pg Hog-2
35 — Ibid
36 — Mason, J., and Singer, P., as per note 16, pgs 23-24
37 — "Tail-Biting is Really Anti-Comfort Syndrome," *Hog Farm Management*, March 1976, pg 94
38 — Sterkel, H., "Cut Light and Clamp down on Tail-Biting," Farm Journal, March 1976, pg Hog-6
39 — Singer, P., as per note 17, pg 114
40 — Butler, F., personal communication to author

41 — Mason, J., and Singer, P., as per note 16, pg 45
42 — Byrnes, J., "Stacking 3 Decks of Pigs," *Hog Farm Management*, Jan. 1978, pg 16
43 — *An Enquiry into the Effects of Modern Livestock Production on the Total Environment*, The Farm and Food Society, London, 1972, pg 12
44 — Koltveit, A., *Confinement*, Nov-Dec 1976, pg 3
45 — Schell, O., as per note 6, pg 95
46 — Mason, J., and Singer, P., as per note 16, pg 63
47 — Ibid, pg 49
48 — Ibid
49 — "Pig Health Losses Total $187 Million," *Farm Journal*, Sept 1978, pg Hog-2
50 — "Pseudorabies Eradication Plan Drafted," *National Hog Farmer*, March 1977, pg 136
51 — Byrnes, J., "Demand Grows for PRV Vaccine," *Hog Farm Management*, May 1977, pgs 18-20
52 — "Area Depopulation Plan Suggested for Dominican," *National Hog Farmer*, Dec. 1978, pg 34
53 — Rhodes, R., "Watching the Animals," *Harper's*, March 1970

Chapter Four—Holy Cow

1 — Story adapted from Grant, J., *Lord of the Horizon*, Avon Books, 1969, pgs 73-75
2 — Ibid, pg 79
3 — Story adapted from Grant, J., *Winged Pharoah*, Ariel Press, 1985, pg 78
4 — Hudson, W.H., *Afoot in England*, cited in *The Extended Circle*, ed. Wynne-Tyson, J., Centaur Press, 1985, pg 130
5 — Ovid, *Metamorphoses*, cited in Wynne-Tyson ed., as per note 4, pg 232
6 — "Livestock Auction—An Arena of Animal Abuse," *Mainstream*, Spring 1985, pg 16
7 — Singer, P., *Animal Liberation*, Avon Books, 1975, pg 148
8 — *Official Proceedings*, 58th Annual Meeting Livestock Conservation, Inc., Omaha, Nebraska, May 1974, pgs 44, 93
9 — Ibid
10 — Wallace, I., et al, *The Book of Lists #2*, Bantam Books, 1979, pg 240
11 — "Chloramphenicol Use by Cattlemen Said to be Dangerous," *Veg Times*, pg 6
12 — Singer, P., as per note 7, pg 150
13 — Battaglia and Mayrose, *Handbook of Livestock Management Techniques*, Burgess Publishers, 1981
14 — *Pig Farming*, September 1973
15 — Battaglia and Mayrose, as per note 13
16 — Ibid
17 — Smith, R., quoted in *Farm Journal*, Dec. 1973
18 — Schell, O., *Modern Meat*, Vintage Books, 1985
19 — Singer, P., as per note 7, pg 129
20 — Giehl, D., *Vegetarianism*, Harper and Row, 1979, pgs 119-120
　　Hightower, J., *Eat Your Heart Out*, Crown Publishers, 1975, pg 99
　　Hunter, B., *Consumer Beware*, Simon and Schuster, 1971, pgs 113-114
　　Lappe, F.M., *Diet for a Small Planet*, Ballantine, 1982, pgs 67-68
　　Schell, O., as per note 18, pgs 125-6, 137, 143, 148-9, 167, 179-80
　　Singer, P., as per note 7, pg 129
　　Mason, J., and Singer, P., *Animal Factories*, Crown Publishers, 1980, pgs 29-30, 48-9, 72
　　Sussman, V., *The Vegetarian Alternative*, Rodale Press, 1978, pgs 173-4

21 — "What Tells Cattle to Stop Eating?" *Beef*, Nov. 1976, pg 33
22 — *Farm Journal*, Dec 1971
23 — Beard, J., *American Cookery*, Little, Brown and Co., 1972, pgs 331-2
24 — quoted in Singer, P., as per note 7, pg 126
25 — Food Animals Concern Trust (FACT, Inc.) Newsletter
26 — "Sentenced for Life to a Factory Farm," Food Animals Concern Trust newsletter
27 — Food Animals Concern Trust, FACT sheet no. 55, June 1984
28 — Ibid
29 — Ibid
30 — Food Animals Concern Trust, FACT sheet no. 23, August 15, 1982

Chapter Five—Any Way You Slice It, It's Still Balogna

1 — Kupfer, E., *Animals My Brethren*, quoted in Braunstein, M., *Radical Vegetarianism*, Panjandrum Books, 1981, pgs 133-135
2 — Braunstein, M., as per note 1, pg 113
3 — *Meat Board Report 1974-1975*, National Livestock and Meat Board, 1975, pg 23
4 — Salt, H., *Seventy Years Among Savages*, George Allen and Unwin, 1921, pg 9
5 — Singer, I.B., "The Slaughterer," from *The Seance*, Avon Books, 1969, pg 24
6 — Gullo, K., "An Inside Look at the American Meat-Packing Industry," *Veg Times*, Sept 1983, pgs 46-47, adapted from a 5-part series by Ackland, L., *Chicago Tribune*, June 5-9, 1983
7 — Ibid
8 — Schell, O., *Modern Meat*, Vintage Books, 1985, pgs 308-309
9 — Gullo, K., as per note 6
10 — *Official Proceedings*, 58th Annual Meeting, Livestock Conservation Inc., Omaha, Nebraska, May 1974, pgs 49-50
11 — *Poultry World*, June 14, 1962
12 — Singer, P., *Animal Liberation*, Avon Books, 1975, pg 153
13 — Ibid, pg 155
14 — Ibid
15 — Ibid, pg 156
16 — Braunstein, M., as per note 1, pg 92
17 — Rhodes, R., "Watching the Animals," *Harper's*, March 1970, pg 91

Chapter Six—Different Strokes for Different Folks

1 — Williams, Roger J., *You Are Extraordinary*, Pyramid Books, New York, 1967
2 — Anson, Barry Joseph, *Atlas of Human Anatomy*, Saunders College Publishing, Philadelphia, 1963, pg 376
3 — As per note 1, page 25
4 — Ibid
5 — Ibid
6 — Ibid
7 — As per note 1, page 40
8 — Ibid
9 — Kapleau, Philip, *To Cherish All Life*, Harper and Row, San Francisco, 1981, page 59
10 — McDougall, John, *The McDougall Plan*, New Century Publishers, 1983, page 7
11 — Williams, Roger J., *Nutrition Against Disease*, Bantam Books, 1973, page 12

12 — Ibid, page 189

13 — For one example among many, see *Journal of the American Medical Association*, June 29, 1979, page 2833

14 — Personal communication with author

15 — Hindhede, M., "The Effect of Food Restrictions During War on Mortality in Copenhagen," *Journal of the American Medical Association*, 74 (6):381, 1920

16 — Ibid

17 — Strom, A., and Jensen, R. A., "Mortality From Circulatory Diseases in Norway, 1940-1945", *Lancet*, 260:126-129, 1951

18 — Sussman, Vic, *The Vegetarian Alternative*, Rodale Press, Emmaus, Pa., 1978, page 55

19 — As per note 9, page 67

20 — Ibid

21 — Hur, Robin, *Food Reform: Our Desperate Need*, Heidelberg Publishers, 1975, page 95

22 — Ibid, page 2, 95-6

23 — Leaf, A. *National Geographic*, 143:93, 1973

24 — As per note 21, page 95

25 — Fisher, Irving, "The Influence of Flesh Eating on Endurance," *Yale Medical Journal*, 13(5):205-221, 1907

26 — Ibid

27 — Ibid

28 — Ioteyko, J., et al, *Enquete scientifique sur les vegetariens de Bruxelles*, Henri Lamertin, Brussels, pg 50

29 — Astrand, Per-Olaf, *Nutrition Today* 3:no.2,9-11, 1968

30 — Schouteden, A., *Ann de Soc. Des Sciences Med. et Nat. de Bruxelles* (Belgium) I

31 — Dallman, P., *American Journal of Clinical Nutrition* 33:86, 1980
Murray, M., *American Journal of Clinical Nutrition* 33:697, 1980
Abdulla, M., *American Journal of Clinical Nutrition* 34:2464, 1981

32 — Narins, D., in Bezkorovainy, A., *Biochemistry of Nonheme Iron*, New York, Plenum, 1980, pages 47-126

33 — Weil, A., *Health and Healing*, Houghton Mifflin Co., Boston, 1983, pages 87-88

34 — Diamond, E. G., et al, "Comparison of Internal Mammary Artery Ligation and Sham Operation for Angina Pectoris," *American Journal of Cardiology* 5 (1960), 483

35 — Ibid

Chapter Seven—The Rise and Fall of the Protein Empire

1 — Hausman, Patricia, *Jack Sprat's Legacy*, Richard Marek Publishers, 1981, pgs 16-17, 25-39

2 — Scrimshaw, N., "An Analysis of Past and Present Recommended Dietary Allowances for Protein in Health and Disease," *New England Journal of Medicine*, Jan. 22, 1976, pg 200
Irwin, M., "A Conspectus of Research on Protein Requirements of Man," *Journal of Nutrition*, 101 (1975):385

3 — Hegsted, D., "Minimum Protein Requirements of Adults," *American Journal of Clinical Nutrition*, 21 (1968):3520
Rose, W., "The Amino Acid Requirements of Adult Man, XVI . . . "Jour Biol Chem 217 (1955):997

4 — Stare, F., "Nutrition," *Ann Rev Biochem* 14 (1945):431

5 — "Protein Requirements," Food and Agricultural Organization, World Health Organization Expert Group, United Nations Conference, Rome, 1965

6 — Pfeiffer, C., *Mental and Elemental Nutrients*, New Canaan: Keats, 1975

7 — Food and Nutrition Board, *Recommended Daily Allowances*, Washington, D.D., National Academy of Sciences

8 — National Research Council, *Recommended Dietary Allowances*, 9th ed., Washington, D.C., National Academy of Sciences, 1980, pg 46

9 — Reuben, D., *Everything You Always Wanted to Know About Nutrition*, Avon Books, 1978, page 154-5

10 — Williams, R.J., "We Abnormal Normals," *Nutrition Today*, 1967, 2:19-28

11 — Data from: *Nutritive Value of American Foods in Common Units*, Agriculture Handbook No. 456

See also: Ford Heritage, *Composition and Facts about Foods*, Mokelumne Hill, Cal.: Health Heritage, 1971

12 — Markakis, P., "The Nutritive Quality of Potato Protein," in *Protein Nutritional Quality of Foods and Feeds*, pt. 2, ed. M. Friedman, New York: M. Dekker, 1975

Kofranyi, E., et al, "The Minimum Protein Requirement of Humans . . ." cited in Akers, K., *A Vegetarian Sourcebook*, G.P. Putnam's Sons, New York, 1983, page 205

Kon, S. "The Value of Potatoes in Human Nutrition," *Journal of Biological Chemistry* 22:258, 1928

13 — Osborn, T., "Amino Acids in Nutrition and Growth," *Journal of Biological Chemistry* 17:325, 1914

14 — Rose, W., "Comparative Growth of Diets . . ." *Journal of Biological Chemistry* 176:753, 1948

15 — Sanchez, A., et al, "Nutritive Value of Selected Proteins and Protein Combinations," *American Journal of Clinical Nutrition*, vol. 13, no. 4, Oct. 1963, page 247

McDougall, J., *The McDougall Plan*, New Century Publishers, 1983, pg 96

16 — Vaghefi, S.B., et al, "Lysine Supplementation of Wheat Proteins," *American Journal of Clinical Nutrition*, 27:1231, 1974

17 — Lappe, F.M., *Diet For A Small Planet*, Ballantine Books, 1971

18 — Kofrany, E. "The Minimum Protein Requirements of Humans . . . ", *Journal of Physiological Chemistry*, 351:1485, 1970

19 — Pritikin, Nathan, quoted in *Vegetarian Times*, issue 43, pg 22

20 — Lappe, F.M., *Diet For A Small Planet*, Ballantine Books, 1982

21 — Ibid, page 162, 172

22 — Ibid, page 162

23 — Ibid

24 — Editorial, *The Lancet*, London, 2:956, 1959

25 — Hardinge, M., et al, "Nutritional Studies of Vegetarians: Part V, Proteins . . . ", *Journal of the American Dietic Association*, Vol. 48, no. 1, Jan 1966, pg 27

Hardinge, M., et al, "Nutritional Studies of Vegetarians: Part I, . . ." *Journal of Clinical Nutrition*, Vol. 2, no. 2, March-April, 1984, pg 81

Hausman, P., "Protein: Enough is Enough," *Nutrition Action*, Oct. 1977, pg 4

26 — Food and Nutrition Board, "Vegetarian Diets," Washington, D.C.: National Academy of Sciences, 1974, pg 2

27 — Hegsted, D., cited in Register, U.D., et al, "The Vegetarian Diet," *Journal of the American Dietetic Association*, 62(3):255, 1973

28 — Hardings, M., et al, op cit note 25

29 — Ibid

30 — Scharffenberg, J., *Problems With Meat*, Woodbridge Press, 1982, pg 90

31 — Pritikin, N., quoted in *Vegetarian Times*, issue 43, pg 21

32 — Hardinge, M. op cit note 25
McLaren, D., "The Great Protein Fiasco," *Lancet* 2:93, 1974

33 — Nicol, B., et al, "The Utilization of Proteins and Amino Acids in Diets Based on Cassava
. . . "*British Journal of Nutrition* 39(2):271, 1978

34 — Gopalan, C., "Effect of Calorie Supplementation on Growth of Undernourished Children," *American Journal of Clinical Nutrition*, 26:563, 1973
Golden, M., "Protein Deficiency, Energy Deficiency, and the Oedema of Malnutrition," *Lancet*, 2:93, 1974
Lopez de Romana, G., "Prolonged Consumption of Potato-Based Diets by Infants and Small Children," *Journal of Nutrition* 111:1430, 1981
Lopez de Romana, G., "Utilization of the Protein and Energy of the White Potato by Human Infants," *Journal of Nutrition* 110:1849, 1980

35 — McLaren, D., op cit note 32, page 95
Gopalan, C., op cit note 36
Holt, E., *Protein and Amino Acid Requirements in Early Life*, University Press, N.Y., 1960, pg 12
McLaren, D., "A Fresh Look at Protein-Calorie Malnutrition," *Lancet* 2:485, 1966

36 — Schwarzenegger, A., *Arnold's Body-Building For Men*, Simon and Schuster, 1981

37 — National Academy of Sciences, *Recommended Dietary Allowances*, 8th ed. Washington, D.C. 1974, pg 43

38 — Bodansky, O., *Biochemistry of Disease*, McMillan, 2nd ed. 1952, pg 784

39 — Barzel, V., *Osteoporosis*, Grune and Stratton, New York, 1970

40 — Ibid

41 — Heaney, R., "Calcium Nutrition and Bone Health in the Elderly," *American Journal of Clinical Nutrition*, 36:986, 1982
Paterson, C. "Calcium Requirements in Man: A Critical Review," *Postgrad Medical Journal* 54:244, 1978
Walker, A., "The Human Requirement of Calcium: Should Low Intakes Be Supplemented?", *American Journal of Clinical Nutrition*, 25:518, 1972
Symposium on Human Calcium Requirements: Council on Foods and Nutrition, *Journal of the American Medical Association*, 185:588, 1963

42 — Johnson, N., et al, "Effect of Level of Protein Intake on Urinary and Fecal Calcium and Calcium Retention . . ." *Journal of Nutrition*, 100:1425, 1970
Allen, L., et al, "Protein-Induced Hypercalcuria: A Longer-Term Study," *American Journal of Clinical Nutrition*, 32:741, 1979

43 — Solomon, L., "Osteoporosis and Fracture of the Femoral Neck in the South African Bantu," *Journal of Bone and Joint Surgery* 50B:2, 1968
McDougall, J., *McDougall's Medicine*, New Century Publishing 1985, pgs 61-96

44 — Allen, L., et al, op cit note 42
Altchuler, S., "Dietary Protein and Calcium Loss: A Review," *Nutritional Research* 2:193, 1982
McDougall, J., op cit note 15, pg 101

45 — Solomon, L., op cit note 43
Hegsted, M., "Urinary Calcium and Calcium Balance in Young Men as Affected by Level of Protein and Phosphorus Intake," *Journal of Nutrition*, 111:553, 1981
Anand, C., "Effect of Protein Intake on Calcium Balance in Young Men Given 500 Mg Calcium Daily," *Journal of Nutrition*, 104:695, 1974

Walker, R., "Calcium Retention in the Adult human Male as Affected by Protein Intake," *Journal of Nutrition*, 102:1297, 1972

Johnson, N., "Effect of Level of Protein Intake on Urinary and Fecal Calcium and Calcium Retention . . ." *Journal of Nutrition*, 100:1425, 1970

Linkswiler, H. "Calcium Retention of Young Adult Males As Affected by Level of Protein and Calcium Intake," *Transcripts of New York Academy of Science*, 36:333, 1974

Altchuler, S., op cit note 44

46 — McDougall, J., op cit note 43, pg 75

47 — Chalmers, J., "Geographic Variations of Senile Osteoporosis," *Journal of Bone and Joint Surgery*, 52B:667, 1970

48 — Walker, A., op cit note 41

McDougall, J., op cit note 43, pg 67

49 — Pritikin, N., quoted in *Vegetarian Times*, Issue 43, pg 22

50 — Walker, A., "Osteoporosis and Calcium Deficiency," *American Journal of Clinical Nutrition*, 16:327, 1965

51 — Smith, R., "Epidemiologic Studies of Osteoporsis in Women of Puerto Rico and Southeaster Michigan . . ." *Clin Ortho* 45:32, 1966

52 — Solomon, L., op cit note 43

Walker, A., op cit note 41

Walker, A., "The Influence of Numerous Pregnancies and Lactations on Bone Dimensions in South African Bantu and Caucasian Mothers," *Clinical Science*, 42:189, 1972

Walker, A., op cit note 50

53 — Mazess, R., "Bone Mineral Content of North Alaskan Eskimos, *Journal of Clinical Nutrition*, 27:916, 1974

54 — Ibid

55 — Ibid

56 — Ellis, F., et al, "Incidence of Osteoporosis in Vegetarians and Omnivores," *American Journal of Clinical Nutrition*, 25:555, 1972

57 — *American Journal of Clinical Nutrition*, March 1983

58 — Ellis, F., et al, op cit note 56

Wachman, Amnon, et al, "Diet and Osteoporosis," *Lancet*, May 4, 1968, pg 958

59 — Anon., *Vegetarian Times*, April 1984, pg 32

60 — McCance, R. and Widdowson, E., *The Composition of Foods*, Her Majesty's Stationary Office, 1960

61 — Hur, R., *Food Reform: Our Urgent Need*, Heidelberg Press, 1975, pgs 98-107

Shah, B.G., et al, *Journal of Nutrition*, 92(1):30, 1967

62 — Hur, op cit note 61, pg 102

63 — Ibid, pg 103; from USDA Handbook No. 8, 1963

64 — Recker, R., "The Effect of Milk Supplements on Calcium Metabolism, Bone Metabolism and Calcium Balance," *American Journal of Clinical Nutrition*, 41:254, 1985

65 — Nilas, L. "Calcium Supplementation and Postmenopausal Bone Loss," *British Medical Journal*, 289:1103, 1984

66 — Wachman, A., et al, op cit note 58

67 — Robertson, W., "Should Recurrent Calcium Oxalate Stone Formers Become Vegetarians?" *British Journal of Urology*, 51:427, 1979

Coe, F., "Eating Too Much Meat Called Major Cause of Renal Stones," *Internal Medicine News*, 12:1, 1979

Anon., "Urinary Calcium and Dietary Protein," *Nutritional Review*, 38:9, 1980

Anon., "Diet and Urinary Calculi," *Nutr Rev*, 38:74, 1980

Shah, P., "Dietary Calcium and Idiopathic Hypercalcuria," *Lancet*, 1:786, 1981

68 --- Brenner, B., "Dietary Protein Intake and the Progressive Nature of Kidney Disease . . .", *New England Journal of Medicine*, 307:652, 1982

Walser, M., "Nutritional Support in Renal Failure: Future Directions," *Lancet*, 1:340, 1983

69 --- Shilling, E., *Nutr Abstr and Rev* 33:114, 1963

70 --- Brenner, B., op cit note 68

Walser, M., op cit note 68

Walser, M., "Does Dietary Therapy Have a Role in the Predialysis Patient?" *American Journal of Clinical Nutrition*, 33:1629, 1980

71 --- McDougall, J., op cit note 15, pg 103-104

72 --- Ross, M.H., "Protein, Calories and Life Expectancy," *Fed Proc.*, 18:1190-1207, 1959

Exton-Smith, A., "Physiological Aspects of Aging: Relationship to Nutrition," *American Journal of Clinical Nutrition*, 25:853-59, 1972 Krohn, P., "Rapid Growth, Short Life," *Journal of the American Medical Association*, 171:461, 1959

Sherman, H., *Chemistry of Food and Nutrition*, MacMillan Co., N.Y., 1952, pg 208

Sherman, H., *The Science of Nutrition*, Columbia Univ. Press, N.Y., 1943, pgs 177-98

73 --- Krohn, P., op cit note 72

74 --- Campbell, T.C., quoted in Lang, S., "Diet and Disease," *Food Monitor*, May/June 1983, pg 24

75 --- Winick, M., quoted in Goodman, D., "Breaking the Protein Myth," *Whole Life Times*, July/Aug. 1984, pg 26

Chapter Eight—Food for the Caring Heart

1 --- Gordon, T., "Premature Mortality from Coronary Heart Disease: The Framingham Study," *Journal of the American Medical Association*, 215:1617, 1971

Bainton, C., "Deaths From Coronary Heart Disease . . ." *New England Journal of Medicine*, 268:569, 1963

Kannel, W., "Incidence and Prognosis of Unrecognized Myocardial Infarction—An Update on the Framingham Study," *New England Journal of Medicine*, 311:1144, 1984

Ornish, D., "Effects of Stress Management Training and Dietary Changes in Treating Isochemic Heart Disease," *Journal of the American Medical Association*, 249:54, 1983

Thuesen, L., "Beneficial Effect of a Lowfat Low-Calorie Diet on . . . Angina Pectoris," *Lancet*, 2:59, 1984

Ellis, F., "Angina and Vegan Diet," *American Heart Journal*, 93:803, 1977

Pritikin, N., "Diet and Exercise as a Total Therapeutic Regimen for . . . Severe Peripherial Vascular Disease," 52nd Annual Session of the American Congress of Rehabilitation Medicine, Atlanta, 1975

Ribeiro, J., "The Effectiveness of a Low Lipid Diet . . . Coronary Artery Disease," *American Heart Journal*, 108:1183, 1984

Goldman, L., "The Decline in Ischemic Heart Disease Mortality Rates . . ." *Annals of Internal Medicine*, 101:825, 1984

Editorial: "Trials of Coronary Heart Disease Prevention," *Lancet*, 2:803, 1982

Gordon, T., "Diet and its Relation to Coronary Heart Disease . . ." *Circulation*, 63:500, 1981

Kallio, V., "Reduction in Sudden Deaths . . . After Acute Myocardial Infarction," *Lancet*, 2:1091, 1979

Lipid Research Clinics Program. The Lipid Research Clinics Coronary Primary Prevention Trial Results, I. Reduction in Incidence of Coronary Heart Disease, *Journal of the American Medical Association*, 251:351, 1984

Lipid Research Clinics Program. The Lipid Research Clinics Coronary Primary Prevention Trial Results, II. The Relationship of Reduction in Incidence of Coronary Heart Disease to Cholesterol Lowering, *Journal of the American Medical Association*, 251:365, 1984 Connor, W., "The Key Role of Nutritional Factors in the Prevention of Coronary Heart Disease," *Preventive Medicine*, 1:49, 1972

Taylor, C., "Spontaneously Occurring . . . of Cholesterol," *American Journal of Clinical Nutrition*, 32:40, 1979

Welch, C., "Cinecoronary Arteriography . . . , "*Circulation*, 42:647, 1970

Page, I., "Prediction of Coronary Heart Disease . . . ," *Circulation*, 42:625, 1970

Zampogna, A., "Relationship Between Lipids and Occlusive Coronary Artery Disease," *Archives of Internal Medicine*, 140:1067, 1980

Cohn, P., "Serum Lipid Levels . . . Coronary Artery Disease," *Annals of Internal Medicine*, 84:241, 1976

Jenkins, P., "Severity of Coronary Artherosclerosis . . . ," *British Medical Journal*, 2:388, 1978

Kannel, W., "Cholesterol in the Prediction of Atherosclerotic Disease: New Perspectives Based on the Framingham Study," *Annals of Internal Medicine*, 90:85, 1979

Anderson, J., "The Dependence of the Effects of Cholesterol . . . ," *American Journal of Clinical Nutrition*, 29:1784, 1976

Jackson, R., "Influence of Polyunsaturated and Saturated Fats . . . ", *American Journal of Clinical Nutrition*, 39:589, 1984

Flynn, M., "Serum Lipids in Humans Fed Diets Containing Beef or Fish and Poultry," *American Journal of Clinical Nutrition*, 34:2734, 1981

Flynn, M., "Dietary 'Meats' and Serum Lipids," *American Journal of Clinical Nutrition*, 35:935, 1982

O'Brien, B., "Human Plasma Lipid Responses to Red Meat, Poultry, Fish and Eggs," *American Journal of Clinical Nutrition*, 33:2573, 1980

Acheson, R., "Does Consumption of Fruit and Vegetables Protect Against Stroke?" *Lancet*, 1:1191, 1983

Shekelle, R., "Diet, Serum Cholesterol and Death From Coronary Heart Disease," *New England Journal of Medicine*, 304:65, 1981

Burkitt, D., "Some Diseases Characteristic of Modern Western Civilization," *British Medical Journal*, 1:274, 1973

Mattson, F., "Effect of Dietary Cholesterol on Serum Cholesterol in Man," *American Journal of Clinical Nutrition*, 25:589, 1972

Keys, A., "Serum Cholesterol Response to Changes in Dietary Lipids," *American Journal of Clinical Nutrition*, 19:175, 1966

Carroll, K., "Hypocholesterolemic Effect of . . . ," *American Journal of Clinical Nutrition*, 31:1312, 1978

Kritchevsky, D., "Dietary Fiber and Other Dietary Factors in Hypercholesterema," *American Journal of Clinical Nutrition*, 30:979, 1977

Taik Lee, Kyu, "Geographic Studies of Atherosclerosis: The Effect of a Strict Vegetarian Diet . . ." *Archives of Environmental Health*, 4:14, 1962

Walden, R., "Effect of . . . Among Seventh Day Adventists," *American Journal of Medicine*, 36:271, 1964

Hardinge, M., "Nutritional Studies of Vegetarians: IV. Dietary Fatty Acids and Serum Cholesterol Levels," *American Journal of Clinical Nutrition*, 10:522, 1962

Barrow, J., "Studies in Atherosclerosis . . . ," *Annals of Internal Medicine*, 52:372, 1960

Keys, A., "Serum Cholesterol . . . The Effect of Cholesterol in the Diet," *Metabolism*, 14:759, 1965

Keys, A., "Serum Cholesterol . . . Particular Saturated Fatty Acids," *Metabolism*, 14:776, 1965

Hegsted, D., "Quantitative Effects of Dietary Fat on Serum Cholesterol in Man," *American Journal of Clinical Nutrition*, 17:281, 1965

Mahley, R., "Alterations in . . . Plasma Cholesterol, Induced by Diets High in Cholesterol," *Lancet*, 2:807, 1978

Kannel, W., "Serum Cholesterol, Lipoproteins, and the Risk of Coronary Heart Disease," *Annals of Internal Medicine*, 74:1, 1971

Castelli, W., "HDL-Cholesterol . . . in Coronary Heart Disease," *Circulation*, 55:767, 1977

Robertson, T., "Epidemiologic Studies of Coronary Heart Disease and Stroke . . . ," *American Journal of Cardiology*, 39:244, 1977

Miettinen, M., "Effect of Cholesterol-Lowering Diet on Mortality from Coronary Heart Disease . . . ," *Lancet*, 2:835, 1972

2 — Enos, W., "Pathogenesis of Coronary Disease in American Soldiers Killed in Korea," *Journal of the American Medical Association*, 158:912, 1955

Collens, W., "Atherosclerotic Disease: An Anthropologic Theory," *Medical Counterpoint*, pg 54, Dec 1969

3 — Taik Lee, Kyu, "Chemicopathologic Studies . . . ," *Archives of Internal Medicine*, 109:426, 1962

Hausman, P., *Jack Sprat's Legacy - The Science and Politics of Fat and Cholesterol*, Richard Mauk Publishers, NY, 1981, pgs 28, 196

4 — Hausman, P., as per note 3, pg 53

5 — Ibid, pgs 53-61, 68, 85-86

6 — Marmot, M., "Epidemiologic Studies of Coronary Heart Disease and Stroke in Japanese Men . . . ," *American Journal of Epidemiology*, 102:511, 1975

7 — Keys, A. (ed) "Coronary Heart Disease in Seven Countries," *American Heart Association* Monograph No. 29, *Circulation*, 41, Supplement 1, pg 211, 1970

Keys, A. (ed) *Seven Countries—A Multivariate Analysis of Death and Coronary Heart Disease in Ten Years*, Harvard University Press, Cambridge, 1980

8 — As per note 7

9 — Wissler, R., "Studies of Regression of Advanced Atherosclerosis in Experimental Animals and Man," *Annals of the New York Academy of Science*, 275:363, 1976

10 — Armstrong, M., "Regression of Coronary Atheromatosis in Rhesus Monkeys," *Circ Res* 27:59, 1970

11 — Collens, W., as per note 2

12 — Phillips, R., "Coronary Heart Disease Mortality Among Seventh Day Adventists with Differing Dietary Habits," Abstract American Public Health Association Meeting, Chicago, Nov 16-20, 1975

13 — Ruys, J., "Serum Cholesterol . . . in Australian Adolescent Vegetarians," *British Medical Journal*, 6027:87, 1976

Sacks, F., "Plasma Lipids and Lipoproteins in Vegetarians and Controls," *New England Journal of Medicine*, 292:1148, 1975

Sacks, F., "Blood . . . in Vegetarians," *American Journal of Epidemiology*, 100:390, 1974

Armstrong, B., "Blood . . . ," *American Journal of Epidemiology*, 105:444, 1977

Sirtori, C., "Soybean Protein Diet . . . ," *Lancet*, 8006:275, 1977

Barrow, J., as per note 1

Phillips, R., as per note 12

Phillips, R., "Coronary Heart Disease . . . Differing Dietary Habits: A Preliminary Report," *American Journal of Clinical Nutrition*, 31:181, 1978

14 — Walles, C., "Hold the Eggs and Butter: Cholesterol is Proved Deadly and Our Diet May Never Be the Same," *Time*, March 26, 1984, pg 62

15 — Norum, K., "What is the Expert's Opinion on Diet and Coronary Heart Diseases? "*Journal of the Norwegian Medical Association*, Feb 12, 1977; Cited by Sen. Edward Kennedy in testimony to Senate Select Committee on Nutrition and Human Needs, March 24, 1977

16 — Imperato, P., and Mitchell, G., *Acceptable Risks*, Viking, New York, 1985, pgs 9-24

Coleman, M., "The Research Smokescreen: Moving from Academic Debate to Action on Smoking," *New York State Journal of Medicine*, 13:1280, 1983

Cummins, K., "The Cigarette Makers: How They Get Away with Murder, with the Press as an Accessory," *Washington Monthly*, 3:14, 1984

Blum, A., (ed) "The Cigarette Pandemic," *New York State Journal of Medicine*, 83:13, 1983

Hartz, A., "Smoking, Coronary Artery Occlusion . . ." *Journal of the American Medical Association*, 246:851, 1981

Kannel, W., "Cigarettes, Coronary Occlusions and Myocardial Infarction," (editorial), *Journal of the American Medical Association*, 246:871, 1981

17 — Koch, T., "The Mad Nasty Book," *Mad*, Super-Special Winter 1985, pg 56

18 — Jacobson, M., preface to Hausman, P., as per note 3, pg 13-19

19 — Imperato, P., as per note 16, pg 69

20 — "Hubbards Awarded for Worst Ads of the Year," Associated Press, Washington, *Santa Cruz Sentinel*, June 14, 1985, pg. A-6

21 — Liebman, B., The Center for Science in the Public Interest, in *Nutrition Action*, cited in Vegetarian Times, July, 1985

22 — Oski, F., *Don't Drink Your Milk*, Wyden Books, 1977, pg 6

23 — cited in Giehl, D., *Vegetarianism*, Harper and Row, New York, 1977, pg 3

24 — Mayer, J., "Egg vs. Cholesterol Battle," *New York Daily News*, Oct 9, 1974, pg 48

25 — Hausman, P., as per note 3, pg 218

26 — Ibid

27 — Ibid, pg 219

28 — "Orders a Stop on Egg Claims," *New York Daily News*, Dec 12, 1975, pg 62

29 — Ibid

30 — cited in Hausman, P. as per note 3, pg 219

31 — Flynn, M., "Effect of Dietary Egg on Human Serum Cholesterol and Tryglycerides," *American Journal of Clinical Nutrition*, 32:1051, 1979

Slater, G., "Plasma Cholesterol and Triglycerides in Men with Added Eggs in the Diet," *Nutrition Rep Int*, 14:249, 1976

Dawber, T., "Eggs, Serum Cholesterol and Coronary Heart Disease," *American Journal of Clinical Nutrition*, 36:617, 1982

Porter, M., "Effect of Dietary Egg on Serum Cholesterol and Triglyceride of Human Males," *American Journal of Clinical Nutrition*, 30:490, 1977

Flaim, E., "Plasma Lipid . . ." *American Journal of Clinical Nutrition*, 34:1103, 1981

32 --- McDougall, J., *The McDougall Plan*, New Century Publishers, 1983, pg 56

33 --- O'Brien, B., as per note 1

Roberts, S., "Does Egg Feeding (i.e. Dietary Cholesterol) Affect Plasma Cholesterol Levels in Humans? The Results of A Double Blind Study," *American Journal of Clinical Nutrition*, 34:2092, 1981

McMurry, M., "Dietary Cholesterol and the Plasma Lipids . . ." *American Journal of Clinical Nutrition*, 37:741, 1982

Mattson, F., as per note 1

34 --- Hausman, P., as per note 3, pg 214

35 --- Ibid

36 --- Sacks, F., "Ingestion of Egg Raises Plasma Low Density Lipoproteins in Free-Living Subjects," *Lancet*, 1:647, 1984

37 --- U.S. Senate Select Committee on Nutrition and Human Needs, Hearing: "Diet Related to Killer Diseases, Volume 6, Response Regarding Eggs," July 26, 1977

38 --- Hausman, P., as per note 3, pg 221

39 --- Levy, R., quoted in Hausman, P., as per note 3, pg 215

40 --- Task Force to the American Society of Clinical Nutrition, quoted in Hausman, P., as per note 3, pg 93-4

41 --- Hausman, P., as per note 3, pg 216

42 --- Ibid, pg 214-16

43 --- Roberts, S., as per note 33

O'Brien, B., as per note 1

Mattson, F., as per note 1

Connor, W., "The Interrelated Effects of Dietary Cholesterol and Fat Upon Human Serum Lipid Levels," *Journal Clin Invest* 43:1691, 1964

44 --- Mattson, F., as per note 1

45 --- Imperato, P., as per note 16, pg 65-66

46 --- quoted in Hausman, P., as per note 3, pg 205

47 --- "Milk Still Makes a Difference," National Dairy Council, quoted in Hausman, P., as per note 3, pg 206

48 --- Jacobson, M., as per note 18, pg 17

49 --- Harty, S., *Hucksters in the Classroom*, Center for Study of Responsive Law, 1979, pg 23

50 --- National Dairy Council, Nutrition Education Materials, 1985-1986 (Catalog), pg 16-22

51 --- Ibid, pg 16, reference no. 0920N

52 --- Ibid, pg 17, reference no. 0921N

53 --- quoted in Hausman, P., as per note 3, pg 207

54 --- Harty, S., as per note 49, pg 24

55 --- quoted in Hausman, P., as per note 3, pg 207

56 --- cited in Hausman, P., as per note 3, pg 207

57 --- Ibid

58 --- Ibid

59 --- Harty, S., as per note 49, pg 24

60 --- Ibid

61 --- Hausman, P., as per note 3, pg 40-49

62 --- Ibid, pg 44-45

63 — "Myths and Facts About Meat Products," Oscar Mayer, Inc.
64 — "Dietary Fitness—A Meat Lover's Guide," Oscar Mayer Inc.
65 — Ibid
66 — Ibid
67 — Imperato, P., as per note 16, pg 75
68 — Hausman, P., as per note 3, pg 194
69 — Hausman, P., as per note 3, pg 82
70 — McDougall, J., as per note 32, pg 65
71 — Connor, W., as per note 1
     Kannel, W., as per note 1
72 — Ibid
73 — McDougall, J., as per note 32, pg 117
74 — Pritikin, N., quoted in *Vegetarian Times*, Issue 43
75 — Elliot, J., "An 'Ideal' Serum Cholesterol Level?" *Journal of the American Medical Association*, 241:1979, 1979
76 — quoted in Hausman, P., as per note 3, pg 180
77 — Ibid, pg 180-181
78 — Tall, A., "Current Concepts; Plasma High-Density Lipoproteins," *New England Journal of Medicine*, 299:1232, 1978
     Flanagan, M., "The Effects of Diet on High Density Lipoprotein Cholesterol," *Journal of Human Nutrition*, 34:43, 1980
     Bradby, G., "Serum High-Density Lipoproteins in Peripheral Vascular Disease," *Lancet*, 2:1271, 1978
79 — Barndt, R., "Regression and Progression . . ." *Annals of Internal Medicine*, 86:139, 1977
     Basta, L., "Regression of Atherosclerotic . . ." *American Journal of Medicine*, 61:420, 1976
     Hubbard, J., "Nathan Pritikin's Heart," *New England Journal of Medicine*, 313:52, 1985
     Ornish, D., as per note 1
80 — Barndt, R., as per note 79
81 — Blakesless, A., and Stamler, J., *Your Heart Has Nine Lives*, Prentice-Hall, New York, pg 67-69
82 — Hausman, P., as per note 3, pg 90
83 — Ellis, F. and Sanders, T., "Angina and Vegetarian Diet," letter to the editor, *Lancet*, May 29, 1976
     Ellis, F. and Sanders, T., "Angina and Vegan Diet," *American Heart Journal*, June, 1977, 93:803
84 — quoted in Imperato, P., as per note 16, pg 78
85 — "Eating the Moderate Fat and Cholesterol Way," (Deleted Chapter), *Food 2*, Washington, D.C., U.S.D.A., 1982
86 — Hausman, P., as per note 3, pg 151
87 — Imperato, P., as per note 16, pg 70-71
     Hausman, P., as per note 3, pgs 202-204
88 — As per note 87
89 — quoted in Hausman, P., as per note 3, pg 203
90 — As per note 87
91 — quoted in Hausman, P., as per note 3, pg 204
92 — Lipid Research Clinics Program. The Lipid Research Clinics Coronary Primary Prevention Trial Results, I. Reduction in Incidence of Coronary Heart Disease, *Journal of the American Medical Association*, 251:351, 1984

Lipid Research Clinics Program. The Lipid Research Clinics Coronary Primary Prevention Trial Results, II. The Relationship of Reduction in Incidence of Coronary Heart Disease to Cholesterol Lowering, *Journal of the American Medical Association*, 251:365, 1984

93 — Walles, C., as per note 14, pg 56

94 — As per note 92

95 — Ibid

96 — Walles, C., as per note 14, pg 58

97 — Ibid

98 — Hausman, P., as per note 3, pg 90-91

99 — quoted in Imperato, P., as per note 16, pg 79

100 — Gordon, T., "Diabetes, Blood Lipids and the Role of Obesity in Coronary Heart Disease Risk . . . ," *Annals of Internal Medicine*, 87:393, 1977

Wood, P., "Plasma Lipoprotein Distributions in Male and Female Runners," *Annals of New York Academy of Science*, 301:748, 1977

Price, J., *Coronaries, Cholesterol and Chlorine*, Jove Publishers, New York, 1981

Forde, O., "The Tromso Heart Study: Coffee Consumption and . . . ," *British Medical Journal*, 290:893, 1985

Little, J., "Coffee and Serum-Lipids in Coronary Heart Disease," *Lancet*, 1:732, 1966

Hartz, A., as per note 16

Kannel, W., as per note 16

101 — "Diet and Stress in Vascular Disease," *Journal of the American Medical Association*, Vol. 176, No. 9, June 3, 1961, pg 806

Chapter Nine—Losing a War We Could Prevent

1 — "85 Million for Research on Cancer," *San Francisco Chronicle*, March 26, 1986

2 — Pauling, L., quoted in Chowka, P., "Cancer Research —The $20 Billion Failure," *Vetegarian Times*, Dec 1981, pg 32

3 — Henderson, I., "Cancer of the Breast—The Past Decade," Parts 1 & 2, *New England Journal of Medicine*, 302:17-78, 1980

Baum, M., "The Curability of Breast Cancer," *British Medical Journal*, 1:439, 1976

Costanza, M., "Adjuvant Chemotherapy: Eight Years Later," *Journal of the American Medical Association*, 252:2611, 1984

Kerbel, R., "Facilitation of Tumour Progression by Cancer Therapy," *Lancet*, 2:977, 1982

Greenberg, D., "'Progress' In Cancer Research—Don't Say it Isn't So." *New England Journal of Medicine*, 292:707, 1975

Mueller, C., "Bilateral Carcinoma of the Breast—Frequency and Mortality," *Journal of Surgery*, 21:459, 1978

Stehlin, J., "Treatment of Carcinoma of the Breast," *Surg Gynecol Obstet*, 149:911, 1979

Langlands, A., "Long Term Survival of Patients with Breast Cancer: A Study of the Curability of the Disease," *British Medical Journal*, 2:1247, 1979

McDougall, J., *McDougall's Medicine*, New Century Press, 1985, pg 6

Vorherr, H., "Adjuvant Chemotherapy of Breast Cancer: Reality, Hope, Hazard?" *Lancet*, 2:1413, 1981

Cancer Surveillance, Epidemiology and End Results (SEER) Program, *Cancer Patient Survival*—Report No. 5, Dept. of Health, Education and Welfare publication no. (NIH) 77-992, 1976

Vorherr, H., "Adjuvant Chemotherapy of Breast Cancer: Tumour Kinetics and Survival," *Lancet*, 2:690, 1981

4 — U.S. "War on Cancer a Failure, Says Former Scientist," *Animals' Agenda*, Sept 1985, pg 14

5 — Ibid

Skrabanek, P., "False Premises and False Promises of Breast Cancer Screening," *Lancet*, 2:316, 1985

Mueller, C., "Breast Cancer in 3,558 Women . . ." *Surgery*, 83:123, 1978

6 — McDougall, J., as per note 3, pg 7

7 — Chowka, P., as per note 2

8 — Statement by Arthur Upton, Director—National Cancer Institute: Status of the Diet, Nutrition and Cancer Program before the Subcommittee on Nutrition, Oct. 2, 1972

9 — Committee on Diet, Nutrition and Cancer: Assembly of Life Sciences, *National Research Council*, "Diet, Nutrition and Cancer," National Academy Press, Washington, D.C., 1982

"Nutrition and Cancer: Cause and Prevention," *An American Cancer Society Special Report*, CA 34:121, 1984

U.S. Senate Report: *Dietary Goals for the United States*, Govt Printing Office, Washington, 1977

Reddy, B., "Nutrition and Its Relationship to Cancer," *Advances in Cancer Research* 32:237, 1980

Tannenbaum, A., "The Genesis and Growth of Tumours, III: Effects of a High-Fat Diet," *Cancer Research*, 2:468, 1942

"Nutrition in the Causation of Cancer," *Cancer Research*, 35:3231, 1975

Carroll, K., "Dietary Fat in Relation to Tumour Genesis," *Progress in Biochemical Pharmacology*, 10:308, 1975

Armstrong, B., and Doll, R., "Environmental Factors and Cancer Incidence and Mortality in Different Countries," *International Journal of Cancer*, 15:617, 1975

10 — Reddy, B., as per note 9

11 — Gori, G., quoted in Chowka, P., as per note 2, pg 34

12 — Gori, G., quoted in Sussman, F., *The Vegetarian Alternative*, Rondale Press, 1978

13 — Hausman, P., *Jack Sprat's Legacy—The Science and Politics of Fat and Cholesterol*, Richard Marek Publishers, New York, 1981, pgs 103-119

14 — Ibid, pg 116

15 — Hirayama, T., "Epidemiology of Breast Cancer with Special Reference to the Role of Diet," *Prev Med*, 7:173, 1978

Wynder, E., "Dietary Fat and Colon Cancer," *Journal of the National Cancer Institute*, 54:7, 1975

Berg, J., "Can Nutrition Explain the Pattern of International . . . Cancers?" *Cancer Research*, 35:3345, 1975

Wynder, E., "The Dietary Environment and Cancer," *Journal of the American Dieticians Association*, 71:385, 1977

Weisburger, J., "Nutrition and Cancer—On the Mechanisms Bearing on Causes of Cancer of the Colon, Breast, Prostate, and Stomach," *Bulletin of the New York Academy of Medicine*, 56:673, 1980

Mann, G., "Food Intake and Resistance to Disease," *Lancet*, 1:1238, 1980

Committee on Diet, Nutrition and Cancer, Assembly of Life Sciences, as per note 24

American Cancer Society Special Report, as per note 9

U.S. Senate Report, as per note 9

Reddy, B., and Wynder, E., "Large Bowel Carcinogenisis: Fecal Constituents of Populations with Diverse Incidence of Colon Cancer," *Journal of the National Cancer Institute*, 50:1437, 1973

Hill, M., "Bacteria and the Aetiology of Cancer of the Large Bowel," *Lancet*, 1:95, 1971

Reddy, B., as per note 9

Reddy, B., "Metabolic Epidemiology of Large Bowel Cancer," *Cancer*, 42:2832, 1978

Hill, M., "Colon Cancer: A Disease of Fiber Depletion or of Dietary Excess," *Digestion*, 11:289, 1974

Walker, A., "Colon Cancer and Diet with Special References to Intakes of Fat and Fiber," *American Journal of Clinical Nutrition*, 34:2054, 1981

Cummings, J., "Progress Report: Dietary Fiber," *Gut*, 14:69, 1983

Phillips, R., "Role of Lifestyle and Dietary Habits in Risk of Cancer . . ." *Cancer Research*, 35:3513, 1975

Hardinge, M., "Nutritional Studies of Vegetarians: III. Dietary Levels of Fiber," *American Journal of Clinical Nutrition*, 6:523, 1958

Weisburger, J., "Colon Cancer—Its Epidemiology . . . ," *Cancer*, 40:2414, 1977

16 — *Science*, Feb 1974, pg 416

17 — Reddy, B., as per note 9

New York Times, Sept 29, 1972, pgs 24

Haenszel, W., "Studies of Japanese Migrants, I. Mortality from Cancer . . ." *Journal of the National Cancer Institute*, 40:43, 1968

18 — *Journal of the National Cancer Institute*, Dec 1973, pg 1771

19 — Reddy, B., "Metabolic Epidemiology of Large Bowel Cancer," *Cancer*, 42:2832, 1978

Walker, A., as per note 15

Wynder, E., as per note 15

Berg, J., as per note 15

Weisburger, J., as per note 15

20 — Berg, J., as per note 15

Wynder, E., as per note 15

Weisburger, J., as per note 15

Hill, M., as per note 15

Walker, A., as per note 15

Cummings, J., as per note 15

Phillips, R., as per note 15

Hardinge, M., as per note 15

Liu, K., "Dietary Cholesterol, Fat, and Fiber and Colon-Cancer Mortality," *Lancet*, 2:782, 1979

Cruse, J., "Dietary Fiber . . . and Experimental Colon Cancer," *Gut*, 19:A983, 1978

Burkitt, D., "Epidemiology of Cancer of the Colon and Rectum," *Cancer*, 28:3-13, July 1971

Burkitt, D., "Some Diseases Characteristic of Modern Western Civilization," *British Medical Journal*, 1:274, 1973

Trowell, H., "Ischemic Heart Disease and Dietary Fiber," *American Journal of Clinical Nutrition*, 25:926, 1972

21 — McDougall, J., *The McDougall Plan*, New Century Publishers, 1983, pg 120

22 — Hepner, G., "Altered Bile Acid Metabolism in Vegetarians," *American Journal of Digestive Diseases*, 20:935, 1975

Hill, M., "The Effect of Some Factors on the Fecal Concentration of . . . ," *Journal of Pathology*, 104:239, 1971

Reddy, B., and Wynder, E., as per note 15

Reddy, B., as per note 15

Wynder, E., as per note 15

23 --- Hoye, Dr. Martin, personal communication with author

24 --- As per note 15

25 --- Pearce, M., "Incidence of Cancer in Men on a Diet High in Polyunsaturated Fat," cited in Hausman, P. as per note 13, pg 173

26 --- Bennion, "Risk Factors for the Development of Cholethiasis in Man," *New England Journal of Medicine*, 299:1221, 1978

Broitman, S., "Polyunsaturated Fats, Cholesterol and Large Bowel Tumorigenesis," *Cancer*, 40:2455, 1977

Carroll, K., "Dietary Polyunsaturated Fat Versus Saturated Fat in Relation to Mammary Carcinogenisis," *Lipids*, 14:155, 1979

27 --- Nestel, P., "Lowering of Plasma Cholesterol . . . with Consumption of Polyunsaturated Ruminant Fats," *New England Journal of Medicine*, 288:379, 1973

28 --- "Meat-Packer Defends Beef," *Riverside Herald*, Pg A-1, May 8, 1976

29 --- Obituary Column, pg C-11, *Riverside Herald*, March 14, 1982

30 --- Lea, A., "Dietary Factors Associated with . . . ," *Lancet*, 2:332, 1966

Hirayama, T., as per note 15

McDougall, J., as per note 3, pgs 18-50

Morrison, A., "Some International Differences in Treatment and Survival in Breast Cancer," *International Journal of Cancer*, 18:269, 1976

Nemoto, T., "Differences in Breast Cancer Between Japan and the United States," *Journal of the National Cancer Institute*, 58:193, 1977

Armstrong, B., "Environmental Factors and Cancer Incidence and Mortality . . . ," *International Journal of Cancer*, 15:617, 1975

31 --- Hirayama, T., Paper presented at Conference on Breast Cancer and Diet, U.S.-Japan Cooperative Cancer Research Program, Fred Hutchinson Cancer Center, Seattle, WA, March 14-15, 1977

32 --- Ibid

33 --- Kagawa, Y., "Impact of Westernization on the Nutrition of Japanese: Changes in Physique, Cancer . . . ," *Prev Med*, 7:205, 1978

Hill, P., "Diet, Life-Style, and Menstrual Activity," *American Journal of Clinical Nutrition*, 33:1192, 1980 Staszewski, J., "Age at Menarche and Breast Cancer," *Journal of the National Cancer Institute*, 47:935, 1971

34 --- Frommer, D., "Changing Age of the Menopause," *British Medical Journal*, 2:349, 1964

Armstrong, B., "Diet and Reproductive Hormones, A Study of Vegetarian and Non-Vegetarian Postmenopausal Women," *Journal of the National Cancer Institute*, 67:761, 1981

Hill, P., "Environmental Factors of Breast and Prostatic Cancer," *Cancer Research*, 41:3817, 1981

Trichopoulos, D., "Menopause and Breast Cancer Risk," *Journal of the National Cancer Institute*, 48:605, 1972

35 --- As per note 34

36 --- As per note 9

37 --- Hur, R., *Food Reform, Our Desperate Need*, Heidelberg Publishers, Austin, TX, 1975, pg 24

38 --- McDougall, J., as per note 3, pgs 60-89

39 — Zeil, H., "Increased Risk of Endometrial Carcinoma . . . "New England Journal of Medicine, 293:1167, 1975

    Smith, D., "Association of Exogenous Estrogen and Endometrial Carcinoma," *New England Journal of Medicine*, 294:1262, 1976

    Mack, T., "Estrogens and Endometrial Cancer . . ." *New England Journal of Medicine*, 294:1262, 1976

40 — Berg, J., as per note 15

    Wynder, E., "The Dietary Environment and Cancer," as per note 15

41 — Phillips, R., as per note 15

    Hardinge, M., as per note 15

    Malhotra, S., "A Comparison of . . . Diet in the Management of Duodenal Ulcer," *Postgrad Medical Journal*, 54:6, 1978

    MacDonald, W., "Histological Effect . . ." *Canadian Medical Association Journal*, 96:1521, 1967

    Wynder, E., "Epidemiology of Adenocarcinoma of the Kidney," *Journal of the National Cancer Institute*, 53:1619, 1974

    "Nutrition in the Causation of Cancer," as per note 9

    Bennion, L., as per note 26

    Stuverdant, R., "Increased Prevalence of Cholethiasis in Men Ingesting a Serum Cholesterol Lowering Diet," *New England Journal of Medicine*, 288:24, 1973

    "Nutrition in the Causation of Cancer," as per note 9

42 — Hill, P., as per note 34

43 — Breslow, N., "Latent Carcinoma of Prostate at Autopsy in Seven Areas," *International Journal of Cancer*, 20:680, 1977

44 — Virag, R., "Is Impotence an Arterial Disorder?" *Lancet*, 1:181, 1985

45 — McDougall, J., as per note 3, pgs 96-126

46 — Lemon, F., "Death from Respiratory Disease," *Journal of the American Medical Association*, 198:117, 1966

47 — Stamler, J., "Elevated Cholesterol May Increase Lung Cancer Risk in Smokers," *Heart Research Letter*, 14:2, 1969

48 — Lemon, F., as per note 46

Chapter Ten—An Ounce of Prevention

1 — Walford, R., *Maximum Life Span*, Norton and Co., 1983, pg 11.

    Tokuhata, G., "Diabetes Mellitus: An Underestimated Public Health Problem," *Journal of Chronic Diseases*, 28:23, 1975

    Kaplan, S., "Diabetes Mellitus," *Annals of Internal Medicine*, 96:635, 1982

    Kannel, W., "Diabetes and Cardiovascular Risk Factors: The Framingham Study," *Circulation*, 59:8, 1975

2 — Ibid

    Cohen, A., "Myocardial Infarction and Carbohydrate Metabolism," *Geriatrics*, 23:158, 1968

    Editorial, "The Complications of Diabetes Mellitus," *New England Journal of Medicine*, 298:1250, 1978

3 — Hur, R. *Food Reform: Our Desperate Need*, Neidelberg Publishers, 1975, pgs 67-73

    McDougall, J., *McDougall's Medicine*, New Century Publishers, 1985, pgs 203-230

4 — Report of the National Commission on Diabetes to Congress. Vol III, pt 2; Dept. of Health, Education and Welfare Publication no. (NIH) 76-1022, 1975

5 — Singh, I., "Low-Fat Diet and Therapeutic Doses of Insulin in Diabetes Mellitus," *Lancet*, 263:422, 1955

6 — Kipnis, D., "Insulin Secretion in Normal and Diabetic Individuals," *Advances in Internal Medicine*, 16:103, 1970

7 — Himsworth, H., "The Physiological Activation of Insulin," *Clinical Science*, 1:1, 1933
  Sweeney, J., "Dietary Factors that Influence the Dextrose Tolerance Test . . ." *Archives of Internal Medicine*, 40:818, 1927 Olefsky, J., "Reappraisal of the Role of Insulin in Hypertriglyceridemia," *American Journal of Medicine*, 57:551, 1974
  Davidson, P., "Insulin Resistance in Hyperglyceridemia," *Metabolism*, 14:1059, 1965

8 — Anderson, J., "High Carbohydrate, High-Fiber Diets for Insulin Treated Men With Diabetes Mellitus," *American Journal of Clinical Nutrition*, 32:2312, 1979

9 — Asmal, A., "Oral Hypoglycaemic Agents . . . ," *Drugs*, 28:62, 1984
  Kiehm, T., "Beneficial Effects of a High Carbohydrate, High Fiber Diet on Hyperglycemic Diabetic Men," *American Journal of Clinical Nutrition*, 29:895, 1976
  Simpson, H., "A High Carbohydrate Leguminous Fiber Diet Improves All Aspects of Diabetes Control," *Lancet*, 1:1, 1981
  Anderson, J., as per note 8
  Simpson, R., "Improved Glucose Control in Maturity-Onset Diabetes Treated with High-Carbohydrate Modified-Fat Diet," *British Medical Journal*, 1:1753, 1979
  Singh, I., as per note 5
  Brunzell, J., "Improved Glucose Tolerance with High Carbohydrate Feeding in Mild Diabetes," *New England Journal of Medicine*, 284(10):521, 1971

10 — McDougall, J., as per note 3, pg 210

11 — Editorial, "Acute Mishaps During Insulin Pump Treatment," *Lancet*, 1:911, 1985
  Rosenstock, J., "Insulin Pump Therapy: A Realistic Appraisal," *Clinical Diabetes*, 3:25, 1985
  Dahl-Jorgensen, K., "Rapid Tightening of Blood Glucose Control Leads to Transient Deterioration of Retinopathy in Insulin Dependent Diabetes Mellitus," *British Medical Journal*, 290:811, 1985

12 — Anderson, J., "Hypolipidemic Effects of High-Carbohydrate, High-Fiber Diets," *Metabolism*, 29:551, 1980
  Blanc, M., "Improvement of Lipid Status in Diabetic Boys . . ." *Diabetes Care*, 6:64, 1983
  Van Eck, W., "The Effect of a Lowfat Diet on the Serum Lipids in Diabetes," *American Journal of Medicine*, 27:196, 1959

13 — McDougall, J., as per note 3

14 — Kawate, R., "Diabetes Mellitus and Its Vascular Complications in Japanese Migrants on the Island of Hawaii," *Diabetes Care*, 2:161, 1979
  Trowell, H., "Dietary Fiber Hypothesis of the Etiology of Diabetes Mellitus," *Diabetes*, 24:762, 1975
  Ringrose, H., "Nutrient Intakes in an Urbanized Micronesian Population with a High Diabetes Prevalence," *American Journal of Clinical Nutrition*, 32:1334, 1979

15 — As per note 14

16 — Statement by Snowden, D., quoted in *Vegetarian Times*, Aug 1985

17 — Ibid

18 — McDougall, J., "Healthy By Choice," *Vegetarian Times*, Dec 1985

19 — Sweeney, J., as per note 7

20 — Hollenbeck, C., "The Effects of Variations . . ." *Diabetes*, 34:151, 1985
  Olefsky, J., as per note 7

Haber, G., "Depletion and Disruption of Dietary Fiber, Effects on Satiety, Plasma-Glucose and Serum-Insulin," *Lancet*, 2:679, 1977

Anderson, J., as per note 8

Miranda, P., "High-Fiber Diets in the Treatment of Diabetes Mellitus," *Annals of Internal Medicine*, 88:482, 1978

21 --- Baker, R., *Lancet*, 1:26, 1963

22 --- Agranoff, B. "Diet and the Geographical Distribution of Multiple Sclerosis," *Lancet*, 2:1061, 1974

Alter, M., "Multiple Sclerosis and Nutrition," *Archives of Neurology*, 23:460, 1970

23 --- Dept of Health and Social Security, "Present-Day Infant Feeding Practice Report," No. 9, 1974

Crawford, M. "Essential Fatty Acids Requirements in Infancy," *American Journal of Clinical Nutrition*, 31:2181, 1978

Agranoff, B., as per note 22

USDA Home Economics Report No 7, "Fatty Acids in Food Fats" 24 --- Swank, R., and Grimsgaard, A., *Low-Fat Diet: Reasons, Rules and Recipes*, Univ.of Oregon, 1959

24 --- Swank, R., "Multiple Sclerosis: Twenty Years on a Low-Fat Diet," *Archives of Neurology*, 23:460, 1970

Swank, R., *A Biochemical Basis of Multiple Sclerosis*, Thomas, 1961, pgs 3, 44-45

25 --- Cheraskin, E., *New Hope for Incurable Diseases*, Arco, 1971, pg 32

26 --- As per notes 22, 23, 24, 25

27 --- Ibid

28 --- McDougall, J., "Healthy by Choice," *Vegetarian Times*

29 --- Malhotra, A., "A Comparison of Unrefined Wheat and Rice Diet in the Management of Duodenal Ulcer," *Postgraduate Medical Journal*, 54:6, 1978

Rydning, A., "Prophylactic Effect of Dietary Fiber in Duodenal Ulcer Disease," *Lancet*, 2:736, 1982

Childs, P., "Peptic Ulcer, Pylorplasty and Dietary Fat . . . ," *Annals of the Royal College of Surgeons*, 59:143, 1977

Trowell, H., "Definition of Dietary Fiber," *American Journal of Clinical Nutrition*, 29:417, 1976

Burkitt, D., "Dietary Fiber and Disease," *Journal of the American Medical Association*, 229:1068, 1974

30 --- Ippoliti, A., "The Effect of Various Forms of Milk on Gastric-Acid Secretions, Studies in Patients with Duodenal Ulcers . . . ," *Annals of Internal Medicine*, 84:286, 1976

Hur, R., as per note 3, pg 118

31 --- Hartroft, W., "The Incidence of Coronary Heart Disease in Patients Treated with the Sippy Diet," *American Journal of Clinical Nutrition*, 15:205, 1964

Briggs, R., "Myocardial Infarction in Patients Treated with Sippy and Other High Milk Diets," *Circulation*, 21:538, 1960

32 --- Hur, R., as per note 3, pg 118

33 --- Gray, R., *The Colon Health Handbook*, Rockridge Publishing Co.

34 --- Burkitt, D., *Lancet* 2:1408, 1972

35 --- Burkitt, D., "Varicose Veins, Deep Vein Thrombosis and Haemorrhoids: Epidemiology and Suggested Aetiology," *British Medical Journal*, 2:556, 1972

36 --- Holt, R. *Hemorrhoids*, California Health Publications, 1980

Thompson, W., "The Nature of Hemorrhoids," *British Journal of Surgery*, 62:542, 1975

37 — Burkitt, D., "Dietary Fiber and Disease," *Journal of the American Medical Association,* 229:1068, 1974

Prasad, G., "Studies on Etipathogenesis of Hemorrhoids," *American Journal of Proctology,* June 1976

Burkitt, D., as per note 35

McDougall, J., *The McDougall Plan,* New Century Publishers, 1984, pg 117

38 — Burkitt, D., "Hiatus Hernia: Is it Preventable?" *American Journal of Clinical Nutrition,* 34:428, 1981

39 — Burkitt, D., "Some Diseases Characteristic of Modern Western Civilization," *British Medical Journal,* 1:274, 1973

40 — Editorial, "Keep Taking Your Bran," *Lancet,* 1:1175, 1979

Robinson, C., *Normal and Therapeutic Nutrition,* MacMillan, 13th ed., 1967, pg 386

Painter, N., "The High Fiber Diet in the Treatment of Diverticular Disease of the Colon," *Postgraduate Medical Journal,* 50:629, 1974

McDougall, J., as per note 37, pgs 117-119

41 — Berman, P., *American Journal of Digestive Disorders,* 17:741, 1972

42 — Painter, N., "Fiber Deficiency and Diverticular Disease of the Colon," in *Fiber Deficiency and Colonic Disorders,* Reilly, R. & Kirsner, J. (ed.) Plenum Books, 1975

43 — Piepmeyer, J., "Use of Unprocessed Bran in Treatment of Irritable Bowel Syndrome," *American Journal of Clinical Nutrition,* 27:106, 1974

Manning, A., "Wheat Fiber and Irritable Bowel Syndrome," *Lancet,* 2:417, 1977

Editorial, "Management of the Irritable Bowel," *Lancet,* 2:557, 1978

McDougall, J., as per note 37, pg 119

44 — Burkitt, D., "Appendicitis," in Burkitt, D. and Trowell, H. (ed.) *Refined Carbohydrate Foods and Disease,* Academic Press, N.Y. 1978

Westlake, C. "Appendectomy and Dietary Fiber," *Journal of Human Nutrition,* 34:267, 1980

Walker, A., "Appendicitis, Fiber Intake and Bowel Behavior in Ethnic Groups in South Africa," *Postgraduate Medical Journal,* 49:243, 1973

45 — Friday, S., *The Food Sleuth Handbook,* Athenum Publishers, 1982

46 — Mayer, J. and Goldberg, J., "Nutrition," (a syndicated column), *Washington Post,* July 26, 1981

47 — Tartter, P., "Cholesterol and Obesity as Prognostic Factors. . . ." *Cancer,* 47:2222, 1981

Donegan, W., "The Association of Body Weight with Recurrent Cancer . . . ," *Cancer,* 41:1590, 1978 Editorial, "Obesity—The Cancer Connection," *Lancet,* 1:1223, 1982

48 — Hur, R., as per note 3, pg 74

49 — Ellis, F., "Veganism, Clinical Findings and Investigations," *American Journal of Clinical Nutrition,* 23(3):249, 1970

Sacks, F., "Plasma Lipids and Lipoproteins in Vegetarians and Controls," *New England Journal of Medicine,* 292(22):1148, May 1975

Ellis, F., "Angina and Vegan Diet," *American Heart Journal,* 93(6):803, June 1977

Hardinge, M., "Nutritional Studies of Vegetarians . . . ," *American Journal of Clinical Nutrition,* 2:73, 1974

50 — Hur, R., as per note 3, pg 76-77

51 — Blaw, S., and Schultz, D., *Arthritis,* Doubleday, 1974

Kellgren, J., "Osteo-arthrosis . . ." *Annals of Rheumatic Disease,* 17:388, 1958

McDougall, J., as per note 3, pg 237

52 — McDougall, J., as per note 3, pgs 231-250

53 — Lucas, P., "Dietary Fat Aggravates Active Rheumatoid Arthritis," *Clinical Research*, 29:754A, 1981

54 — Parke, A., "Rheumatoid Arthritis and Food . . ." *British Medical Journal*, 282:2027, 1981

55 — Valkenburg, H., "Osteoarthritis in Some Developing Countries," *Journal of Rheumatology*, 10:20, 1983

Solomon, L., "Rheumatic Disorders in the South African Negro," Pt. I, *South African Medical Journal*, 49:1292, 1975

Solomon, L., "Rheumatic Disorders in the South African Negro," Pt. II, *South African Medical Journal*, 49:1737, 1975

Beasley, R., "Low Prevalence of Rheumatoid Arthritis in Chinese . . . ," *Journal of Rheumatology*, 10:11, 1983

56 — Beighton, "Rheumatoid Arthritis in a Rural South African Negro Population," *Annals of Rheumatic Diseases*, 34:136, 1975

57 — Solomon, L., as per note 55

58 — Williams, R., *Nutrition Against Disease*, Bantam Books, 10th ed, 1981, pg 134

59 — Zollner, N., "Diet and Gout," Proceedings of the Ninth International Congress on Nutrition, 1:267, 1975

60 — Hall, A., "Epidemiology of Gout and Hyperuricemia," *American Journal of Medicine*, 42:27, 1967

Berkowitz, D., "Blood Lipid and Uric Acid . . ." *Journal of the American Medical Association*, 190:856, 1964

61 — Healey, L., "Hyperuricemia in Filipinos . . ." *American Journal of Human Genetics*, 19:81, 1967

62 — Derrick, F., "Kidney Stone Disease: Evaluation and Medical Management," *Postgraduate Medical Journal*, 66:115, 1979

63 — Robertson, W., "Dietary Changes and the Incidence of Irinary Calculi . . ." *Journal of Chronic Diseases*, 32:469, 1979

64 — Heaton, K., "Gallstones and Cholecystitis," in *Refined Carbohydrate Foods and Diseases*, as per note 44

Sarles, H., "Diet and Cholesterol Gallstones," *Digestion*, 17:121, 1978

65 — Hill, M., "Colon Cancer and Diet with Special Reference to Intakes of Fat and Fiber," *American Journal of Clinical Nutrition*, 29:1417, 1976

Walker, A., "Colon Cancer and Diet with Special Reference to Intakes of Fat and Fiber," *American Journal of Clinical Nutrition*, 29:1417, 1976

66 — Boston Collaborative Drug Surveillance Program, "Surgically Confirmed Gallbladder Disease . . . ," *New England Journal of Medicine*, 290:15, 1974

Grache, W., "The Natural History of Silent Gallstones," *New England Journal of Medicine*, 307:798, 1982

67 — Baum, C., "Drug Use in the United States In 1981," *Journal of the American Medical Association*, 251:1293, 1984

68 — Kannel, W., "Should All Mild Hypertension Be Treated? Yes," in *Controversies in Therapeutics*, Lasagna, L. (ed), W. B. Saunders Co., 1980, pg 299

McDougall, J., as per note 3

Evans, P., "Relation of Longstanding Blood Pressure Levels to Atherosclerosis," *Lancet*, 1:516, 1965

69 --- Freis, E., "Salt, Volume and the Prevention of Hypertension," *Circulation*, 53:589,1976
    Editorial, "Why Does Blood Pressure Rise with Age?" *Lancet*, 2:289, 1981
    Kuller, L., "An Explanation for Variations in Distribution of Stroke and Arteriosclerotic
        Heart Disease Among Populations and Racial Groups," *American Journal of Epide-
        miology*, 93:1, 1971

70 --- Freis, E., as per note 69

71 --- Freis, E., "Hemodynamics of Hypertension," *Physiol Review*, 40:27, 1960
    Parfrey, P., "Relation Between Arterial Pressure, Dietary Sodium Intake . . ." *British
        Medical Journal*, 283:94, 1981

72 --- Kaplan, N., "Mild Hypertension: When and How to Treat," *Archives of Internal Medi-
        cine*, 143:255, 1985
    McAlister, N., "Should We Treat 'Mild' Hypertension?" *Journal of the American Medi-
        cal Association*, 249:379, 1983
    Boyd, G., "The Pressure to Treat," *Lancet*, 2:1134, 1980
    Kaplan, N., "Therapy for Mild Hypertension—Toward a More Balanced View," *Jour-
        nal of the American Medical Association*, 249:365, 1983

73 --- Editorial, "Fatigue as an Unwanted Effect of Drugs," *Lancet*, 1:123, 1985
    Stone, R., "Proximal Myopathy During Beta-Blockade," *British Medical Journal*,
        2:1583, 1979

74 --- Holme, I., "Treatment of Mild Hypertension with Diuretics . . ." *Journal of the Ameri-
        can Medical Association*, 25:1298, 1984

75 --- Curb, J., "Long-Term Surveillance for Adverse Effects of Antihypertensive Drugs,"
        Journal of the American Medical Association, 253:3263, 1985

76 --- Stamler, J., "Hypertension Screening . . . ," *Journal of the American Medical Association*,
        235:2299, 1976
    McGill, H., "Persistent Problems in the Pathogenesis of Atherosclerosis," *Atherosclero-
        sis*, 4:443, 1984

77 --- Hartoft, W., "The Incidence of Coronary Heart Disease in Patients Treated with the
        Sippy Diet," *American Journal of Clinical Nutrition*, 15:205, 1964
    Oski, F. "Is Bovine Milk a Health Hazard?" *Pediatrics* 75 (suppl.)182, 1985
    Belizan, J., "Reduction of Blood Pressure with Calcium Supplementation in Young
        Adults," *Journal of the American Medical Association*, 249:1161, 1983
    Johnson, N., "Effects on Blood Pressure of Calcium Supplementation of Women,"
        American Journal of Clinical Nutrition, 42:12, 1985
    Sowers, M., "The Association of . . . Calcium with Blood Pressures Among Women,"
        American Journal of Clinical Nutrition, 42:135, 1985

78 --- Friedman, M., "Serum Lipids and Conjunctival Circulation After Fat Ingestion . . . ,"
        Circulation, 29:874, 1984
    Friedman, M., "Effect of Unsaturated Fats upon Lipemia and Conjunctival Circula-
        tion," *Journal of the American Medical Association*, 198:882, 1976
    O'Brien, J., "Acute Platelet Changes After Large Meals of Saturated and Unsaturated
        Fats," *Lancet*, 1:878, 1976

79 --- Burr, M., "Plasma Cholesterol and Blood Pressure in Vegetarians," *Journal of Human
        Nutrition*, 35:437, 1981
    Sacks, F., "Blood Pressure in Vegetarians," *American Journal of Epidemiology*, 100:390,
        1974
    Armstrong, B., ". . . Blood Pressure in Vegetarians," *American Journal of Clinical Nutri-
        tion*, 32:2472, 1979

Ophir, O., "Low Blood Pressure in Vegetarians," *American Journal of Clinical Nutrition*, 37:755, 1983

Kaplan, N., "Non-Drug Treatment of Hypertension," *Annals of Internal Medicine*, 102:359, 1985

Editorial, "Lowering Blood Pressure Without Drugs," *Lancet*, 2:459, 1980

Rouse, I., "Blood Pressure Lowering Effect of a Vegetarian Diet . . . ," *Lancet*, 1:5, 1983

80 --- Armstrong, B., "Blood Pressure in Seventh Day Adventists," *American Journal of Epidemiology*, 105:444, 1977

81 --- Dallman, P., *American Journal of Clinical Nutrition*, 33:86, 1980

Murray, M., *American Journal of Clinical Nutrition*, 33:697, 1980

Abdulla, M., *American Journal of Clinical Nutrition*, 34:2464, 1981

82 --- Wilson, J., *Journal of Pediatrics*, 84:335, 1974

83 --- Lindahl, O., "Vegan Regimen with Reduced Medication in the Treatment of Bronchial Asthma," *Journal of Asthma*, 22:44, 1985

84 --- National Academy of Sciences, "An Evaluation of the Salmonella Problem," a report to the United States Department of Agriculture and Federal Drug Administration, prepared by the Committee on Salmonella, National Research Council, 1969

85 --- Giehl, D., *Vegetarianism*, Harper and Row, 1979

86 --- as per note 84, pg 125

87 --- Statement by Richard Novick, Hearings before the Subcommittee on Agricultural Research and General Legislation of the Committee on Agriculture, Nutrition and Forestry, Sept 21, 1977

88 --- "Salmonellae in Slaughter Cattle," *Journal of the American Veterinary Medical Association*, 160(6):884, 1972

89 --- "Salmonella Contamination in a Commercial Poultry Processing Operation," *Poultry Science*, 53:814-21, 1974

90 --- Wellford, H., *Sowing the Wind*, Bantam Books, 1973, pgs 133-134

91 --- Molotsky, Irvin, "Antibiotics in Animal Feed Linked to Human Ills," *New York Times*, Feb 22, 1987

92 --- New Jersey State Health Department, Division of Environmental Health, cited in Scharffenberg, J., *Problems with Meat*, Woodbridge Press, 1982, pg 60

Stoller, K., "Feeding an Epidemic," *Animals' Agenda*, May 1987, pg 32-33

Chapter Eleven—America the Poisoned

1 --- Williams, R., "The Trophic Value of Foods," Proceedings of the National Academy of Science, 70:3, March, 1973, pgs 710-713

Tolan, A., "The Chemical Composition of Eggs Produced under Battery, Deep Litter and Free Range Conditions," *British Journal of Nutrition*, 30:181, pgs 185

2 --- Crawford, M. A., "A Re-evaluation of the Nutrient Role of Animal Products," Proceedings of the Third World Conference on Animal Production, ed. Reid, R. L., Sydney University Press, 1975, pg 24

3 --- Schell, O., *Modern Meat*, Vintage Books, Random House, 1985, pg 283-284

4 --- Saenz de Rodriguez, Dr. C.A., *Journal of the Puerto Rican Medical Association*, Feb 1982, cited in Schell, O., as per note 3, pgs 286-287

5 --- Schell, O., as per note 3, pg 287

6 --- Quoted in "Drugs in Animals Affect Human Growth," *Health Bulletin*, Nov 6, 1965, pg 6

Cited in Hunter, B., *Consumer Beware*, Simon and Schuster, New York, 1971, pg 116

7 — Schell, O., as per note 3, pg 197

8 — Ibid, pg 198

9 — Hadlow, W., "Stilbestrol-Contaminated Feed and Reproductive Disturbances in Mice," *Science*, 122:3171, 1955, pgs 643-644

10 — Verrett, J., and Carper, J., *Eating May Be Hazardous to Your Health*, Simon and Schuster, 1974, pg 170

11 — Schell, O., as per note 3, pgs 254

12 — Ibid, pgs 257-268

13 — Carson, R., *Silent Spring*, Crest Books, 1962

14 — Ibid, pg 97

15 — "Pesticide Safety: Myths and Facts," *National Coalition Against the Misuse of Pesticides*

16 — Regenstein, L., *How to Survive in America the Poisoned*, Acropolis Books, 1982, pg 103

17 — Carson, R., as per note 13, pgs 35-37

18 — Carson, R., cited in Regenstein, L, as per note 16, pg 106

19 — Duggan, R., "Dietary Intake of Pesticide Chemicals in the United States (11), June 1966-April 1968," *Pesticides Monitoring Journal*, 2:140-52, 1969

20 — Harris, S., "Organochlorine Contamination of Breast Milk," *Environmental Defense Fund*, Washington, D.C., Nov 7, 1979

Balbien, J., Harris, S., and Page, T., "Diet as a Factor Affecting Organochlorine Contamination of Breast Milk," *Environmental Defense Fund*, Washington, D.C.

21 — Severo, R., *New York Times*, May 6, 1980

22 — Barringer, F., "Thirty More Regulations Targeted for Review," *Washington Post*, Aug 13, 1981, pg A-27

Brown, M., "Reagan Wants to Ax Product Safety Agency," *Washington Post*, May 10, 1981

"Stockman Moves to Kill Consumer Safety Panel," *New York Times*, May 9, 1981

23 — "True or False," Leage of Conservation Voters, Washington, D.C., 1980

24 — Regenstein, L, as per note 16, pg 348

25 — "Environmental Quality - 1975," The Sixth Annual Report of the Council on Environmental Quality, Washington, D.C., Dec 1975, pg 369

26 — "DDT and the Dolphin," *Animals' Agenda*, Sept. 1985

27 — Longgood, *The Darkened Land*, Simon and Schuster, 1972, pg 143

28 — Carson, R., as per note 13

Highland, J., "Corporate Cancer," Environmental Defense Fund, Washington, D.C.

29 — "Environmental Quality—1975," as per note 25

"A Brief Review of Selected Environmental Contamination Incidents with a Potential for Health Effects," Prepared by the Library of Congress for the Committee on Environment and Public Works, U.S. Senate, August 1980, pgs 173-174

"Aldrin/Dieldrin," Criteria Document, *United States Environmental Protection Agency*, Washington, D.C., 1976

30 — Highland, J., as per note 28

31 — Regenstein, L, as per note 16, pg 355

32 — Carson, R., as per note 13, pgs 33-34, 88

33 — Regenstein, L, as per note 16, pgs 352-353

34 — Boyle R., and Environmental Defense Fund, *Malignant Neglect*, Alfred Knopf, 1979, pg 128

"Environmental Quality—1974," *The Fifth Annual Report of the Council on Environmental Quality*, Washington, D.C. Dec 1974, pg 161

35 — Associated Press, "Banquet Foods Recall Turkey," *Washington Post*, June 27, 1980, pg A-8

36 — Cimons, M., "Veterans Gaining Ground in Agent Orange Struggle," *Los Angeles Times*, Dec 27, 1979

37 — Regenstein, L, as per note 16, pg 58
Hornblower, M., "A Sinister Drama of Agent Orange Opens in Congress," *Washington Post*, June 27, 1979
"Effects of 2,4,5-T on Man and the Environment," Hearings before the Subcommittee on Energy, Natural Resources and the Environment, U.S. Senate, April, 1970, pg 1

38 — Hornblower, M., as per note 37

39 — Regenstein, L, as per note 16, pg 19

40 — Courtney, Dr. D., testimony before Senate Commerce Committee Subcommittee on the Environment, Aug 9, 1974

41 — Federal Register, Dec 13, 1979, pg 72,325

42 — "A Plague . . ." as per note 44

43 — Regenstein, L, as per note 16, pg 48

44 — "Environmental Quality—1979," *The Tenth Annual Report of the Council on Environmental Quality*, Washington, D.C., Dec 1979
"A Plague on Our Children," NOVA, WGBH Educational Foundation, Boston, 1979
Severo, R., "Two Studies for National Institute Link Herbicide to Cancer in Animals," *New York Times*, June 27, 1980

45 — Nordland, R. and Friedman, J., "Poison at our Doorstep," *Philadelphia Inquirer*, reprint of Sept 23-28, 1979

46 — Graham, F., *Since Silent Spring*, Crest Books, 1970, pgs 59-66

47 — Denton, H., "Contaminated Pork Shipped to Schools," *Washington Post*, May 24, 1980, pg A-1

48 — "Train Suspends Major Uses of Chlordane/Heptachlor . . . ," *Environmental News*, United States Environmental Protection Agency, Washington, D.C., Dec 24, 1979

49 — Butler, W., and Warren, J., "Petition for Suspension and Cancellation of Chlordane/Heptachlor," *Environmental Defense Fund*, Washington, D.C., Oct 1974

50 — Regenstein, L, as per note 16, pg 368
"Environmental Protection Agency, Vesichol Chemical Co. et al, Consolidated Heptachlor/Chlordane Hearing," Federal Register, Feb 19, 1976, pg 7556

51 — "The EPA and the Regulation of Pesticides," Staff Report to the Subcommittee on Administrative Practice and Procedure," U.S. Senate, Dec 1976, pg 24

52 — "Environmental Protection Agency, Pesticide Products Containing Heptachlor or Chlordane," Federal Register, Nov 26, 1974, pg 41300 "Report on Export of Products Banned by U.S. Regulatory Agencies," Committee on Government Operations, U.S. House of Representatives, Oct 4, 1978, pg 8
Denton, H., as per note 47

53 — Denton, H., as per note 47, pgs A-1, A-8

54 — "New Danger in Mother's Milk," *Time*, April 7, 1986, pg 31

55 — "Schools Ground Beef Blocked Over Pesticides," *San Francisco Chronicle*, April 7, 1986, pg 31

56 — "New Danger . . ." as per note 54

57 — "Breast Milk Contamination," *Birth Defect Prevention News*, Jan-March, 1986

58 — Mason, J., and Singer, P., *Animal Factories*, Crown Publishers, 1980, pgs 59-60

59 — "Corporate Crime," Subcommittee on Crime, U.S. House of Representatives, May 1980, pgs 25-28

60 — Grzech, E. and Warbelow, K., *Detroit Free Press*, "Distribution Hid Facts of PBB Peril,
       March 13, 1977; "State Knew But Did Not Warn Farmers of PBB-Tainted Feed,"
       March 14, 1977; "How State Leaders Ducked PBB Issue," March 15, 1977
61 — Brody, J., "Farmers Exposed to a Pollutant Face Medical Study . . ." *New York Times*,
       Aug 12, 1976, pg C-20
     "PBB Michigan Contamination Continues," *Guardian*, May 4, 1977, pg 2
     Gzech, E. and Warbelow, K., as per note 60
     "Corporate Crime," as per note 59
     Associated Press, "Michigan Study Indicates 97% Have Traces of PBB," *Washington
       Post*, Dec 31, 1981
62 — As per note 61
63 — cited in Regenstein, L, as per note 16, pg 341
64 — Longgood, as per note 27, pgs 132-134
65 — *Whole Earth Review*, #48, Fall 1985, pg 51
66 — "Surveillance, Epidemiology and End Results: Incidence and Mortality Data, 1973-
       1977," *National Cancer Institute*, Monograph 57, U.S. Department of Health and
       Human Services, National Institute of Health, Bethesda, Maryland, June 1981, pg 4
67 — Regenstein, L, as per note 16, pg 74
68 — Whiteside, R., *The Pendulum and the Toxic Cloud*, Yale University Press, 1979, pg 134
69 — Hoffman, R., Webb, K., and Schramm, W., "Health Effects of Long-term Exposure to
       2,3,7,8-Tetrachlorodibenzo-P-Dioxin," *Journal of the American Medical Association*,
       255:2031, April 18, 1986
70 — Perlman, D., "New Evidence Reported on Dioxin as Health Hazard," *San Francisco
       Chronicle*, April 18, 1986, pgs A-1, A-4
71 — *British Medical Journal*, 290:808, 1985
     Regenstein, Lewis, personal correspondence
72 — Boyle, R., as per note 34, pgs 59, 62
     "A Plague . . ." as per note 44
     Culhane, J., "PCB's: The Poisons That Won't Go Away," *Reader's Digest*, Dec. 1980,
       pgs 113, 115
     "Toxic Chemicals and Public Protection," A Report to the President by the Toxic Sub-
       stances Strategy Committee, Council on Environmental Quality, 1980, pg 3
     Nader, R., et al, *Who's Poisoning America*, Sierra Club Books, 1981, pg 177
     "Pesticides Found in Wild Polar Bears," *Animals' Agenda*, Sept. 1985
73 — Culhane, J., as per note 72
74 — Regenstein, L, as per note 16, pg 293
75 — "A Plague . . ." as per note 44
76 — Ibid
77 — Richards, B., "Drop in Sperm Count is Attributed to Toxic Environment," *Washington
       Post*, Sept 12, 1979
     Brody, J., "Sperm Found Especially Vulnerable to Environment," *New York Times*,
       March 10, 1981
     "Unplugging the Gene Pool," *Outside*, Sept 1980
     Jansson, E., "The Impact of Hazardous Substances Upon Infertility Among Men in the
       U.S., and Birth Defects," Friends of the Earth, Washington, D.C., Nov 17, 1980
78 — As per note 77
79 — Ibid
80 — Ibid
81 — Regenstein, as per note 16, pg 295

82 — "Environmental Quality—1979", as per note 54, pgs 11, 99-100, 448-449

83 — Regenstein, L, as per note 16, pg 298

84 — Longgood, as per note 27, pgs 132, 134

85 — "Environmental Quality—1975," as per note 25, pgs 368, 375, 387
     "A Brief Review . . ." as per note 29, pg 223

86 — Graham, F., as per note 46, pg 113
     Wurster, C., "DDT Reduces Photosynthesis by Marine Phytoplankton," *Science*, 1968,
     pgs 1474-1475
     Longgood, as per note 27, pg 137

87 — Holt, S., "The Food Resources of the Ocean," *Scientific American*, 221:178-194, 1969

88 — Borgstrum, G., *The Hungry Planet*, Collier Books, 1967, pg 311

89 — "A Brief Review . . ." as per note 29, pg 284
     Nelson, B., "PCB Pollution Grave Question, US Says," *Los Angeles Times*, Oct 7, 1979
     Congressional Quarterly, Sept 6, 1980, pg 2643
     Associated Press, "PCB's Discovered in Foods in West," *Washington Star*, Sept 15, 1979

90 — Frederickson, G., personal communication with author, Jan 13, 1986

91 — "A Brief Review . . ." as per note 29, pgs 284-287
     Longgood, as per note 27, pg 495
     Boyle, R., as per note 34, pg 77

92 — As per note 91

93 — "A Brief Review . . ." as per note 29

94 — Regenstein, L, as per note 16, pg 304

95 — "Toxic Chemicals . . ." as per note 72, pg 2
     "Chemical First Strike," Editorial, *Washington Post*, May 17, 1980, pg A-18

96 — Ibid

97 — "The Global Environment and Basic Human Needs," A Report to the Council on Envi-
     ronmental Quality by the Worldwatch Institute, Council on Environmental Quality,
     Washington, D.C. 1978, pg 20
     "Toxic Chemicals . . ." as per note 72, pg xiv
     "EPA is Slow to Carry Out Its Responsibility to Control Harmful Chemicals," U.S.
     General Accounting Office, Washington, D.C., Oct 28, 1980, pg 1

98 — Boyle, R., as per note 34, pg 7
     "Environmental Quality—1979," as per note 44, pg 198

99 — Grzech, E. and Warbelow, K., as per note 60

100 — Cavalieri, L., "Carcinogens and the Value of Life," *New York Times*, July 20, 1980
      Regenstein, L, as per note 16, pg 232

101 — Boyle, R., as per note 34, pgs 196-198

102 — Pimentel, D., "Pesticides . . ." *BioScience 27*, March 1977
      Turner, J., *A Chemical Feast: Report on the Food and Drug Administration*, Grossman,
      1970
      Pimentel, D., "Realities of a Pesticide Ban," *Environment*, March, 1973

103 — Regenstein, L, as per note 16, pg 275

104 — "Infant Abnormalities Linked to PCB Contaminated Fish," *Vegetairan Times*, Nov 1984,
      pg 8

105 — Jacobson, S., "The Effect of Intrauterine PCB Exposure on Visual Recognition Mem-
      ory," *Child Development*, Vol 56, 1985

106 — Regenstin, L., as per note 16, pg 233

107 — "Toxaphene: Position Document 1," Toxaphene Working Group, United States Envi-
      ronmental Protection Agency, Washington, D.C., April 19, 1977, pg 19-20

108 — Ibid

109 — Taylor, R., "Cattle Deaths Stir Pesticide Debate," *Los Angeles Times*, Nov 5, 1979
110 — Regenstein, L, as per note 16, pg 336
111 — Taylor R., as per note 109
      Bradley, E., "60 Minutes," CBS News, Nov 22, 1981
112 — Schell, O., as per note 3, pg 155
113 — Ibid
114 — Ibid, pgs 164-165
115 — USDA Food Processing/Marketing Report, 1965, cited in Hunter, B., as per note 6, pg 155
116 — "Effects, Uses, Control and Research of Agricultural Pesticides," A Report by the Surveys and Investigations Staff, USDA; Presented at Hearings before a Subcommittee on Appropriations, 89th Congress, first session, House of Representatives, Department of Agricultural Appropriations, part 1, pg 174
117 — *Mainstream*, Summer 1983, pg 17
118 — Ibid
119 — USDA Statistical Summary: Federal Meat and Poultry Inspection for 1976, Jan 1977, pg 3
120 — "U.S. Meat Banned for Export Through The Common Market," *Vegetarian Times*, Oct 1984, pg 17
121 — Regenstein, L, as per note 16, pgs 86, 272
122 — United Press, "Food and Drug Administration: Meat Dye May Cause Cancer," *Washington Post*, April 6, 1973
123 — Luck, R., "Chemical Insect Control," *BioScience*, Sept 1977
124 — Lappe, F.M. and Collins, J., *Food First—Beyond the Myth of Scarcity*, Ballantine Books, 1977, pg 63
125 — Ibid, pg 64
126 — Ibid, pg 71
127 — Bottrell, D., "Integrated Pest Management," Council on Environmental Quality, 1980, pgs iv-viii, 39, 99
128 — "What One Bird Can Do," Garden Club of America, cited in Regenstein, L., as per note 16, pg 127
129 — Fillip, J., "American Farmers and USDA Start to Take Organic Seriously," *Not Man Apart*, Sept 1980
130 — Ibid
131 — Weir, D., and Schapiro, M., *Circle of Poison*, Institute for Food and Development Policy, 1981
      Weir, D., and Schapiro, M., "The Corporate Crime of the Century," *Mother Jones*, Nov 1979
      Weir, D., "The Boomerang Crime," *Mother Jones*, Nov 1979
      Smith, R.J., "US Beginning to Act on Banned Pesticides," *Science*, June 29, 1979
132 — Regenstein, L., as per note 16, pg 273
133 — "Environmental Quality—1975," as per note 25, pg 375
134 — cited in Regenstein, L., as per note 16, pg 250
135 — "A Brief Review . . ." as per note 29, pg 289
136 — Boyle, R., as per note 34, pgs 206-207
      Harris, S., and Highland, J., "Birthright Denied," EDF, 1977, pg 11
      Regenstein, L, as per note 16, pg 297
137 — "A Brief Review . . . ," as per note 29, pg 289
138 — Harris, S., as per note 20, pg 2
139 — "Environmental Quality—1975," as per note 25, pg 375
      Harris, S., and Highland, J., as per note 136, pg 2

140 — Boyle, R., as per note 34, pgs 206-207

141 — "A Brief Review . . ." as per note 29, pg 289

142 — Katz, D., "PCB's Found in Milk in All Michigan Mothers Tested," *Detroit Free Press*, Feb 1, 1981

143 — "Environmental Quality—1975," as per note 25, pg 375

144 — Harris, S. as per note 20, and as per note 177

145 — *New England Journal of Medicine*, March 26, 1981

146 — "A Brief Review . . . ," as per note 29, pg 289

147 — Regenstein, L., as per note 16, pgs 255-256

148 — Hilts, P., "Chemicals at Parents' Job May Cause Child's Tumor," *Washington Post*, July 3, 1981

149 — "Chemical Hazards to Human Reproduction," Council on Environmental Quality, Jan 1981, pgs II-3, 12

150 — "Politics of Poison," KRON-TV, San Francisco, 1979

151 — Gofmann, J. and Tamplin, A., quoted in Brand S., "Human Harm to Human DNA," *Co-Evolution Quarterly*, Spring 1979, pg 11

Chapter Twelve—All Things Are Connected

1 — Bralove, Mary, "The Food Crisis: the Shortages May Pit the 'Have Nots' Against the 'Haves,'" *Wall Street Journal*, October 3, 1974, pg 20

2 — Maidenburg, H.J. "The Livestock Population Explosion," *New York Times*, July 1, 1973, pg 1 Finance section

   Brody, Jane E. "The Quest for Protein," from *Give Us This Day*, Arno Press, 1975, pg 222

3 — Lappe, Frances Moore, *Diet for a Small Planet*, Tenth Anniversary Edition, Ballantine Books, New York, 1982, pg 69

   Altschul, Aaron, *Proteins: Their Chemistry and Politics*, Basic Books, 1965, pg 264

   Doyring, Folke, "Soybeans," *Scientific American*, February 1974

4 — "The World Food Problem," a report by the *President's Science Advisory Committee*, Vol. II, May, 1967; FACT SHEET, *Food Animals Concern Trust*, Issue No. 26, November 1982, Chicago

5 — As per note 3

6 — Resenberger, Boyce, "Curb on U.S. Waste Urged to Help World's Hungry," *New York Times*, October 25, 1974

7 — *Acres, U.S.A.*, Kansas City, Missouri, Volume 15, No. 6, June 1985, pg 2

8 — Rensberger, Boyce, "World Food Crisis: Basic Ways of Life Face Upheaval from Chronic Shortages," *New York Times*, November 5, 1974, pg 14

9 — as per note 3

10 — MacKay, Alastair, *Farming and Gardening in the Bible*, Spire, 1970, pg 224

   Genesis 13:5-7

   Numbers 31:32-33

   Deuteronomy 12:20

11 — Plato, *The Republic*, Book II, translated B. Jowett, pg 233

12 — Ibid

13 — Carter, Vernon Gill, and Dale, Tom, *Topsoil and Civilization*, Rev. ed., Norman, Univ. of Oklahoma Press, 1974

14 — Brune, William, State Conservationist, Soil Conservation Service, Des Moines, Iowa, testimony before Senate Committee on Agriculture and Forestry, July 6, 1976

King, Seth, "Iowa Rain and Wind Deplete Farmlands," *New York Times*, December 5, 1976, pg 61

Harnack, Curtis, "In Plymouth County, Iowa, the Rich Topsoil's Going Fast, Alas," *New York Times*, July 11, 1980

15 --- Hur, Robin, "Six Inches from Starvation; How and Why America's Topsoil is Disappearing," *Vegetarian Times*, March, 1985, pgs 45-47

16 --- Ibid

17 --- cited in Hur, as per note 15

18 --- Harnack, as per note 14

19 --- Hur, as per note 15

Pimental et al, "Land Degradation: Effects on Food and Energy Resources," in *Science*, Vol 194, Oct. 1976

National Association of Conservation Districts, Washington, D.C. *Soil Degradation: Effects on Agricultural Productivity*, Interim Report Number Four, National Agricultural Lands Study, 1980, pg 20

King, Seth, "Farms Go Down the River," *New York Times*, December 10, 1978, citing Soil Conservation Service

As per estimates cited in Lappe, op cit note 4, calculated from estimates by Medard Gabel for the Cornucopia Project, c/o Rodale Press, Inc., Emmaus, PA

20 --- Harnack, as per note 14

21 --- Hur, as per note 15

22 --- Hur, Robin quoted in Lappe, as per note 3, pg 80

Soil and Water Resources Conservation Act—Summary of Appraisal, USDA Review Draft, 1980, pg 18

Pimental, as per note 19

Soil Degradation . . . , as per note 19

USDA, Economics and Statistics Service, *Natural Resource Capital in U.S. Agriculture: Irrigation, Drainage and Conservation Investments Since 1900*, ESCS Staff Paper, March, 1979

23 --- Gagel, Medard, Cornucopia Project, Preliminary Report, Rodale, Inc., Emmaus, PA

Wolfbauer, C.A., "Mineral Resources for Agricultural Use," in *Agriculture and Energy*, ed. William Lockeretz, New York, Academic Press, 1977, pgs 301-314

U.S. Bureau of Mines, *Facts and Problems*, 1975, pgs 758-868

General Accounting Office, *Phosphates: A Case Study of a Valuable Depleting Mineral in America*, Report to the Congress by the Comptroller General of the United States, EMD-80-21, November 30, 1979

24 --- as per note 3

25 --- Chief Seattle's Testimony, an 1854 oration, cited in *The Extended Circle*, ed., Jon Wynne-Tyson, Centaur Press, Fontwell Sussex 1985

26 --- Hur, Robin, and Fields, Dr. David, "Are High-Fat Diets Killing Our Forests?" *Vegetarian Times*, Feb 1984

27 --- Ibid

28 --- Ibid

29 --- Ibid

30 --- cited in Hur and Fields, op cit note 26

31 --- as per note 26

32 --- Ibid

33 --- Ibid

34 --- Parsons, James, "Forest to Pasture: Development or Destruction?" *Revista de Biologia Tropical*, Vol 24, Supplement 1, 1976

Myers, Norman, "Cheap Meat Vs. Priceless Rainforests," *Vegetarian Times*, May 1982
DeWalt, Billie, "The Cattle Are Eating the Forest," *Bulletin of the Atomic Scientists*
The World Conservation Stragegy: "The World Conservation Strategy in Brief," World Wildlife Fund, 1980

35 --- *Acres, U.S.A.*, as per note 7

36 --- Ibid

37 --- Ibid

38 --- Ibid

39 --- Lappe, as per note 3

40 --- Borgstrom, Georg, presentation to the Annual Meeting of the American Association for the Advancement of Science, 1981

41 --- Altschul, as per note 3

42 --- Erlich, Paul and Anne, *Population, Resources, Environment*, W.H. Freeman, 1972, pgs 75-76

43 --- "The Browning of America," *Newsweek*, February 22, 1981, pg 26

44 --- Fields, David and Hur, Robin, "America's Appetite for Meat is Ruining Our Water," *Vegetarian Times*, Jan 1985

45 --- Ibid

46 --- Ibid

47 --- Ibid

48 --- Ibid

49 --- Ibid

50 --- cited in Fields and Hur, as per note 44

51 --- Raup, Philip, "Competition for Land and the Future of American Agriculture," in *The Future of American Agriculture as a Strategic Resource*, edited by Sandra Batle and Robert Healy, A Conservation Foundation Conference, July 14, 1980, Washington, D.C.

Lagrone, William, "The Great Plains," in *Another Revolution in US Farming?*, Schertz et al, USDA, ESCS, Agricultural Economic Report No. 441, December 1979

Harris, Joe, resource economist part of four-year government-sponsored study, "The Six State High Plains Ogallala Aquifer Agricultural Regional Resource Study," cited in Lappe, op cit note 4, pg 466

Fields and Hur, as per note 45

52 --- Lagrone, as per note 51

"Report: Nebraska's Water Wealth is Deceptive," *Omaha World-Herald*, May 28, 1981

53 --- Pimental, David, "Energy and Land Constraints in Food Protein Production," *Science*, November 21, 1975

Jasiorowski, H.A., "Intensive Systems of Animal Production," *Proceedings of the III World Conference on Animal Production*, ed. R. L. Reid, Sydney, Sydney University Press, 1975, pg 384

Robbins, Jackie, *Environmental Impact Resulting From Unconfined Animal Production*, Environmental Protection Technology Series, Cincinnati, U.S.E.P.A., Office of Research and Development, Environmental Research Information Center, February 1978, pg 9

Environmental Science and Technology, Vol. 4, No. 12, 1970, pg 1098, cited in Lappe, as per note 3

54 --- Mason, Jim and Singer, Peter, *Animal Factories*, Crown Publishers, New York, 1980, pg 84

55 --- Loehr, Raymond, *Pollution Implications of Animal Wastes—A Forward Oriented Review*, Water Pollution Control Research Series, Washington, D.C.: Office of Research and Monitoring, U.S.E.P.A., 1968, pg 26, table 7, cited in Singer and Mason, as per note 54

56 --- Myles, Bruce, "U.S. Antipollution Laws May Boost Cattle-Feeders' Cost—and Meat Prices," *Christian Science Monitor*, March 11, 1974, pg 3A

57 --- *Newsweek*, November 8, 1971, pg 85

58 --- Borgsrum, Georg, cited in Lappe, Frances Moore, *Diet for a Small Planet*, 1975 edition, pg 22

59 --- Ibid

60 --- *Raw Materials in the United States Economy 1900-1977*, Technical paper 47, Vivian Spencer, U.S. Department of Commerce, U.S. Department of Interior, Bureau of Mines, pg 3; cited in Lappe, as per note 3, pg 66

61 --- Reid, J.T. "Comparative Efficiency of Animals in the Conversion of Feedstuffs to Human Foods," *Confinement*, April 1976, pg 23

62 --- Hur, Robin and Fields, David, "How Meat Robs America of its Energy," *Vegetarian Times*, April 1985

63 --- Ibid

64 --- Roller, W.L. et al, "Energy Costs of Intensive Livestock Production," American Society of Agricultural Engineers, June 1975, St. Joseph, Michigan, paper no. 75-4042, table 7, pg 14, cited in Singer and Mason, *Animal Factories*, as per note 54

65 --- Pimental et al, as per note 53

66 --- *Scientific American*, February 1974, pgs 19-20

67 --- Hur and Fields, as per note 62

68 --- Ibid

69 --- Ibid

70 --- Ibid

INDEX

2, 4-D, 321
2, 4, 5-T, 321

Ulcers, 282-284

Veal calves, 112-121
Vegetarians, athletes, 158-163
  and B-12, 300
  breast milk of, 344-347
  health of. *See* specific diseases
  iron deficiency in, 164-165. *See also*
    Anemia
  longevity of, 154-155
  protein sufficiency of, 174, 176
  strength and stamina of, 155-158
Velsicol Chemical Corporation, 322-323
Verot, Pierreo, 161
Verret, Jacqueline, 312
Violet dye –1, 338
Virginia Polytechnic Institute, 51-52
Vitamin B-12, 300
Vitamin U, 283
Vladislavich, Yvonne, 24

War and meat, 354-356
Watchman, Dr. Aaron, 199
Water pollution and meat, 371-373
Water use and meat, 366-371
Watson, E. L., 49
Webb, Harry, 372
White, Dr. Paul Dudley, 215
Williams, Roger, 150, 174
Winick, Myron, 202
Wissler, Dr. Robert, 214
Wolves, 39

NOTICE

If you feel touched by the message of DIET FOR A NEW AMERICA, you may well be interested in the work of the EarthSave Foundation, founded by John Robbins.

To receive more information, please write:
EARTHSAVE FOUNDATION
Post Office Box 949
Felton, CA 95018-0949

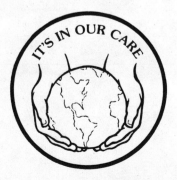